P. Altmeyer S. el-Gammal
K. Hoffmann (Eds.)

Ultrasound in Dermatology

With 470 Figures, including 95 colour pictures
and 20 Tables

Springer-Verlag
Berlin Heidelberg New York
London Paris Tokyo
Hong Kong Barcelona
Budapest

Prof. Dr. med. PETER ALTMEYER
Dr. med. STEPHAN EL-GAMMAL
Dr. med. KLAUS HOFFMANN
Dermatologische Klinik der Ruhr-Universität Bochum
St. Josef-Hospital
Gudrunstraße 56
4630 Bochum 1, FRG

ISBN 3-540-53750-3 Springer-Verlag Berlin Heidelberg New York
ISBN 0-387-53750-3 Springer-Verlag New York Berlin Heidelberg

Library of Congress Cataloging-in-Publication Data
Ultrasound in dermatology / P. Altmeyer, S. el-Gammal, K. Hoffmann (Hrsg.).
  ISBN (invalid) 3-540-53750-3 (alk. paper) -- ISBN 0-387-53750-3 (alk. paper)
1. Skin--Ultrasonic imaging. I. Altmeyer, Peter. II. El-Gammal, S. (Stephan),
1957-   III. Hoffmann, K. (Klaus), 1961-   .
  [DNLM: 1. Skin Diseases--ultrasonography. WR 140 U47] RL 106.U48U48 1991
616.5'07543--dc20   91-38709 CIP

This work is subject to copyright. All rights are reserved, whether the whole or part of the material is concerned, specifically the rights of translation, reprinting, reuse of illustrations, recitation, broadcasting, reproduction on microfilm or in other ways, and storage in data banks. Duplication of this publication or parts thereof is permitted only under the provisions of the German Copyright Law of September 9, 1965, in its current version, and permission for use must always be obtained from Springer Verlag. Violations are liable for prosecution under the German Copyright Law.

© Springer-Verlag Berlin Heidelberg 1992
Printed in Germany

The use of general descriptive names, registered names, trademarks, etc. in this publication does not imply, even in the absence of a specific statement, that such names are exempt from the relevant protective laws and regulations and therefore free for genereal use.

Product liability: The publisher cannot guarantee the accuracy of any information about dosage and application contained in this book. In every individual case the user must check such information by consulting the relevant literature.

Typesetting, printing and binding: Druckhaus Beltz, Hemsbach/Bergstr.
27/3145-543210 – Printed on acid-free paper

Preface

Until May 1990, when the First International Congress on Ultrasound in Dermatology was held, high-resolution ultrasound was employed at only a few centers worldwide. The intensive communication and discussion at this congress between dermatologists, engineers, and physicists resulted in intensive clinical research in the past 2 years. More than 200 different dermatological departments all over the world are now using high-resolution ultrasound.

In 1990, the International Society for Ultrasound and the Skin was founded, which among other activities has been organizing a second international congress which was held in Modena, Italy, in 1991, and is planning the Third International Congress on Ultrasound and the Skin to be held in Copenhagen in Denmark in 1993. The intensive scientific communication between the members of this society has been significantly enhancing the knowledge about ultrasound phenomena in dermatology.

This book introduces the reader to the activities of these different international ultrasound research groups (e.g., physics of ultrasound, image formation, and interpretation). Furthermore, traditional ultrasound applications such as lymph node analysis and duplex sonography of blood vessels are reviewed. Clinical good practice and the interpretation of 20–50 MHz B-scan images in over 50 different skin tumors and inflammatory diseases are thoroughly discussed. Finally, future prospects (e.g., intravascular ultrasound, three-dimensional modelling) and the limits of high-resolution ultrasound are outlined and evaluated; experts in ultrasound will particularly appreciate the detailed subject index.

November, 1991
                                                                                                                        PETER ALTMEYER
                                                                                                                       STEPHAN EL-GAMMAL
                                                                                                                         KLAUS HOFFMANN

Contents

The Physics of Ultrasound

Physical Ultrasound Phenomena in Tissues
H. KUTTRUFF 3

A- and B-Scan Techniques of Conventional Ultrasound Units.
A Survey
G. KREITZ 12

High Frequency Ultrasonic Imaging Systems
A. HÖSS, H. ERMERT, S. EL-GAMMAL, and P. ALTMEYER 22

A Procedure to Improve the Resolution of Superposed Ultrasound
Signals
R. TAUTE, H. J. HEIN, and K. V. JENDERKA 32

General Ultrasound Phenomena

Ten Years' Experience with High-Frequency Ultrasound
Examination of the Skin:
Development and Refinement of Technique and Equipments
J. SERUP 41

General Phenomena of Ultrasound in Dermatology
P. ALTMEYER, K. HOFFMANN, M. STÜCKER, S. GOERTZ,
and S. EL-GAMMAL 55

Automatic Measurement of Skin Thickness
A. PECH, E.-G. LOCH, and W. VON SEELEN 80

Lymphnodes in 5- to 7.5-MHz Ultrasound

B-Scan Ultrasound of Regional Lymph Nodes
in Different Dermatological Diseases
B. RIEDL, D. HILLER, and N. STOSIEK 87

Comparison of Ultrasound with Clinical Findings in the
Early Detection of Regional Metastatic Lymph Nodes in Patients
with Malignant Melanoma
R. LOOSE, J. WEISS, W. KÜHN, R. SIMON, J. TEUBNER,
and M. GEORGI 93

The Value of Sonography in Diagnosis and Follow-Up of Lymph
Nodes in HIV-Patients
U. MENDE, W. TILGEN, U. PEKAR, and M. HARTMANN 100

Tumors in 5- to 7.5-MHz Ultrasound

Efficacy of Sonography in Differential Diagnosis of Soft-Tissue
Tumors
H. MERK, D. ESSER, G. MERK, and L. LANGEN 111

Sonography: The Ideal Imaging Method for Staging and Follow-Up
of Malignant Melanoma
U. MENDE, D. PETZOLDT, W. TILGEN, and P. SCHRAUBE 119

Observations and Experiences in Sonographic Grading and Staging
of Malignant Melanomas
G. MERK, H. MERK, J. ULRICH, K.-H. KÜHNE,
and C. WILLGEROTH 130

Doppler Ultrasound and Ultrasound Duplex

Basis and Clinical Application of Ultrasound Doppler Systems
P. A. PAYNE, A. AYATOLLAHI, and R. Y. FADDOUL 139

Duplex Sonography and Color Encoded Blood Flow Imaging
P. SCHLICHTING, D. BRECHTELSBAUER, and L. HEUSER 147

The Value of Duplex Sonography
in Diagnosing Phlebologic Diseases
G. HESSE 156

Bi-planar Transesophageal Echocardiography
R. HAMMENTGEN, S. EL-GAMMAL, M. HAUSMANN, K. HOFFMANN,
M. BERGBAUER, and D. RICKEN 161

Skin Tumors in 20 MHz Ultrasound

Sonographic Structure of Benign Skin Tumors
E. W. BREITBART and P. MOHR 171

Skin Tumours in High-Frequency Ultrasound
K. HOFFMANN, S. EL-GAMMAL, K. WINKLER, J. JUNG,
K. PISTORIUS, and P. ALTMEYER 181

Assets and Limitations of High-Frequency Ultrasound
in the Analysis of Basal Cell and Squamous Cell Carcinomas
D. VIELUF and H. C. KORTING 202

The Acoustic Characteristics of the Basal Cell Carcinoma
in 20-MHz Ultrasonography
M. STÜCKER, K. HOFFMANN, S. EL-GAMMAL, and P. ALTMEYER .. 207

Value of High-Frequency Sonography in Determination of Maximal
Vertical Tumor Thickness in Primary Malignant Melanoma of the
Skin
G. GASSENMEIER, F. KIESEWETTER, and H. SCHELL 221

Inflammatory Diseases in 20 MHz Ultrasound

Examination of Circumscribed Scleroderma Using 20-MHz B-Scan
Ultrasound
K. HOFFMANN, S. EL-GAMMAL, U. GERBAULET, H. SCHATZ,
and P. ALTMEYER 231

Examination of Psoriasis Vulgaris Using 20-MHz B-Scan Ultrasound
K. HOFFMANN, S. EL-GAMMAL, H. SCHWARZE, T. DIRSCHKA,
and P. ALTMEYER 244

Ultrasound Assessment of the Comparative Atrophogenicity
of Potent Fluorinated and Nonfluorinated Topical Glucocorticoids

H. C. KORTING, D. VIELUF, and M. KERSCHER 250

Ultrasound: Applications in the Study of Human Skin Disorders
and the Response to Treatment

H. SCHATZ, T. STOUDEMAYER, and A. M. KLIGMAN 256

Experimental Approaches in 20 MHz Ultrasound

Ultrasound Evaluation of Wound Volume as a Measure of Wound
Healing Rate

P. T. PUGLIESE, F. MONCLOA, and R. T. MCFADDEN 267

Possibilities for Application of High-Frequency Ultrasound
in Clinical Research

K. HOFFMANN, S. EL-GAMMAL, T. DIRSCHKA, K. WINKLER,
S. FELDMANN, and P. ALTMEYER 273

Intravascular Ultrasound

R. HAMMENTGEN, V. GODDER, S. EL-GAMMAL, M. MEINE,
M. BERGBAUER, and D. RICKEN 289

50 MHz Ultrasound

A 50-MHz High-Resolution Ultrasound Imaging System
for Dermatology

S. EL-GAMMAL, K. HOFFMANN, T. AUER, M. KORTEN,
P. ALTMEYER, A. HÖSS, and H. ERMERT 297

GHz Ultrasound Microscopy and Ultrastructure

Scanning Acoustic Microscopy:
A New Procedure to Examine Skin Sections

N. BUHLES, P. ALTMEYER, and J. BEREITER-HAHN 325

Acoustic Microscopy in Dermatology:
Normal Skin Structures and Tumours

U. MATTHES, S. HÖXTERMANN, K. HOFFMANN, S. EL-GAMMAL,
E. BRUSCHKE, and P. ALTMEYER 328

From Ultrasound to Ultrastructure

K. SCHMIDT, M. BACHARACH-BUHLES, N. BUHLES, K. HOFFMANN,
and P. ALTMEYER 341

Three-Dimensional Computer Reconstructions

Principles of Three-Dimensional Reconstructions
from High-Resolution Ultrasound in Dermatology

S. EL-GAMMAL, K. HOFFMANN, J. KENKMANN, P. ALTMEYER,
A. HÖSS, and H. ERMERT 355

Three-Dimensional Reconstruction of Serial Ultrasound Images of
the Skin

F.-M. PAWLAK, K. HOFFMANN, S. EL-GAMMAL, and P. ALTMEYER   385

New Developments

New Concepts and Developments in High-Resolution Ultrasound

S. EL-GAMMAL, K. HOFFMANN, A. HÖSS, R. HAMMENTGEN,
P. ALTMEYER, and H. ERMERT 399

Appendix: Principles of Image Processing 420

Subject Index 443

List of Contributors

Altmeyer, P.
 Dermatologische Klinik der Ruhr-Universität Bochum, St. Josef-Hospital,
 Gudrunstraße 56, W-4630 Bochum 1, FRG

Auer, T.
 Dermatologische Klinik der Ruhr-Universität Bochum, St. Josef-Hospital,
 Gudrunstraße 56, W-4630 Bochum 1, FRG

Ayatollahi, A.
 Department of Instrumentation and Analytical Science,
 University of Manchester, Institute of Science and Technology,
 P.O. Box 88, Manchester M60 1QD, UK

Bacharach-Buhles, M.
 Dermatologische Klinik der Ruhr-Universität Bochum, St. Josef-Hospital,
 Gudrunstraße 56, W-4630 Bochum 1, FRG

Bereiter-Hahn, J.
 Arbeitskreis kinematische Zellforschung, F. B. Biologie der Johann
 Wolfgang Goethe-Universität, W-6000 Frankfurt/Main, FRG

Bergbauer, M.
 Medizinische Klinik der Ruhr-Universität Bochum, St. Josef-Hospital,
 Gudrunstraße 56, W-4630 Bochum 1, FRG

Brechtelsbauer, D.
 Institut für Radiologie und Nuklearmedizin, Ruhr-Universität Bochum,
 Knappschaftskrankenhaus, W-4630 Bochum 1, FRG

Breitbart, E. W.
 Dermatologische Klinik, Universität Hamburg, Martinistraße 52,
 W-2000 Hamburg 20, FRG

Bruschke, E.
 Dermatologische Klinik der Ruhr-Universität Bochum, St. Josef-Hospital,
 Gudrunstraße 56, W-4630 Bochum 1, FRG

Buhles, N.
Dermatologische Abteilung der Nordseeklinik Westerland,
Norderstraße 81, W-2280 Westerland/Sylt, FRG

Dirschka, T.
Dermatologische Klinik der Ruhr-Universität Bochum, St. Josef-Hospital,
Gudrunstraße 56, W-4630 Bochum 1, FRG

el-Gammal, S.
Dermatologische Klinik der Ruhr-Universität Bochum, St. Josef-Hospital,
Gudrunstraße 56, W-4630 Bochum 1, FRG

Ermert, H.
Institut für Hochfrequenztechnik, Ruhr-Universität Bochum,
Universitätsstraße 150, W-4630 Bochum 1, FRG

Esser, D.
Klinik für HNO, Medizinische Akademie Magdeburg, Leipziger Straße
44, O-3090 Magdeburg, FRG

Faddoul, R. Y.
Department of Instrumentation and Analytical Science,
University of Manchester, Institute of Science and Technology,
P.O. Box 88, Manchester M60 1QD, UK

Feldmann, S.
Dermatologische Klinik der Ruhr-Universität Bochum, St. Josef-Hospital,
Gudrunstraße 56, W-4630 Bochum 1, FRG

Gassenmeier, G.
Dermatologische Klinik, Universität Erlangen-Nürnberg,
Hartmannstraße 14, W-8520 Erlangen, FRG

Georgi, M.
Institut für Klinische Radiologie, Klinikum Mannheim der Universität
Heidelberg, Postfach 10 00 23, W-6800 Mannheim 1, FRG

Gerbaulet, U.
Dermatologische Klinik der Ruhr-Universität Bochum, St. Josef-Hospital,
Gudrunstraße 56, W-4630 Bochum 1, FRG

Godder, V.
Herzzentrum Nordrhein-Westfalen, Ruhr-Universität Bochum,
Georgstraße 11, W-4970 Bad Oeynhausen, FRG

Goertz, S.
 Dermatologische Klinik der Ruhr-Universität Bochum, St. Josef-Hospital,
 Gudrunstraße 56, W-4630 Bochum 1, FRG

Hammentgen, R.
 Herzzentrum Nordrhein-Westfalen, Ruhr-Universität Bochum,
 Georgstraße 11, W-4970 Bad Oeynhausen, FRG

Hartmann, M.
 Hautklinik der Universität Heidelberg, Voßstraße 2, W-6900 Heidelberg,
 FRG

Hausmann, M.
 Medizinische Klinik der Ruhr-Universität Bochum, St. Josef-Hospital,
 Gudrunstraße 56, W-4630 Bochum 1, FRG

Hein, H. J.
 Institut für angewandte Biophysik, Medizinische Fakultät der Martin-
 Luther-Universität Halle-Wittenberg, Straße der deutsch-sowjetischen
 Freundschaft 81, O-4014 Halle, FRG

Hesse, G.
 Romanplatz 10a, W-8000 München 19, FRG

Heuser, L.
 Institut für Radiologie und Nuklearmedizin, Ruhr-Universität Bochum,
 Knappschaftskrankenhaus, W-4630 Bochum 1, FRG

Hiller, D.
 Dermatologische Klinik, Universität Erlangen-Nürnberg,
 Hartmannstraße 14, W-8520 Erlangen, FRG

Hoffmann, K.
 Dermatologische Klinik der Ruhr-Universität Bochum, St. Josef-Hospital,
 Gudrunstraße 56, W-4630 Bochum 1, FRG

Höß, A.
 Institut für Hochfrequenztechnik, Ruhr-Universität Bochum,
 Universitätsstraße 150, W-4630 Bochum 1, FRG

Höxtermann, S.
 Dermatologische Klinik der Ruhr-Universität Bochum, St. Josef-Hospital,
 Gudrunstraße 56, W-4630 Bochum 1, FRG

Jenderka, K. V.
Institut für angewandte Biophysik, Medizinische Fakultät
der Martin-Luther-Universität Halle-Wittenberg,
Straße der deutsch-sowjetischen Freundschaft 81, O-4014 Halle, FRG

Jung, J.
Dermatologische Klinik der Ruhr-Universität Bochum, St. Josef-Hospital,
Gudrunstraße 56, W-4630 Bochum 1, FRG

Kenkmann, J.
Dermatologische Klinik der Ruhr-Universität Bochum, St. Josef-Hospital,
Gudrunstraße 56, W-4630 Bochum 1, FRG

Kerscher, M.
Dermatologische Klinik und Poliklinik der Universität München,
Frauenlobstraße 9–11, W-8000 München 2, FRG

Kiesewetter, F.
Dermatologische Klinik, Universität Erlangen-Nürnberg,
Hartmannstraße 14, W-8520 Erlangen, FRG

Kligmann, A. M.
University of Pennsylvania, 422 Curie Boulevard, Philadelphia, PA 19104,
USA

Korten, M.
Dermatologische Klinik der Ruhr-Universität Bochum, St. Josef-Hospital,
Gudrunstraße 56, W-4630 Bochum 1, FRG

Korting, H. C.
Dermatologische Klinik und Poliklinik der Universität München,
Frauenlobstraße 9–11, W-8000 München 2, FRG

Kreitz, G.
Siemens AG, UB Med, Marketing Ultraschall, Henkestraße 127,
W-8520 Erlangen, FRG

Kühn, W.
Hautklinik, Klinikum Mannheim der Universität Heidelberg,
Postfach 10 00 23, W-6800 Mannheim 1, FRG

Kühne, K. H.
Klinik für Hautkrankheiten, Medizinische Akademie Magdeburg,
Leipziger Straße 44, O-3090 Magdeburg, FRG

Kuttruff, H.
Institut für Technische Akustik der Rheinisch-Westfälischen Technischen
Hochschule Aachen, Templergraben 55, W-5100 Aachen, FRG

Langen, L.
Klinik für Urologie, Medizinische Akademie Magdeburg,
Leipziger Straße 44, O-3090 Magdeburg, FRG

Loch, E. G.
Deutsche Klinik für Diagnostik, Aukammallee 33, W-6200 Wiesbaden,
FRG

Loose, R.
Institut für Klinische Radiologie, Klinikum Mannheim der Universität
Heidelberg, Postfach 10 00 23, W-6800 Mannheim 1, FRG

Matthes, U.
Dermatologische Klinik der Ruhr-Universität Bochum, St. Josef-Hospital,
Gudrunstraße 56, W-4630 Bochum 1, FRG

McFadden, R. T.
Peter T. Pugliese MD & Associates, Rte 183, Rd#1, Bernville, PA 19506,
USA

Meine, M.
Herzzentrum Nordrhein-Westfalen, Ruhr-Universität Bochum,
Georgstraße 11, W-4970 Bad Oeynhausen, FRG

Mende, U.
Radiologische Klinik der Universität Heidelberg, Abteilung Klinische
Radiologie, Im Neuenheimer Feld 400, W-6900 Heidelberg, FRG

Merk, G.
Klinik für Hautkrankheiten, Medizinische Akademie Magdeburg,
Leipziger Straße 44, O-3090 Magdeburg, FRG

Merk, H.
Klinik für Orthopädie, Medizinische Akademie Magdeburg,
Leipziger Straße 44, O-3090 Magdeburg, FRG

Moncloa, F.
Angio-Medical Corporation, 1350 Avenue of the Americas, New York,
NY 10019, USA

Mohr, P.
Dermatologische Klinik, Universitäts-Krankenhaus Eppendorf,
Martinistraße 52, W-2000 Hamburg 20, FRG

Pawlak, F. M.
Dermatologische Klinik der Ruhr-Universität Bochum, St. Josef-Hospital,
Gudrunstraße 56, W-4630 Bochum 1, FRG

Payne, P. A.
Department of Instrumentation and Analytical Science,
University of Manchester, Institute of Science and Technology,
P.O. Box 88, Manchester M60 1QD, UK

Pech, A.
Systemhaus für Automation und technische Informatik GmbH,
Nordendstraße 32, W-6082 Mörfelden-Walldorf, FRG

Peskar, U.
Hautklinik der Universität Heidelberg, Voßstraße 2, W-6900 Heidelberg,
FRG

Petzoldt, D.
Hautklinik der Universität Heidelberg, Voßstraße 2, W-6900 Heidelberg,
FRG

Pistorius, K.
Dermatologische Klinik der Ruhr-Universität Bochum, St. Josef-Hospital,
Gudrunstraße 56, W-4630 Bochum 1, FRG

Pugliese, P. T.
Peter T. Pugliese MD & Associates, Rte 183, Rd#1, Bernville, PA 19506,
USA

Ricken, D.
Medizinische Klinik der Ruhr-Universität Bochum, St. Josef-Hospital,
Gudrunstraße 56, W-4630 Bochum 1, FRG

Riedl, B.
Hautklinik, Universität Erlangen-Nürnberg, Hartmannstraße 14,
W-8520 Erlangen, FRG

Schatz, H.
Dermatologische Klinik der Ruhr-Universität Bochum, St. Josef-Hospital,
Gudrunstraße 56, W-4630 Bochum 1, FRG

Schell, H.
 Dermatologische Klinik, Universität Erlangen-Nürnberg,
 Hartmannstraße 14, W-8520 Erlangen, FRG

Schlichting, P.
 Institut für Radiologie und Nuklearmedizin, Ruhr-Universität Bochum,
 Knappschaftskrankenhaus, W-4630 Bochum 1, FRG

Schmidt, K.
 Dermatologische Klinik der Ruhr-Universität Bochum, St. Josef-Hospital,
 Gudrunstraße 56, W-4630 Bochum 1, FRG

Schraube, P.
 Radiologische Klinik der Universität Heidelberg, Abteilung Klinische
 Radiologie, Im Neuenheimer Feld 400, W-6900 Heidelberg, FRG

von Seelen, W.
 Institut für Neuroinformatik, Ruhr-Universität Bochum,
 Universitätsstraße 150, W-4630 Bochum 1, FRG

Serup, J.
 Department of Dermatology, Bispebjerg Hospital, Bispebjerg Bakke 23,
 2400 Copenhagen, Denmark

Simon, R.
 Institut für Klinische Radiologie, Klinikum Mannheim der Universität
 Heidelberg, Postfach 10 00 23, W-6800 Mannheim 1, FRG

Stosiek, N.
 Hautklinik, Universität Erlangen-Nürnberg, Hartmannstraße 14,
 W-8520 Erlangen, FRG

Stoudemayer, T.
 Biosearch Inc., 3408-50 "B" Street, Philadelphia, PA 19134, USA

Stücker, M.
 Dermatologische Klinik der Ruhr-Universität Bochum, St. Josef-Hospital,
 Gudrunstraße 56, W-4630 Bochum 1, FRG

Taute, R.
 Institut für angewandte Biophysik, Medizinische Fakultät
 der Martin-Luther-Universität Halle-Wittenberg,
 Straße der deutsch-sowjetischen Freundschaft 81, O-4014 Halle, FRG

Teubner, J.
Institut für Klinische Radiologie, Klinikum Mannheim der Universität Heidelberg, Postfach 10 00 23, W-6800 Mannheim 1, FRG

Tilgen, W.
Hautklinik der Universität Heidelberg, Voßstraße 2, W-6900 Heidelberg, FRG

Ulrich, J.
Klinik für Hautkrankheiten, Medizinische Akademie Magdeburg, Leipziger Straße 44, O-3090 Magdeburg, FRG

Vieluf, D.
Dermatologische Klinik und Poliklinik der Universität München, Frauenlobstraße 9–11, W-8000 München 2, FRG

Weiß, J.
Hautklinik, Klinikum Mannheim der Universität Heidelberg, Postfach 10 00 23, W-6800 Mannheim 1, FRG

Willgeroth, C.
Klinik für Hautkrankheiten, Medizinische Akademie Magdeburg, Leipziger Straße 44, O-3090 Magdeburg, FRG

Winkler, K.
Dermatologische Klinik der Ruhr-Universität Bochum, St. Josef-Hospital, Gudrunstraße 56, W-4630 Bochum 1, FRG

The Physics of Ultrasound

Physical Ultrasound Phenomena in Tissues

H. KUTTRUFF

Introduction

Medical diagnostics with ultrasound, known as sonography, is based upon a principle which is also employed in several technical methods of ranging. These are nondestructive testing of materials, i.e., ranging underwater by means of sound. In all these methods a short wave train is emitted in a certain direction, and from the reflected and received echoes conclusions are drawn about the objects which have reflected the ranging beam, in particular their distance and also their speed if the Doppler effect is exploited. However, no reliable information on the nature and the size of the objects is obtained in this way.

The objects to be detected and displayed in sonography are the boundaries between different tissues and the interior structures of the tissues themselves. Thus, in sonography the medium itself is the object of investigation, whereas in other fields it plays rather an inferior role. The physical properties of the objects and the processes taking place in them under the influence of sound are therefore of particular importance for the quality and significance of sonographic representation.

At sufficiently high sound intensities, permanent changes in a tissue, i.e., tissue damage, may occur; this potential for causing damage must also be taken into consideration.

In this chapter, the following phenomena will be discussed:
1. Reflection and refraction of sound incident on boundaries (boundaries of tissues)
2. Absorption of sound in tissues, and the heating caused by it
3. Scattering of sound by tissues
4. Tissue damage caused by heat and cavitation.

Reflection and Refraction

If a sound ray hits the boundary between two different media (Fig. 1), for example between two different organs or tissues, part of the sound energy will be reflected while the other part will be transmitted through the boundary.

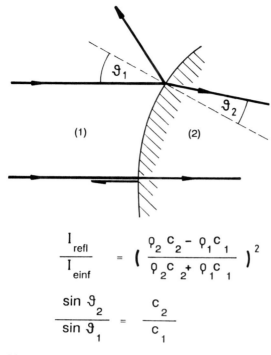

Fig. 1. Reflection and refraction of sound at a boundary

The strength of the echo, characterized by its intensity, depends on the ratio of the characteristic impedances Z_0 by which we mean the product of the densitiy ϱ and the sound velocity c:

$$\frac{I_r}{I_0 I_0} = \left(\frac{Z_{02} - Z_{01}}{Z_{02} + Z_{01}}\right)^2 ; \quad Z_{01} = \varrho_i \, c_i$$

In the usual impulse echo method, the echo will not contribute to the image unless the ray hits the boundary perpendicularly, otherwise it is not reflected towards the transducer but in a different direction. The ray penetrating the boundary from which we expect further information will be refracted, i.e., it will continue in a somewhat different direction:

$$\frac{\sin \vartheta_1}{\sin \vartheta_2} = \frac{c_i}{c_2}$$

Therefore, all subsequent echoes are attributed to a direction, strictly speaking, which does not agree with the actual direction of propagation. This leads to geometrical distortion of the image. As we shall see, the sound

Table 1. Acoustical properties of biological tissues

Tissue	Sound velocity at 1 MHz (m/s)	Characteristic impedance (10^6 N s/m^3)
Blood	1530	1.62
Spleen	1550	1.6
Liver	1560	1.65
Fat	1450	1.38
Brain	1560	1.6
Muscle	1545–1630	1.65–1.74
Bone	2700–4100	3.2–7.4
Lung	650–1160	0.26–0.46
(Water)	1492	1.49

velocities of soft tissues do not differ very much, so these distortions are not too dramatic, but they are present.

Table 1 lists sound velocities and characteristic impedances of some tissues [1, 5]. Obviously, the values do not show strong differences in most cases. Accordingly, the directional deviations due to refraction will hardly exceed 5°. Furthermore, the energy reflection coefficients are typically 1% or less. For this reason, the ranging beam can usually traverse several tissue boundaries. Exceptions are the lung, which has a comparatively small characteristic impedance because it is filled with gas, and also the bones, which have a high characteristic impedance. Ultrasound can not penetrate any of them under the usual conditions of observation.

Absorption of Ultrasound

The second effect to be discussed here is sound absorption within tissues, i.e., attenuation caused by various dissipative processes which effect continuous conversion of sound energy into heat (Fig. 2). This definitely constitutes a disadvantage for sonography since it limits the reach of sound rays and hence the depth accessible to examination; the heat produced may damage the tissue in extreme cases, and thus defines an upper limit for applicable sound energy. This point will be discussed below. The attenuation of sound rays can be partially compensated by electronic time gain control Although its efficiency is limited by the inevitable background noise, this method has proved extremely valuable.

It should be noted that absorption is not the only cause of sound attenuation. Another cause is scattering caused by tissue inhomogeneity; this will be discussed in more detail in the next section. Differentiation between these attenuation processes is quite difficult, and their relative significance is largely unknown. Therefore, the data presented in Table 2, namely the damping constants and the penetration depths of sound at 1 MHz, represent

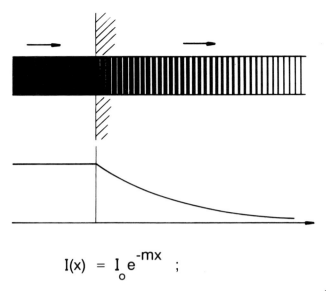

$$I(x) = I_o e^{-mx} ;$$

in-depth signal penetration (10 dB): $h = \dfrac{2{,}3}{m}$

Fig. 2. Absorption of sound in a dissipative medium

Table 2. Acoustical properties of biological tissues

Tissue	Attenuation at 1 MHz (dB/cm)	Penetration depth at 1 MHz (cm)
Blood	0.2	50
Spleen	0.4	25
Liver	0.7	15
Fat	0.8	12
Brain	0.8	12
Muscle	1.5–2.5	4–8
Bone	11	1
Lung	40	0.25
(Water)	0.002	5000

both effects [1, 5]. The penetration depth is defined as the path length along which the intensity of a sound wave drops to one-tenth its initial value. Of course, these figures are only approximate since the physical properties of biological tissues are subject to strong variations. The highest attenuation occurs in the lung and in bones due to their porous structure. The modest penetration depth of other tissues clearly indicates the need of electronic time gain control. Furthermore, the attenuation of ultrasound in tissues increases significantly with frequency, i.e., at higher frequencies the penetration depth is smaller than at lower frequencies. The frequency dependence differs for the various tissues, and cannot be described by a general statement.

Scattering of Ultrasound by Inhomogeneities

Because of the interior structure of each biological tissue, there are local variations in sound velocity and density, both of which cause a disturbance of sound propagation known as scattering.

If a limited obstacle is hit by a sound wave, a secondary wave, the „scattering wave" will emerge from it in more or less every direction. Part of the sound will be back-scattered, another scattered in forward direction, forming a "shadow" by superimposition with the primary wave provided that the obstacle is opaque and sufficiently large. The strength of the scattering wave depends, of course, on the size of the object, in particular compared to the acoustical wavelength. The total energy per second for small obstacles increases to the fourth power of the sound frequency.

If there are many obstacles or inhomogeneities in the insonified region (Fig. 3), each of them will scatter a certain amount of energy from the primary wave, accordingly the latter undergoes additional attenuation. This component of attenuation follows the same law of distance as that caused by absorption, namely an exponential law, making it difficult if not impossible to differentiate both factors.

On the other hand, the scattering waves from the various objects interfere with each other in a complicated way. If the scattering objects were arranged in a regular pattern, the total scattered radiation would also show a regular directional distribution. If the scattered waves are randomly distributed, the

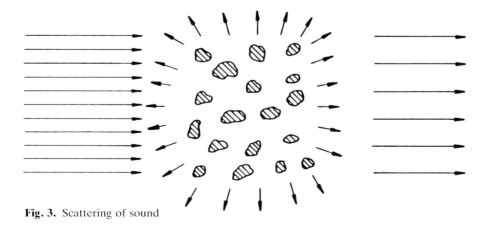

Fig. 3. Scattering of sound

directional distribution does not show regularities but is statistical in character. Since biological tissue often has a texture which is not completely regular, the structures of most tissues will be somewhere between periodic and random.

For the purposes of sonography it is important that part of the secondary radiation is back-scattered to the transducer and is indicated as a collection of many tiny echoes. In technical material testing, this effect is quite undesirable, since it makes it difficult or even impossible to detect flaws in the material. The situation is different in sonography, where the back-scattered echoes contribute significantly to the formation of a sonographic image because their distributions – both spatially and with respect to their strength – are quite different for the various tissues and organs. In the irradiation of liquid-filled voids, for instance, no scattering echoes will be observed at all, and that region will appear dark in a B display, which facilitates the detection of its contour. The presence or absence of scattering echoes and also their spation distribution makes it possible to distinquish different tissues even if their boundaries do not produce significant echoes.

It should be emphasized, however, that not every little bright spot in a B display can be attributed to a certain inhomogeneity since the resolution of sonography is not sufficient to image the inhomogeneities themselves. In reality, the speckled structure of the images is due to random interference of many tiny echoes. In certain regions, they can cancel each other, resulting in a dark spot, or they may enhance each other by constructive interference, which leads to a bright spot.

Which of these will occur depends on the mutual phase differences and hence on the random distribution of the inhomogeneities. This shows that the observed brightness pattern is certainly caused by tissue properties, but not in a simple and deterministic way. If the sound wavelength is varied, the details of an echo pattern will completely change, although its general character will be retained. This can be shown very clearly by computer simulation of back-scattering from tissue models [2].

Two further facts may be mentioned in this context. If the density and scattering efficiency of the obstacles is very high, secondary waves which have already been scattered can be scattered again. This further complication is known as multiple scattering. Furthermore, if the scattering objects are not round but have the shape of disks, the scattered radiation will often have a direction of preference. If the disks are perpendicular to the direction of the primary wave and are spaced, the sound can penetrate in a way similar to that of traffic noise coming through a fence or even several fences. If the disks are not separated by gaps, however, they may form a barrier for ultrasound, particularly at high frequencies. This is probably important for the application of ultrasound in dermatology.

Tissue Damage Caused by Ultrasound

From the physical point of view, there are two primary effects which may cause damage to tissues:
a) production of heat by ultrasound absorption, and
b) cavitation.

While the first factor can be measured – at least in principle – by implanted thermoelements, it is extremely difficult to detect damage caused by cavitation.

Heat

Heating of tissue by continuous conversion of sound energy into heat is counteracted by heat conduction in the tissue and by convection, i.e., by flow of heated blood. The higher the temperature difference between the heated tissue and its environment, the greater the heat exchange. Therefore, immediately after starting irradiation, the temperature will rise relatively quickly; then the rate declines. After some time, a thermal equilibrium will be established in which the heat influx is balanced by losses. The interesting question is a which temperature level this equilibrium will be reached.

Estimates based on the thermal properties of biological tissues and neglecting convection lead to the conclusion that at an average sound intensity of 100 mW/cm^2 the maximum rise in temperature will be of the order of a few degrees C [4]. Since the cooling effect of bloodflow is significant, it is safe to assume that no thermally induced tissue damage will occur at this sound intensity.

Cavitation

Tissue damage caused by cavitation results from the formation of voids or cavities in the underpressure phase of a sound wave [6]. These voids behave in different ways depending on whether they are filled with gas, or whether they are formed rapidly enough to prevent the gas dissolved in body fluid from diffusing into the void. In the former case the cavities create periodic pulsations in a sound field, which are probably harmless. In the second, however, they implode very rapidly after the underpressure has vanished, and these collapses are accompanied by strong shock waves, strong microstreaming, and high local temperatures. Therefore, this kind of cavitation concentrates energy into very small regions. From other disciplines it is well known that the surfaces of solid bodies such as metals may be eroded and damaged. Although there is no unambignous proof of damage caused by cavitation, it would be unsafe to assume that it could not occur at sufficiently high intensities.

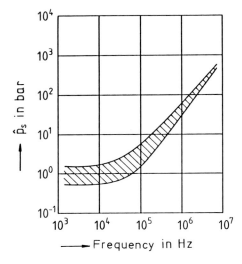

Fig. 4. Cavitation threshold for stationary ultrasonic fields (after Esche [3])

For cavitation to occur, the sound intensity has to exceed a threshold (Fig. 4) that depends on the nature of the irradiated medium and on the shape of the ultrasound signal. It is important to note that it is not the average intensity which determines the onset of cavitation but the peak sound pressure occurring during a sound impulse. An evaluation of the conditions that are typical for sonography leads to the conclusion that the pressure threshold lies in the order of magnitude of 30 atmospheres, corresponding to a peak intensity (in water) of about 300 W/cm^2, i.e., an average intensity of 300 mW/cm^2 if a duty ratio of 1:1000 is assumed. This means that averaged intensities below 100 mW/cm^2 can be considered safe as far as cavitation is concerned.

Conclusions

Many of the questions concerning the propagation and effects of ultrasound in body tissues are still unanswered because the physical properties of these media are not sufficiently known. Some of these questions are unimportant for the practical application of sonography, while others could well contribute to a better differentiation of tissues. It is hoped that more research will be carried out in this interesting field, resulting in still more efficient and useful applications of ultrasound in medicine, and particularly in dermatology.

References

1. Bamber JC (1986) Attenuation and absorption speed of sound. In: Hill CR (ed) Physical principles of medical ultrasonics. Wiley, New York

2. Dickinson RJ (1986) Reflection and scattering. In: Hill CR (ed) Physical principles of medical ultrasonics. Wiley, New York
3. Esche R (1952) Untersuchung der Schwingungskavitation in Flüssigkeiten. Acustica 2: 108
4. Kuttruff H (1991) Ultrasonics – Fundamentals and applications Elsevier Applied Science, London
5. Wells PNT (ed) (1980) Ultrasound in medical diagnostics. Wileey, New York
6. Young FR (1988) Cavitation. McGraw-Hill, London

A- and B-Scan Techniques of Conventional Ultrasound Units. A Survey

G. KREITZ

Introduction

Today, ultrasound diagnostics takes a very important place in clinical and practical medicine. As a noninvasive examination it has been successfully applied for more than 20 years in general medicine, but it has not quite establish ed itself in dermatology despite the fact that, in recent times, very positivve results have been achieved with specialized units.

The most important fields of application of ultrasound diagnostics range from obstetrics to abdominal examinations and cardiology. In cardiology, the Doppler effect is of particular importance since it allows the determination of flow direction and velocity of the blood in the vessels and in the heart.

The introduction of the real time procedure and gray scale recording had a great influence on the broad distribution and acceptance of the method.

Imaging Procedures

The A- and B-scan procedures are frequently used today. A-scan units represent the received (Fig. 1) ultrasound echo signals as a one-dimensional amplitude diagram disgram displayed against the time (Fig. 1). This is referred to as amplitude modulation. The time axis is represented horizontally and corresponds to the field depth in the tissue; the propagation velocity c of the ultrasound waves can be assumed as being constant (c = 1540 m/s). A-scan units are highly suitable, there fore, for distance measurements in tissue.

All the two-dimensional procedures are called B-scan procedures. A two-dimensional ultrasound image consists of single lines (A-lines). Here, the differing amplitudes of the A-lines are represented as brighter or darker pixels. A high signal amplitude corresponds to a bright pixel. This is referred to as "brightness modulation" (Fig. 1). In an image memory the individual ultrasound lines are added to one complete (sectional image).

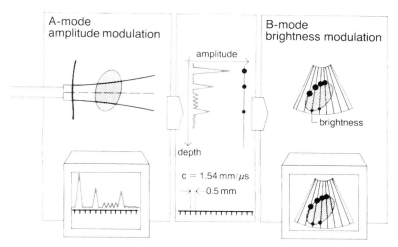

Fig. 1. Imaging procedure. *A-mode (A-scan)* represents the received echo signal as a one-dimensional amplitude diagram displayed against the time. *B-mode (B-scan)* is a two dimensional presentation of different A-lines, where the signal amplitude corresponds to bright pixel.

Image Acquisition and Scanning Methods

One single ceramic element is sufficient as ultrasound transducer for the generation of one A-line. The range of highest definition lies in the focusing region. One single element only has one focus. A two-dimensional sectional image consists of single lines. To produce these it is necessary to detect the echo information a larger region of human tissue, which requires unifrom scanning of the region of interest. To do this, either the sector scan or the linear scan procedure can be used. The sector scan is rather easy to build up: a single element is moved by motor and gears, so that the scan beam of the transducer covers a section of the tissue. Such a swivel of the scan beam can also be generated electronically. So there are two types of sector scanner – mechanical and electronic. Mechanical sector scanners have the best cost-benefit relation, but have only one focusing region. Electronic sector scanners are more sophisticated; they have several channels and permit several foci.

For linear scans there are up-to-date probes containing up to 512 ceramic elements. They are called linear arrays. The higher the number of elements, the higher the number of ultrasound lines to scan the tissue. This leads to an increased information density from the tissue, but also to increased electronic expenditure in the ultrasound unit. In order to achieve a good focus region, single elements are collected in a group (e.g., 16 or 32). In phased array systems groups of 64 to 192 are used.

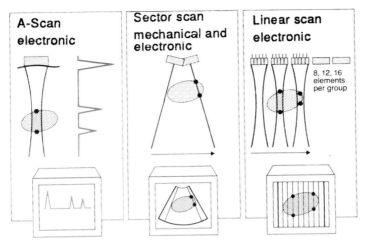

Fig. 2. Image acquisition and scanning method. To generate one A-line, one single element transducer is sufficient. A linear scanner contains up to 512 ceramic elements. For better beam focusing several elements are bundled in groups.

Sector scanners allow easy coupling to the human body since they have a small coupling surface. It is thus possible to reach intercostal spaces (echocardiography). Linear scanners have a large sound window; their application range includes, for example, the thyroid gland where the imaging of the organ in its length is important (Fig. 2).

Technological Limits

In linear or phased array units the information density increases with increasing numbers of channels, i.e., with increasing numbers of elements. These numbers are limited for technological reasons: for frequencies above 7.5 MHz the dimensions of the single elements are already below 0.1 mm. Smaller distances for higher frequencies are not feasible for practical reasons. Thus, linear and phased array units are not suited to very high ultrasound frequencies. This restriction does not apply to single element scanners. Therefore, scanners for super-high frequencies are built up of single element systems. These are mechanical sector scanners with rotating or oscillating single element transducers. In these cases, however, new materials must be used for the ultrasound element (Fig. 3).

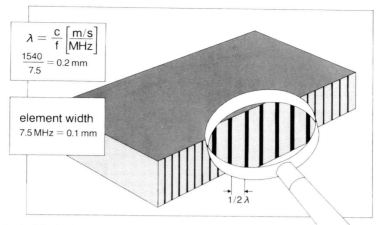

Fig. 3. Technological limitations. It is impossible to build a smaller element width than 0.1 mm, the reason for the limitation by using higher frequencies with linear arrays.

Field Depth and Resolution

The ultrasound unit's most important fields of application cover the representation of abdominal organs both close to the surface and in deeper regions. Ultrasound probes with different frequencies are used in these cases. Absorption in the tissue increases exponentially with the distance covered in the tissue as well as with the ultrasound frequency. As a result, the penetration depth of the ultrasound pulse is restricted.

The resolution is also dependent on the frequency. The highest possible resolution is, for example about 0.44 mm with 3.5 MHz. These values, however, are never achieved in practice.

A distinction is made between axial (in sound propagation direction) and lateral resolution. In axial direction the resolution is determined by the length of the ultrasound pulse and is below 1 mm for 3.5 MHz. The lateral resolution mainly depends on the geometric shape of the sound field and is up to several millimeters.

The ultrasound frequency is selected with regard to the depth of the organ to be examined. The achieved resolution is thus always subject to compromises (Fig. 4).

Damping and Time Gain Control

Signals reflected from a deeper region have a smaller signal height (amplitude) than an echo from a reflector close to the surface. Their direct

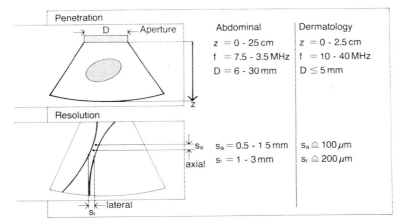

Fig. 4. Resolution. The higher the frequency, the better is axial (s_a) resolution. Lateral resolution (s_l) is related to beam focusing and depends on position of measurement in the ultrasound field.

conversion into brightness signals on the monitor would lead to a representation of echoes close to the surface as bright spots, whereas echoes from deeper regions would be shown as dark spots and thus not be visible. Therefore, vonventional ultrasound units use a time gain control (TGC). Since the damping in human tissue differs widely and is dependent on the patient, the user must carry out the TGC setting manually (Fig. 5).

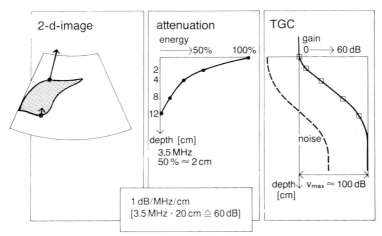

Fig. 5. Attenuation. The attenuation in human tissue differs widely and is dependent on the patient. The user must adjust the TGC-setting manually to get a homogeneous image.

Application of Conventional Ultrasound Units

A-Scan Procedures

Similar to the principle of echo depth sounding, a short ultrasound pulse is insonated in the tissue for the ultrasound-echo-pulse diagnostics. This pulse generates echoes at the boundaries between the different tissues, which, due to their travel time, are sequentially received by the same probe (now working as a receiver). In the unit the echo pulses are processed electronically and displayed as spikes on the monitor. In order to achieve a frozen image this process is repeated about a thousand times per second. This type of display gives information on the location of tissue boundaries along the X-axis (beam direction). It is thus well suited for distance determinations.

Echoencephalography

This method was invented by Leksell in 1954 and introduced in Germany by Schiefer, Kazner and Brückner in 1963.

Echoencephalography is applied in order to detect space-occupying intracranial processes in the region oft the human cerebral hemispheres, e.g., brain tumors, cranio-cerebral trauma, hematoma, ventricular enlargements, and hydrocephalus. In nearly all cases the diagnosis is correct.

The probe is applied above the right or left ear in the region of the temporal lobe and the skull is examined from the left or right.

In the case of an unaffected skull the so-called center-echo is generated at the central structures of the brain (falx cerebri, septum pellucidum, epiphysis, ...) in the echoencephalogram. This center–echo is the most important criterion of echoencephalography and appears at the same image position on

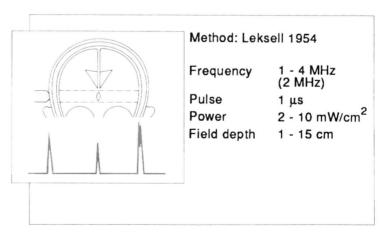

Fig. 6. A-scan echoencephalography. This A-scan method is used to detect a shift of center echo position generated by intracranial processes.

the screen for a healthy person. If there is a space-occupying process, generally a shift of the center-echo away from the image center will occur (Fig. 6).

Echo-ophthalmography

This method was introduced by G.H. Mundt Jr. and W.F. Hughes in 1956. It was popularized in Europe by H. Oksala in 1957. Ophthalmography is used to detect eye diseases, such as retina detachment, tumors, and vitreous opacities, as well as foreign body inclusions, lens thickness and length of the optical axis. These examinations can also be made if other clinical examination techniques, e.g., optical procedures, fail due to corneal clouding or cataracts.

The most important technical difference compared to echoencephalography is the higher ultrasound frequencies used here.

Normally for an examination the probe is placed directly onto the anesthetised eye, a contact stubstance being used.

Due to the application of higher frequencies, the optical axis, for example, can be measured with a preciseness of tenths of a millimeter (Fig. 7).

B-scan Procedures

The most important applications were developed with two-dimensional ultrasound units. Soon after the introduction of ultrasound into internal medicine diagnostics the image display was substantially improved (by the introduction of the gray scale technique). Today's ultrasound units are developed as standard systems; they must meet the requirements of sufficient field depth and high resolution.

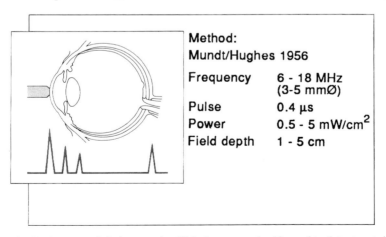

Fig. 7. A-scan ophthalmography. This A-scan method is used to detect certain eye diseases and to measure inside distances of the eye.

This is guaranteed in the first place by a broad selection of probes with different frequencies. The probes are further differentiated with respect to their focusing. In the abdominal examination field organ representations in the range 0–20 cm are needed in most cases, so that here 3.5 MHz and 5 MHz probes are used. Probes for transluminary insonation are of special importance. In recent times, high frequency endoprobes for rectal and vaginal applications have been successfully applied (5 and 7.5 MHz).

Application in Dermatology

The 7.5 MHz probes of conventional ultrasound units are very well suited to represent, for example, lesions in the cervical region if these lie in the centimeter range. However, if the dimensions are in the tenths of a millimeter range, specialized units with frequencies higher than 20 MHz are necessary.

Summary

Today's ultrasound units were developed for a broad range of applications. The probe selection and thus the ultrasound frequency to be used depends on the required organ representation. Characteristic featuers are the number of channels, focusing and resolution. We saw that conventional ultrasound units can also be applied in general dermatologic diagnostics. For the representation of the skin, or for specific questions of dermatologic diagnostics, ultrasound frequencies of 10–50 MHz are specially suitable. The advantage of high-frequency ultrasound is the high resoluton, whereas the depth of penetration is restricted to 2.5–0.5 cm.

References

Introduction
Pätzold J, Krause W, Kresse H, Soldner (1970) Present state of an ultrasonic cross-section procedure with rapid image rate. IEEE Trans Biomed Eng
Rettenmaier G (1971) Ultraschalluntersuchungen im Pankreasgebiet. Fortschr Med 89 (33): 1279–1284
Rettenmaier G (1971) Technik und Kriterien der Ultraschall-Schnittbilduntersuchung der Leber. Electromedica 3
Soldner R, Krause W (1971) Ultraschall-Scanner mit hoher Bildfolge für die medizinische Diagnostik. Biomed Techn 16 (3): 87–89

Imaging Procedures, Image Acquisition and Scanning Methods
Bergmann L (1954) Der Ultraschall, 6th edn. Hirzel, Stuttgart
Borburgh J, Feigt I, Zurinski V (1979) Image artefacts in linear array systems: analysis of phenomena and their elimination. Abstract 2nd meeting of WFUMB and 4th congress on ultrasonics in medicine, Mijazaki/Japan 1979, p 367
Frucht A (1953) Die Schallgeschwindigkeit in menschlichen und tierischen Geweben. Z Ges Exp Med 120: 526–557
Fry W (1978) mechanism of acoustic absorption in tissue. J Acoust (1978) Soc Am 24: 412–415

Fry FJ (1978) Ultrasound: its applications in medicine and biology. Elsevier, Amsterdam
Kossoff G et al. (1968) Ultrasonic two dimensional visualisation for medical diagnosis. JASA 44 (5):
Krause W, Soldner R (1967) Ultraschallbildverfahren (B-scan) mit hoher Bildrequenz für medizinische Diagnostik. Electromedica 35 (4): 8–11
Krautkrämer J, Krautkrämer H (1975) Werkstoffprüfung mit Ultraschall. Springer, Berlin, Heidelberg, New York
Kresse H (1982) Kompendium Elektromedizin. Grundlagen, Anwendungen, Geräte 3rd edn. (1974) Siemens, Berlin
Marini J, Rivenez J (1974) Acoustical fields from rectangular ultrasonic transducers for nondestructive testing and medical diagnosis. Ultrasonics 12: 251–256
Meyer E, Neumann E-G (1967) Physikalische und Technische Akustik. Vieweg Braunschweig
Skudrzyk E (1954) Die Grundlagen der Akustik. Springer, Vienna
Thurstone FL, Ramm OT v (1974) A new ultrasound imaging technique employing two dimensional electronic beam steering. Acoust Hologr 5
Wells P (1969) Physical principles of ultrasonic diagnosis. Academic, London
Zurinski V, Haerten R (1978) Real-Time-Sonographie mit dem Linear-Array-Scanner MULTISON 400. Electromedica 46: 141–148

Application of Conventional Ultrasound Units
A-Scan Procedures
Leksell L (1954) Kirurgisk behandling av skallskador. Paper read at the meeting of Svenska Läkarsällskapet, Stockholm Dezember 1954, p 7
Leksell L (1955/56) Echo-encephalography I. Detection of intracranial complications following head Injury. Acta Chir Scand 110: 301–315
Schiefer W, Kazner E, Brückenr H (1963) The diagnostic possibilities offered by echo-encephalography. Experta Medica, Int Congr Ser 60: 58
Schiefer W, Kazner E, Brücker H (1963) Die Echoencephalographie, ihre Anwendungsweise und klinischen Ergebnisse. Fortschr Neurol Psychiatr 31: 457
Schiefer W (1965) Verbesserte Indikationsstellung zur Kontrastmitteluntersuchung durch vorhergehende Echoencephalographie. Deutscher Röntgenkongreß – Bericht über die 65. Tagung der Dtsch. Röntgengesellschaft. Thieme, Stuttgart
Schiefer W, Kazner E (1966) Methodik und diagnostische Möglichkeiten der Echoencephalographie. Fortschr Med 4
Kazner E, Schiefer W (1964) Das Ultraschall-Echoverfahren (Echoencephalographie), eine Methode zur frühzeitigen Erkennung raumfordernder Prozesse. Med Monatsschr 18: 27
Kazner E, Kunze S, Schiefer W (1965) Die Bedeutung der Echoencephalographie für die Erkennung epiduraler Hämatome. Langenbecks Archiv Klin Chir 310 (4): 267–291
Kazner E, Schiefer W (1966) Echoencephalographische Untersuchungsergebnisse bei Schädel-Hirnverletzungen. Acta Radiol 5: 832–842
Vlieger M de (1964) Echo-encephalographie and extra-cerebral haematoms. In: Gordons D (ed) Ultrasound as a diagnostic and surgical tool. Livingstone, Edinburgh
Echoencephalgraphy
Mundt GH, Jr, Hughes WFH (1956) Ultrasonic in ocular diagnosis. Am J Ophthalmol 41 (3): 488–498
Nover A (1963) Ophthalmol Klinische Ultraschalluntersuchungen bei Netzhautablösung und intraokularen Tumoren. Klin Monatsbl Augenheilkd 142 (1): 176–190
Oksala A, Lehtinen A (1957) Die Ultraschalldiagnostik von Augenkrankheiten. Ophthalmologica 134: 374
Oksala A (1961) Die Ultraschalldiagnostik von Augenkrankheiten Klin Monatsbl Augenheilkd 374
Oksala A (1963) Die Ultraschalldiagnostik von Augenkrankheiten. SRW-Nachrichten 19

Echo-ophthalmography
Edler I, Hertz CH (1954) The use of ultrasonic reflectoscope for the continous recording of the movements of heart walls. Kungl Fysiografiska Sällskapet i Lund Förhandlingar 24: 5
Feigenbaum H (1976) Echocardiography. Lea and Febiger, Philadelphia
Hoffbauer D, Holländer J-J, Weiser P (1966) Neue Möglichkeiten der Ultraschalldiagnostik in der Gynäkologie und Geburtshilfe. Fortschr Med 84: 689–693
Köhler E (1979) Grundriß der Echokardiographie. Enke, Stuttgart
Lutz H (1978) Ultraschalldiagnostik (B-Scan) in der inneren Medizin. Springer, Berlin Heidelberg New York
Meudt RO, Hinselmann M (1975) Ultrasonic differential diagnosis in obstetrics and gynecology. Springer, Berlin Heidelberg New York
Rettenmaier G (1971) Technik und Kriterien der Ultraschallschnittbilduntersuchung der Leber. Electromedica 39: 87–91
Weyns A (1978) Radiation fields of pulsed ultrasonic transducers: plane square, plane annular and spherical radiators. Abstracts 3rd European Congress of ultrasonics in Medicine, Bologna, pp 497–501

High Frequency Ultrasonic Imaging Systems

A. Höss, H. Ermert, S. el-Gammal, and P. Altmeyer

Introduction

In dermatologic examination, structures with details smaller than 100 µm are of interest. Therefore, a high resolution imaging system is necessary to obtain predicable results. Resolution characteristics of ultrasonic imaging systems are mainly determined by both bandwidth and center frequency of the transmitted signals [3, 9]. The higher the bandwidth, the higher the attainable axial resolution will be. Lateral resolution is improved by increasing the center frequency. However, essential problems limiting the usable frequency range occur in realization of rising bandwith imaging systems. Prior to a discussion of these effects, a flexible ultrasound scan system, allowing extremely broadband operation of arbitrary transducers, is described.

Principle of the Imaging System

The entire imaging system is presented in Fig. 1. Figure 2 shows a reduced block diagram. On top of the system a fast personal computer controls several

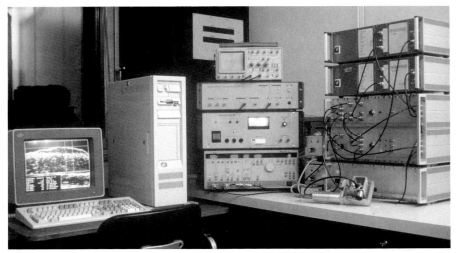

Fig. 1. The imaging system

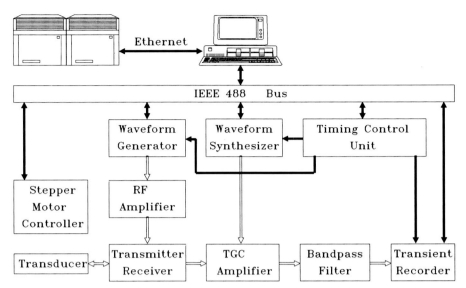

Fig. 2. Block diagram of the imaging system. Host Computer: HP 9000/835; Personal Computer: IBM PS/2 Mod. 80; Waveform Generator: Le Croy AFG 9100; RF-Amplifier: Kalmus Engineering 162 LPS; Transient Recorder: Tektronix RTD 710

measuring units over a standard bus. For starting data acquisition the computer sends an appropriate command to the timing control unit. It triggers the waveform generator, which consequently transmits an arbitrary signal stored previously. Maximum frequency of this analog signal is 100 MHz. As its amplitude is too low for driving an ultrasound transducer, an additional RF power amplifier is necessary.

A transmitter-receiver circuit directs transmitted signals to the transducer. Acoustic pulses generated by the ultrasound transducer are reflected from discontinuities inside a finite layer of skin. The same transducer is used to detect the echo signals. After low noise preamplification the voltage oszillations are directed to a time-gain-controlled (TGC) amplifier. Amplification is controlled by a second programmable waveform synthesizer. Arbitrary gain characteristics allow optimal compensation of the ultrasound attenuation over depth.

According to the Nyquist Criterion the spectrum of reflected signals is limited by a bandpass filter before digitization. In addition, bandpass filtering causes a reduction of high frequency noise in the echo signals.

In a transient recorder, filtered echoes are digitized with 200 MHz sampling rate and 10 bits resolution. Averaging of serveral scans taken at the same transducer position may be applied for further improvement of the signal-to-noise ratio. After transferring the data to the personal computer the ultrasound image is reconstructed. Time expensive algorihms for image

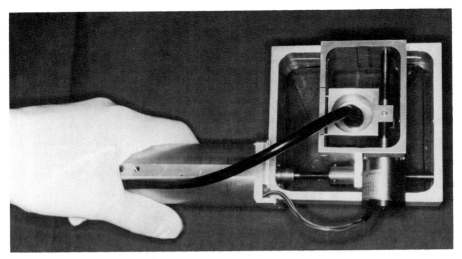

Fig. 3. Top view of the applicator

processing may be calculated using a larger host computer, thus achieving faster results.

As array transducers for high frequencies (more than 20 MHz) presently cannot be realized, single element transducers are employed instead. Therefore, the transducer must be moved mechanically for acquiring an ultrasound B-mode image. Two computer-controlled stepper motors provide transducer movement.

Both transducer and motors are combined in a small-sized applicator for manual application to the skin surface. Figure 3 illustrates the top view of the applicator. In the centre is a mounting head for the ultrasound transducer, which is moved by a stepper-motor-driven spindle. All these parts are located in a second mounting head, which is shifted by a second motor located in the applicator handle. As the third coordinate is calculated from the time delay of the echo signals, this construction permits three-dimensional data acquisition.

First the applicator is positioned on the human body (Fig. 4). For coupling the high frequency transducer to the skin surface, the very small mobile water tank is filled with water. The required distance between transducer and skin is defined by the ultrasound beam profile.

Beam Profile of Ultrasound Transducers

In Fig. 5 a schematic beam profile is outlined. Basically, one can distinguish between near field and far field, separated by the so-called focal zone where

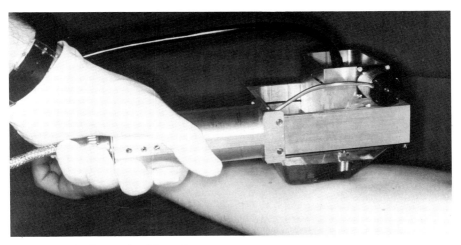

Fig. 4. Application to the skin surface

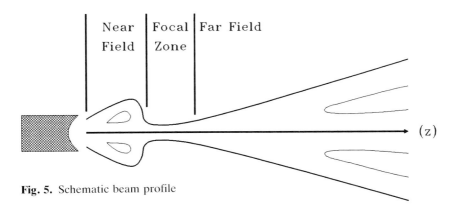

Fig. 5. Schematic beam profile

we find optimal beam profile geometry. Because this region produces maximal lateral resolution, it is of great interest for all B-mode imaging systems. Accordingly, the transducer is fixed in the applicator in such a way that the focal plane is located directly beneath the skin surface.

Transducer geometry determines the distance of the focal plane. We use spherically focused transducers only. Having a radius of curvature of 12 mm and a diameter of 3 mm, the focal plane of the transducer in water is at a distance of 11.5 mm. A calculation of the ultrasonic beam diameter in the focal plane leads to a value of approximately 120 µm.

Polymer Transducer

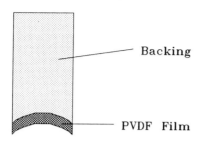

Ceramic Transducer

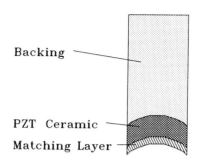

Fig. 6. Principle of PVDF and PZT transducer

Comparison of Polymer and Ceramic Transducers

Various piezoelectric materials applicable for ultrasound transducers are known. Essentially polymer films (PVDF, polyvenylidenedifluoride) and ceramics (PZT, lead-zirconate-titanate) are used. Figure 6 shows the principle of polymer and ceramic transducers. A polymer transducer includes a thin PVDF film. Excited by electrical signals, it operates in thickness vibration mode. Highly attenuating backing loads absorb radiation to the rear of the transducer. Because of its low acoustic impedance, matching of a PVDF transducer to the coupling medium water is rather good. This does not apply for a ceramic transducer; here, an additional matching layer limiting the transducer bandwidth is necessary (Table 1).

The higher the frequencies of transducers, the thinner piezoelectric materials have to be. For flexible PVDF films no problems arise with respect

Table 1. Comparison of PVDF- and PZT transducers

	PVDF film	PZT ceramic
Acoustic impedance	Low	High (matching layer)
Bandwidth	Very high	High
Malleability	High (elastic)	Low (porous)
Transducer size	Small	Small: $f < 25$ MHz Large: $f > 25$ MHz
Electric impedance	High	Low
Signal-to-noise ratio	Low	High

to this requirement. As malleability is very high, small radii of curvature and thereby highly focused transducers are possible. On the other hand, porous ceramic has low malleability. For manufacturing reasons ceramic transducers operating at frequencies higher than 25 MHz can only be realized using plane piezoelectric crystals. Focusing is obtained by a quartz rod containing a lens. Consequently, this method of construction leads to larger transducers. For example, the diameter of a ceramic 50 MHz transducer is more than twice as large as that of an equivalent PVDF transducer and the ceramic transducer is three times langer than the polymer one. Because of these transducer size differences we currently use PVDF transducers.

Ceramic transducers do also offer great advantages. Compared to polymer transducers they have lower electric impedances and are better matched to subsequent electronic circuits. Much more important is the fact that, under the same conditions, the signal-to-noise v-ratio achieved by a ceramic transducer is 10–20 dB higher than that of the corresponding polymer transducer. This is an important consideration – especially in medical applications of ultrasound – when studying the physics of ultrasound in biological tissue [9, 10].

Problems in Broadband Imaging Systems

Roughly, a value of 1 dB/(MHz cm) cm may be assumed for the attenuation of ultrasound in skin. Attenuation of pressure amplitudes obtained from 5 mm depth have been calculated for various frequencies (Fig. 7). Under the same conditions, a 10 MHz signal will lead to a hundred times higher detected amplitude than a 50 MHz signal, and even to a thousand times higher

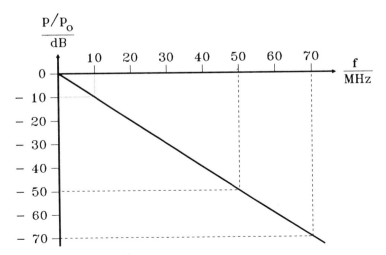

Fig. 7. Attenuation of ultrasound in skin

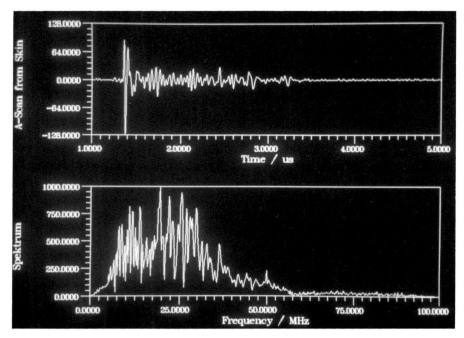

Fig. 8. A-scan of skin

one than a 70 MHz signal. Hence, in addition to very low noise receiving electronics, transducers yielding optimum signal-to-noise ratio are necessary for high frequency ultrasound imaging systems. Therefore, conventional in vivo imaging systems operating at frequencies up to 25 MHz, as well as all array systems, use transducers based on ceramic piezomaterial.

Frequency-dependent attenuation of ultrasound in biological tissue also influences the axial resolution of the imaging system. Figure 8 displays an A-scan of skin. The transducer was excited by a broadband electric pulse. In addition to very short echoes, which are due to several epidermal layers of skin, relatively high but wide echoes at a depth of a few millimeters can be recognized. The lower diagram shows the Fourier spectrum of the A-scan. Distinct falling off to higher frequencies has its cause in the attenuation of ultrasound in skin. Directly beneath skin surface the bandwith is high and thereby the acoustic pulse is short. Here we obtain excellent axial resolution. The larger the depth of invasion, the higher the attenuation of high frequency components. As the pulses get longer, axial resolution decreases. This undesired effect may be tolerated in dermatologic applications because regions of interest are located close to the skin surface.

Moreover, compensation of ultrasound attenuation in skin using a TGC amplifier is necessary. For practical use compensation of 10–15 dB has proved useful. Without any TGC amplification very low echoes are detected at a depth of a few millimeters, while higher compensation leads to an overestimation of those echoes because low frequency spectral components are less attenuated than higher ones.

Some Results

The system described above leads to a penetration depth of about 4 mm. An axial resolution of 24 µm is attainable, while the lateral resolution, mainly influenced by the ultrasonic beam diameter, is about 88 µm. Both values result from thin nylon threads located in the transducer's focal plane. They represent -6 dB measurements of the envelope of the according echoes (Fig. 9).

We have described the principle of three-dimensional data acquisition above. Unfortunately, there is no possibility of a reasonable visualization of three-dimensional recorded data all at once. For this reason, we show the results in various sections (Fig. 10). Both vertical sectional views of skin in

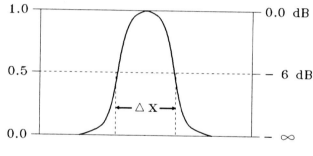

Fig. 9. Measurement of resolution characteristics

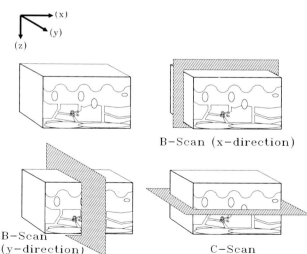

Fig. 10. Graphical illustration of three-dimensional data using various cross-sectional views

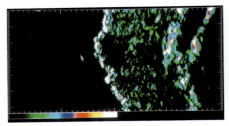
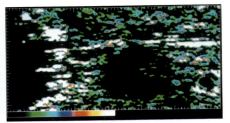

Fig. 11. B-scan of a birthmark

Fig. 12. C-scan of the birthmark

either x or y direction, and sections parallel to skin, are possible. The first two cases result in B-scans while sections parallel to skin are called C-scans.

Some in vivo results are now presented. First, a birthmark approximately 2 mm in diameter was examined. The scanning area was 6.4 mm in x direction and 3.2 mm in y direction. Using scanning steps of 50 μm in both directions we obtained 128 times 64 A-scans each consisting of 1024 points. It should be mentioned that both scanning area and scanning steps may be chosen arbitrarily by setting appropriate parameters in the program. A maximum area of 14 mm in x direction and 17 mm in y direction can be scanned.

Figure 11 displays a B-scan. The depth of invasion is plotted towards the right, and scanning direction x is plotted upwards. The scale shows millimeters and tenths of millimeters. The structure of skin is depicted. Basically, three layers can be recognized. Several epidermal layers produce high intensity echoes. Echoes of medium intensity arise from ultrasonic scattering of various irregularly distributed collagen threads in the second layer of skin. Beneath this layer we find subcutaneous fat tissue which produces low intensity echoes because of vast homogeneity.

There is also a 300 μm thick echo-free area between epidermis and corium which indicates the region of pigments. Observation of several adjacent sectional views of skin guarantees reliable measurement of the birthmark at its greatest depth.

The shape of the birthmark is also of interest. Figure 12 presents a C-scan taken at a depth of 400 μm. Towards the right the scan axis in x direction, and upwards the scan axis in y direction, are displayed. The true-to-scale picture indicates the region of pigments again as an echo-free zone.

As another example, Fig. 13 shows the ultrasonic image of a malignant melanoma. Like a birthmark, the tumor region appears as an area of low echo intensity. With the aid of two cursors, a region of interest has been marked out. This part of the tumor is zoomed out in the bottom right part of Fig. 13. Additional amplification (by a factor of 2.5) as well as algorithms for interpolation and edge enhancement were used in calculating the detail picture. While in the upper total view the tumor nearly appears as a homogeneous black region, the detailed zoom picture indicates structural texture inside the tumor. It seems that differentiation of tumor and a not too

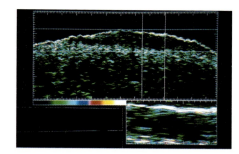

Fig. 13. Ultrasonic image of a malignant melanoma

dense infiltrate as well as characterization of various types of tumors could be possible. Tissue characterization is one focus of our current research. Results will be presented in the near future.

Acknowledgement. The authors are grateful to the Deutsche Forschungsgemeinschaft (DFG), Bonn, for supporting this work (Project No. ER 94/5–1).

Bibliography

1. Cellerame J, Tancrell RH, Wilson DT (1970) Transmitters and receivers for medical ultrasonics. IEEE Ultrason Symp Proc 1: 407–411
2. Dines KA, Sheets PW, Brink JA, Hancke CW, Condra KA, Clendenon JL, Goss SA, Smith DJ, Franklin TD (1984) High frequency ultrasonic imaging of skin: experimental results. Ultrason Imaging 6: 408–434
3. Ermert H (1990) The physics of acoustic wave propagation and engineering concepts of diagnostic imaging. Zentralbl Haut Geschlechtskr 157:317
4. Gammel PM (1981) Improved ultrasonic detection using the analytic signal magnitude. Ultrasonics 2: 73–76
5. Hoess A, Ermert H, el-Gammal S, Altmeyer P (1989) Hochauflösendes Ultraschallsystem für die Untersuchung von Hauterkrankungen und zur Tumordiagnostik in der Dermatologie. Tagung der Deutschen Gesellschaft für Biomedizinische Technik, Kiel
6. Hoess A, Ermert H, el-Gammal S, Altmeyer P (1989) A 50 MHz ultrasonic imaging system for dermatologic application. IEEE Ultrason Symp Proc 2: 849–852
7. Hoess A, Ermert H, el-Gammal S, Altmeyer P (1990) A high frequency ultrasonic imaging system. Zentralbl Haut Geschlechtskr 157:318
8. Krautkraemer J, Krautkraemer H (1986) Werkstoffprüfung mit Ultraschall. Springer, Berlin Heidelberg New York
9. Kuttruff H (1988) Physik und Technik des Ultraschalls. Hirzel, Stuttgart
10. Kuttruff H (1990) The physics of ultrasound in biological tissue. Zentralbl Haut Geschlechtskr 157:317
11. Lucas BG, Muir TG (1982) The field of a focusing source. J Acousut Soc Am 72: 1289–1296
12. Oppenheim A, Schafer R (1975) Digital signal Processing. Prentice-Hall, Inc.
13. Yano T, Fukukita H, Ueno S, Fukumoto A (1987) 40 MHz ultrasound diagnostics system for dermatologic examination. IEEE Ultrason Symp Proc 2: 875–878

A Procedure to Improve the Resolution of Superposed Ultrasound Signals

R. Taute, H.J. Hein, and K.V. Jenderka

Back-scattered ultrasound signals comprise a lot of information on investigated biological tissue. Echo signals are limited by scattering and absorption. This has an important bearing on the characteristics of the spectra of signals. Absorption depends chiefly on frequency; it is greater for higher frequency than for lower. In this way the spectrum is changed by increasing depth of biological tissue. The distances of scatterers, as a characteristic parameter, can be computed from the spectrum [6]. In analyzing distributions of scatterers there often arises the problem of superposition of signals. In the measurement of the scatterer distance, the densities of neighboring components merge more and more with increasing depth. Similar problems occur in A- and B-scan analysis. The decomposition of structures that have small distances along the beam axis is limited by the length of ultrasound pulses (Fig. 1).

The separation of such fused components without increasing expense of measurement is an important factor in obtaining a better estimation of parameters of tissue. The way in which this decomposition of superpositions

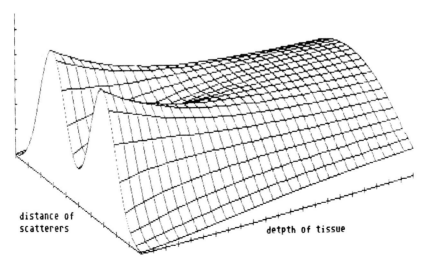

Fig. 1. Fusion of components

A Procedure to Improve the Resolution of Superposed Ultrasound Signals 33

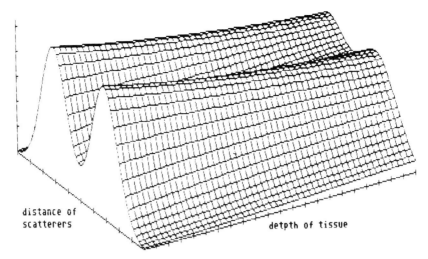

Fig. 2. Separation of components

of components may be achieved is the numerical anlaysis of measured data (Fig. 2.).

A superposition of density functions can be described as follows. In this case, a parametric family of finite mixture density functions, of the form

$$k(x) = \sum_{i=1}^{n} p_i f(x, a_i, b_i) \qquad (0 < b_1 \leq b_2 \leq \ldots \leq b_n), \tag{1}$$

is of interest where each p_i is nonnegative Heaviside, and $\sum_{i=1}^{n} p_i = 1$, and where each f is itself a density function parametrized by expectation a_i and variance b_i, and the number of components N.

Various methods have been described for separating the components of superpositions. Most of them exploit the existence of peaks and shoulders in the graph to define number and position of components, followed by least square fitting of parameters. The powerful feature of these methods is the successful combination of the users subjective intuition in detecting components at the curve with the computer's calculating power to estimate parameters [7]. Another method, well known in traditional statistics, is the maximum-likelihood estimation of parameters. In application at superpositions of components, the problem becomes intricate.

The general approach to determining a maximum-likelihood estimate is first to arrive at a system of likelihood equations satisfied by the maximum-likelihood estimate and then to try to obtain a maximum-likelihood estimate by solving the likelihood equations. These likelihood equations become very intractable because of the increasing number of components. Powerful computers are needed to solve these nonlinear equations.

A good survey of mixture densities and maximum-likelihood estimation is given by Redner and Walker [10]. We apply a combined method for decomposition of superpositions of density functions. The first step is to detect the number and position of components.

The method is called "simple diminishing of the formant" and is described by Doetsch [1, 2] and in detail by Medgyessy [8, 9]. The basic idea of Sen [11] is a transformation of the superposition (e.g., Eg. 1) into a so called test function

$$b(y, \lambda) = \sum_{i=1}^{n} p_i\, g\,(y, a_i, b_i - \lambda) \qquad (0 < \lambda < b_1), \tag{2}$$

with better distinct components (Fig. 3).

For this test function let the following conditions hold:
1. $g(y, a_i, b_i - \lambda)$ is a unimodal transform of increased narrowness of $f(x, a_i, b_i)$ and the analytical relation between $(g(y, a_i, b_i - \lambda)$ and $f(x, a_i, b_i)$ is independent of a_i and b_i.
2. The distance between the abscissae of the peaks of $g(y, a_i, b_i - \lambda)$ and $g(y, a_j, b_j - \lambda)$ is greater than, or equal to, the distance between the abscissae of the peaks of $f(x, a_i, b_i)$ and $f(x, a_j, b_j)$, respectively (Fig. 3).
3. $b(y, \lambda)$ can be constructed by the help of $k(x)$ only, without the knowledge of n, p_i, a_i, b_i and using, eventually, the analytical relation between $g(y, a_i, b_i - \lambda)$ and $f(x, a_i, b_i)$.

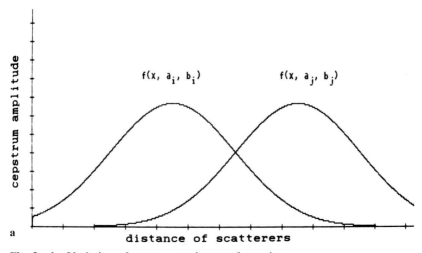

Fig. 3a, b. Variation of components by transformation

A Procedure to Improve the Resolution of Superposed Ultrasound Signals   35

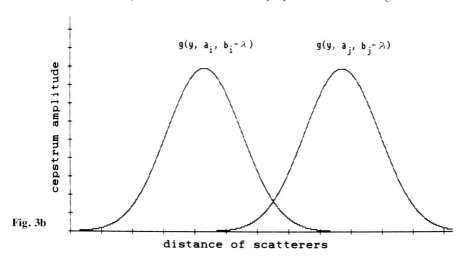

Fig. 3b

The nearer λ lies to b_1, the more peaked the components of $b(y)$, and the better the decomposition that can be expected. In case of a numerical decomposition we do not know the lowest b_k. However, the parameter λ must be less than the lowest b_k. It is necessary to compute the test function for a whole set of λ increasing from 0.

In case of superpositions of normal density functions, the relation of the superposition and the test function is determined by a Fredholm integral equation of the 1-TH-kind. The numerical solution of this equation is, in general an ill-posed problem, but it can be carried out by a series of functions

$$b(y, \lambda) = \sum_{i=0}^{N} \frac{(-\lambda)^i}{i!} k^{(2i)}(y). \tag{3}$$

Medgyessy [9] gives an approximation of, for example, Eg. 3, for measured equidistant datapoints $\hat{k}(y+jh)$ ($j=0, \pm 1, \ldots$; h is distance of datapoints) of $k(x)$ in the form

$$\hat{b}(y, \lambda) = \sum_{j=-m}^{N} c_j^{(m)}(\lambda)\, \hat{k}(y+jh) \qquad (0<\lambda<b_1). \tag{4}$$

$c_j^{(m)}(\lambda)$ is constant, it depends on λ only. The solution of, for example, Egs. 3 and 4, and some other distribution and density functions, is described in detail by Medgyessy [9]. Superpositions of components similiar to normal density functions, for example, Rice and Rayleigh density functions, which are also of importance in ultrasound signal analysis, are described by Dozio et al. [3]. The transformation of a superposition (Eg. 1) into a test function (e.g., Eg. 2) by the method of the simple diminishing of the formant is a fast transformation. It takes only a few seconds with a personal computer for 100 data points. The more separated components can be better discovered in test function than in original superposition. Every peak determines a component of superposition (Fig. 4 and 5).

A second step follows the determination of the unknown variances and weights. These parameters are found and improved together with the expectation of step one, by a nonlinear least squares fitting. Special care must be taken in choosing a suitable, efficient algorithm and good starting parameters. Furthermore, taking into account the linearity of weights, the nonlinear parameters may be reduced to 66%. Golub and Pereyra [4, 5] describe the algorithm of reduced nonlinear least square problems.

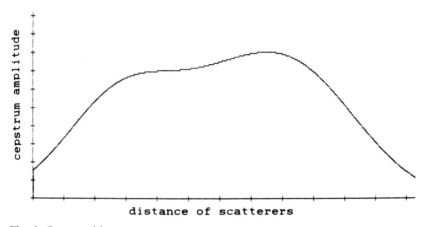

Fig. 4. Superposition

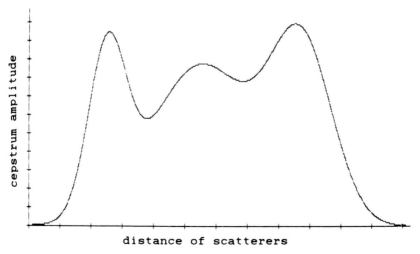

Fig. 5. Test function

As an example, we will give the analysis of back-scattered ultrasound signals of one phantom. The phantom was made of little spheres with diameters of 0.78 mm, 0.99 mm and 1.20 mm. The distribution of measured scatterer distances is shown in Fig. 6.

The transformation was carried out without knowledge of the real diameters of the spheres.

At the region of interest, from minimum at 0.60 mm to minimum at 1.75 mm, the transformation into the test function was applied. In dialog with a computer, the parameter λ was changed to good separation of components, see (Fig. 7).

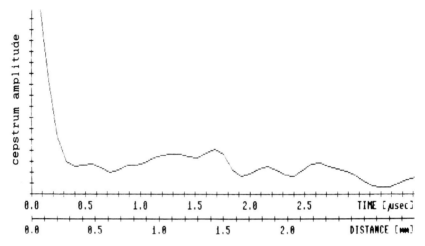

Fig. 6. Measured values

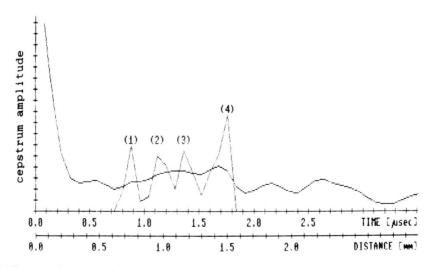

Fig. 7. Separated components

As a result we get:
1. Component measured 0.78 mm,   computed 0.75 mm
2. Component measured 0.99 mm,   computed 0.95 mm
3. Component measured 1.20 mm,   computed 1.15 mm
4. Component   computed 1.50 mm

The incorrect component 4., is the double of the first component.
A good least square fitting was impossible because of 12 parameters at 15 datapoints.

References

1. Doetsch G (1926) Probleme aus der Theorie der Wärmeleitung. III. Mitteilung. Der lineare Wärmeleiter mit beliebiger Anfangstemperatur. Die zeitliche Fortsetzung des Wärmezustandes. Math Z 25: 608–626
2. Doetsch G (1928) Die Elimination des Dopplereffekts bei spektroskopischen Feinstrukturen und exakte Bestimmung der Komponenten. Phys Z 49: 705–730
3. Dozio M, Taute R, Hein HJ, Torrigiani G (1986) Methods of separation of ultrasoundsignal superpositions. Ultraschall Biol Med 6: 57–61
4. Golub GH, Pereyra V (1972) The differentiation of pseudo-inverses and nonlinear least squares problems whose variable separate. Rep STAN C5-72-261 Stanford University, Comput Sc Dp, Stanford Calif
5. Golub GH, Pereyra V (1973) The differentiation of pseudo-inverses and nonlinear least squares problems whose variable separate. SIAM J Numer Anal 10: 413–432
6. Jenderka KV (1989) Die Bestimmung akustischer Parameter aus rückgestreuten Ultraschallsignalen. Phys. Dissertation. University of Halle-Wittenberg, FRG
7. Matthews HR (1985) A curve analyzer for micro-computers. Comput Methods Programs Biomed 20: 261–267
8. Medgyessy P (1961) Decomposition of superpositions of distribution functions. Akademiai Kiado, Budapest
9. Medgyessy P (1977) Decomposition of superpositions of density functions and discrete distribution. Akademiai Kiado, Budapest
10. Redner RA, Walker HF (1984) Mixture densities, maximm likelihood and the EM algorithm. SIAM Review 26: 195–239
11. Sen N (1922) Über den Einfluß des Dopplereffekts auf spektroskopische Feinstrukturen und seine Elimination. Phys Z 23: 397–399

General Ultrasound Phenomena

Ten Years' Experience with High-Frequency Ultrasound Examination of the Skin: Development and Refinement of Technique and Equipment

J. SERUP

Introduction

The real pioneering era of dermatological ultrasound is now over. Due to the availability of a variety of high-quality equipment constructed especially for the study of skin the method can now be more widely used. At the moment, education and traditionalism are the major problems, together with the cost of equipment. Much research work needs to be done, especially in the wide field of applications.

In 1979 a stimulus was given to high-frequency ultrasound examination of skin by Alexander and Miller [1]. Very soon prototype equipments operating at 15–20 MHz were constructed, and the basic principles became validated [2, 3]. This work was carried out in England (Chris Edwards, Ronald Marks, Peter Payne, and Chiun Tan), France (Jean-Luc Leveque and the L'Oréal tam), West Germany (Eckhard Breitbart and Schering AG), Denmark (Jørgen Serup and Allan Northeved) and Japan (Yoshiharu Miki). In at least three of these countries the development of prototypes has resulted in commercially available equipments. Recently a team of researchers in Bochum, Germany, started a dynamic research program, and centers in Berlin, Erlangen, Modena, Munich, Pavia, and Philadelphia are also active, together with many others.

A-mode scanners are unidirectional in principle (Fig. 1) and suitable for skin thickness and in vivo distance measurement between interfaces easy to identify. B-mode scanners are bidirectional (Fig. 1) and allow cross-sectional imaging of skin. C-mode scanners depict a number of automatic and parallel B-scans allowing three-dimensional presentation of a skin lesion. Technically, C-scan may be defined as a bidirectional scan perpendicular to the ultrasound beam direction, i.e., in a plane parallel to the skin surface. In advanced three-dimensional ultrasound scanning a cube of data is obtained for sophisticated processing. M-mode scanning records moving interfaces such as the wall of a larger artery. M-mode can also be used for exclusion of artifacts. Doppler ultrasonography measures moving particles, i.e., blood flow. At the moment A-mode, B-mode, and C-mode ultrasonography are directly relevant in skin research, while M-mode, high-frequency ultrasound Doppler, and advanced three-dimensional scanning are more for the future.

Without giving an extensive review of ultrasound and the skin, this chapter outlines methodology and recent aspects, and describes the contribution of Danish researchers to developments in this field during the 1980s, and their experiences. Thus, the selection of literature is not representative. My purpose is to stimulate and assist researchers who have just entered, or might enter, the fascinating field of dermatological ultrasonography. Reviews, including descriptions of basic ultrasonography, are given elsewhere [4–8].

Ultrasound Examination of Normal Skin

The epidermis and the dermis reflect ultrasound variably, but with well-defined interface echoes toward ambient air (or coupling medium between ultrasound transducer and the skin surface), and toward the underlying subcutaneous fat, which is low-reflect (Fig. 1).

Epidermal echoes may be disturbed by air contained within scales (particularly psoriatic scales), and by the keratotic material of seborrheic keratoses, which causes heavy reflections and shadows that are almost pathognomonic. Observations in psoriasis and acanthosis indicate that the ultrasound interface between epidermis and dermis is mainly determined by the top of the rete papillae.

Epidermis itself is low-reflectant. By A-mode scanning one internal epidermal echo is seen close to the entry echo. This profile is obvious in palms and soles, where the epidermis is thick. The internal epidermal echo probably represents the water barrier of the skin, comparable to the internal echo found in the nailplate [9]. The epidermal thickness is easily measured on palms and soles, where the interface to the low-reflectant dermis of these regions can be reliably defined.

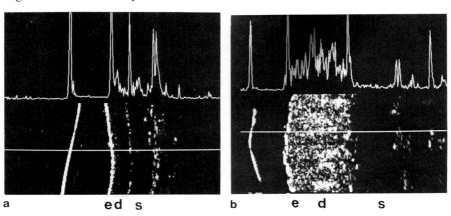

Fig. 1a, b. A-mode and B-mode ultrasound scanning of *a* neonatal skin and *b* adult skin. Neonatal dermis is low-reflectant in contrast to adult skin. *e*, epidermis; *d*, dermis; *s*, subcutaneous fat

Dermal echoes are, in most body regions, many and variable (Fig. 2). They originate from the well-organised fiber network of the dermis, which is also responsible for the tensile properties of skin and the Langer lines. Affections which erode or disturb this network cause low reflectancy. Subepidermal increase of interstitial water in edema is a common cause of low reflectancy. Dermal echoes may be influenced by the distensibility state of the skin and thus by the position of joints. Hair follicles and sebaceous glands are sometimes seen, depending on the body region. Thus, the normal and undisturbed regular fiber network of the dermis is a kind of natural contrast medium in which different pathologies can be outlined if they cause low

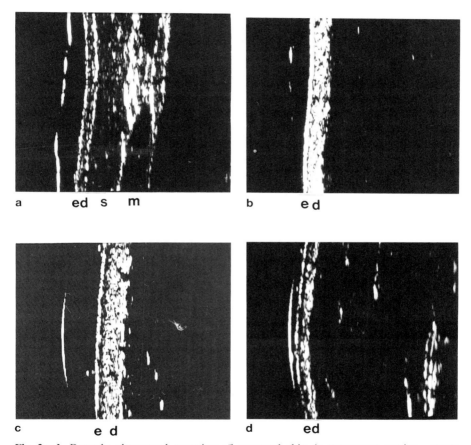

Fig. 2a–d. B-mode ultrasound scanning of neonatal skin (*a* transverse section, upper abdomen in the midline), and adult skin (*b* young individual, *c* older individual, *d* senescence). In older skin a subepidermal band of low reflectancy appears, and this is very prominent in the thin senile skin. *e*, epidermis; *d* dermis; , subcutaneous fat; *m*, rectus muscle

reflectancy, or interfaces and dimensions are disturbed. Palms, soles, and to some extent the face and the scalp are exceptions. In these regions the fiber orientation is variable, and ultrasound reflectancy consequently less. In *neonatal skin*, particularly in premature infants, the whole dermis is low-reflectant or echolucent (Figs. 1 and 2). In the mature infant the dermal echo pattern changes toward a normal or adult pattern within a few months. In *aged skin* a well-defined subepidermal band (Fig. 2) of lowreflectancy appears [10] on sun-exposed sites, such as the forearm. The skin becomes thin, particularly on distal extremities and the dorsum of the hand. Bleeding and suggillation in senile skin progress in this subepidermal zone of low mechanical resistance. In advanced corticosteroid atrophy a similar alteration is seen.

The *subcutaneous space* is normally low-reflectant. Low reflectancy depends, however, on the equipment and the gain. With high gain, subcutaneous veins are seen as dark structures. Other anatomical structures can also be visualized by proper adjustment of the gain. On the neck, chest and back the subcutaneous fascia is often visible.

The *muscle fascia* is easy to define with smooth surfaces, especially toward the muscle, while it may have attachments of retinacula toward the fat. Muscles have few internal echoes if no septal fibrosis. Bone causes heavy reflection.

Ultrasound measurement of in vivo distance can be no more reproducible than the actual biology. Obviously, rete papillae do not constitute a line or a plane, and the interface between dermis and subcutaneous fat is far from smooth due to attachments of subcutaneous retinacula. The anatomical thickness of the subcutaneous fatty layer is even more variable. Thus, the biology itself sets some natural limitations on the necessity of ultrasound equipment to measure with technically extreme precision. There is a popular but incorrect view that, if the frequency of the ultrasound equipment is high enough, all problems of variation are overcome.

Ultrasound Versus Histology and Electron Microscopy as Comparative Techniques

Histology and electron microscopy are, with some limitations, important comparative techniques. One important difference is that microscopy cannot determine tissue elasticity, and in vivo elasticity is an important prerequisite in the acoustic behaviour of tissues. Staining of tissue specimens is a kind of desirable artifact which need not visualize significant alterations of structure demonstrable by other techniques. Thus, sonography is a separate modality not directly comparable to microscopy. There will be structural behavior which is better visualized by ultrasound than histology, and vice versa. An example is the age-band of the papillary dermis [10]. In scleroderma the collagen may stain normal in histology but it may be severely degraded in electron microscopy, and ultrasound may show an echolucent band in accordance with ultrastructure [11]. Punch biopsies are of particularly limited value for comparative study since they undergo retraction and gross change of dimension on cutting [12]. It is a problem for sonography as a new technique that histology, with its long tradition, is a very useful and respected reference in many relations, a golden standard.

In vivo 20 MHz ultrasound examination will not have the resolution of histology. The advantage of ultrasound is noninvasiveness and immediate result, and a large in situ tissue block can be examined easily with a good presentation of the tissue microanatomy and with free choice of body region. Thus, ultrasound is essentially a supplement somewhere in between clinical examination and microscopy, depending on the problem to be evaluated.

Ultrasound Technology and Ultrasound Equipment

In the early 1980s my laboratory developed high-frequency A-mode and B-mode prototype scanners in cooperation with Allan Northeved of the the Danish Institute of Medical Engineering, Academy of Technical Sciences. Some of this initial work has been reviewed [8]. The prototype devices were later put in the hands of Danish industry, and further development and refinement took place, resulting in the Dermascan A and the Dermascan C, which I use in my laboratory today. The ultrasound user of today has the good fortune that a number of high-quality ultrasound devices from different companies are available.

The velocity of longitudinal sound waves in a tissue is determined by the elasticity and density of the tissue. The acoustic impedance is defined as the product of the density of the tissue and the velocity of sound in the medium. It is the difference in acoustic impedance between two adjacent media which determines echogenicity. Ultrasound follows optical laws. Thus, the character of a tissue interface and the incident angle of the ultrasound beam are also prerequisites for an echo to be apparent. The equation necessary to calculate the distance, a, of a reflecting surface from a transducer (or between two interfaces of interest) is:

$$a = 0.5\, c \times \triangle t$$

where c is the assumed average velocity in the tissue and $\triangle t$ the time required by the ultrasound impulse to hit the reflecting interface and return to the transducer (or to the nearer interface of interest). In dermatological sonography the transducer needs to be removed some distance from the skin surface. Normally, water is used as a coupling medium.

It is well known from practical use of ultrasound equipments that a relationship between the center frequency (fo) of the transducer and the axial resolution exists. In theory, however, resolution is not determined by fo but by the bandwidth $\triangle f$ of the system. A thorough theoretical discussion is outside the scope of this chapter, and in a nonideal world with physical limitations, fo does play a role, due to the fact that the achievable $\triangle f$ is a function of fo. A consequence of these considerations is that the center frequency of any ultrasound equipment gives only limited information about the resolution of the system. As mentioned previously, there is a popular but incorrect idea that high frequency is automatically followed by high resolution, and it is often forgotten that, with high frequency, the viewing field in depth becomes too small. General experience has confirmed that 20 MHz provides a good compromise between resolution and viewing depth, and 50 MHz or higher frequencies may only be suitable for scanning of the epidermis.

Resolution and usefulness of a system can only be partly deduced from a list of technical specifications, and skilled use of equipment to solve real problems is the final test. It should be kept in mind that images are qualitative, and are open to subjective or biased evaluation. Thus, modern principles of objective and blinded comparison should be employed whenever possible.

Some Main Parameters to Consider are:
Bandwidth and center frequency
Resolution (axial and lateral)
Scan speed (images per s/s per image/real time)
Swept gain, (fixed/adjustable)
Scanning field (B-mode/C-mode)
Viewing field in depth (fixed/adjustable)
Scan modes (A/B/C/M)
Measuring facilities and image analysis
Image storage facilities
Hard copy facilities
Selection of probes and transducers
Selection of display modes (color scales/split screen/zoom/etc.)

Dermascan A for A-mode Scanning and Skin Thickness Measurement

The transducer is a focused ceramic transducer with a bandwidth of 15 MHz and a center frequency of 20 MHz (Fig. 3). The axial resolution is 50 μm. The gain profile is fixed and adjustable in level. The viewing field is adjustable in depth with a 13 mm maximum width. Cursor controlled measurement with adjustable in vivo ultrasound velocity, zoom and internal memory for four curves are built-in facilities. Hard copy on an external printer, various transducers, and probe front tips are available.

Dermascan C for A-B-C-M-Mode Scanning

The standard unit is equipped with a focused ceramic transducer, bandwidth 15 MHz and center frequency 20 MHz (Fig. 4). The axial resolution is 50 μm,

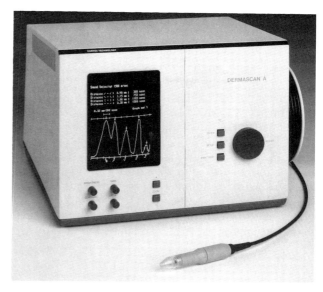

Fig. 3. The Dermascan A 20 MHz A-mode scanner for skin thickness measurements

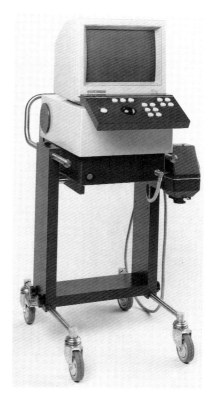

Fig. 4. The Dermascan C 20 MHz A, B, C, M-mode scanner for three-dimensional scanning of skin

and the lateral resolution 300 μm. The selectable inter-slice distances in C-mode are 140, 280 and 560 μm. Each B-mode picture is composed of 224 A-scans. The selectable scan speed/resolution is 4.8 and 12 images per second. Swept gain is fully operator adjustable with respect to slope, level and profile. The scanning field is 22.4 × 2.4 mm, the B-scan position being under full manual control. The maximum width of the viewing field is 13 mm and may be scrolled down to 30 mm in depth. Gain and viewing fields can be adjusted on the live image. The unit has various facilities for in vivo measurement and image analysis. Documentation can be provided on an external video printer. Images may be saved on an external IBM-compatible computer for further analysis and comparison. The unit can be operated with a three- or two-dimensional probe, equipped with different transducers. Display modes include split screen, various operator selectable and definable color scales, and zoom/pan modes. Both scanners are manufactured by Cortex Technology Aps, Hadsund, Denmark.

Ultrasound Velocity of Skin

Estimates of ultrasound velocity are: stratum corneum, 1550 m/s; epidermis, 1540 m/s; dermis, 1580 m/s; and subcutaneous fat, 1440 m/s [13]. The average for normal full-thickness skin is 1577 m/s. Ultrasound velocity of 1580 m/s is commonly used for the calculation of total skin thickness. A recent study found that ultrasound velocity of skin depended on body region (average: 1605 m/s) [14]. From a practical point of view, a minor deviation of ultrasound velocity from the true value of a particular location will not influence significantly the result of the thickness measurement, expressed in millimeters to one decimal point. The ultrasound velocity of the entire nailplate is 2459 m/s, and of the dorsal plate and nail matrix 3101 m/s and 2125 m/s respectively [9].

Ultrasound Examination of Skin Pathologies

Our laboratory introduced high-frequency *A-mode ultrasound* for the quantification of different skin diseases, i.e., psoriasis [15], localized scleroderma in the sclerotic [16, 17] and in the pigmented and atrophic state resembling Pasini-Pierini atrophy [18], and systemic sclerosis of the acral type [19]. A-mode skin thickness measurement can contribute to diagnosis, and it is a useful tool in follow-up and in control of the effect of treatment. We have also found ultrasound useful for the quantification of inflammatory edema of the skin in contact dermatitis and atopic dermatitis. Other laboratories have made similar observations, and more diseases could be added to the list. In the diagnostic spectrum of skin diseases, ultrasound skin thickness measurement has already been shown to have a potential use as a quantitative tool in more than 50 % of diagnoses. It is common to find that skin thickening and skin thinning, as a result of pathological conditions including endocrine discorders, are more pronounced on extremities than on the trunk.

Malignant tumors of the skin are typically low-reflectant [20]. Low reflectancy is of little specificity, and the ultrasound profile is not sufficiently specific to allow differentiation of skin malignancies, including malignant melanoma. Obviously, ultrasound can add information and improve the treatment strategy; and tumor thickness and depth of invasion can be measured. Nevertheless, ultrasound should not be used for the differentiation of benign nevi, dysplastic nevi, and malignant melanoma.

As mentioned, A-mode ultrasound is especially useful for the measurement of nailplate thickneess and epidermal thickness [9]. Nailplate thickness does not change with age as transonychial water loss does [21].

Our laboratory also introduced high-frequency A-mode ultrasound for quantification of allergic patch test reactions [22, 23] and for the measurement of weal thickness as a prerequisite to weal volume calculations [24]. Recent studies conducted by Dr. T. Agner show that ultrasound A-mode scanning is sensitive and accurate for the quantification of the inflammatory edema of irritant patch test reactions [25–30]. Ultrasound can grade both slight and severe edema, and, unlike other methods, such as laser Doppler flowmetry and measurement of transepidermal water loss, it offers the special advantage that seasonal variation and ambient conditions are not a problem. Finally, A-mode ultrasound has been used to measure corticosteroid atrophogeneity and corticosteroid efficacy (five-day chamber test) in the treatment of psoriasis [31, 32].

Thus, as a quantitative tool, A-mode ultrasound measurement of skin thickness has a wide field of applications in experimental as well as clinical dermatology. A-mode measurement is, in comparison with other ultrasound modes, especially useful when the pathology is uniform and no special structural information is required. Probes are smaller, and easy and rapid to handle, and A-mode device are far less expensive. There is with A-mode a risk of measurement of artifact structure but this is overcome by experience. On the other hand, A-mode measurement does not bear the obvious risk of bias of B-mode measurement, when the scan line can be selected from the image. In measurement of skin thickness with A-mode it can be recommended that the median of three recordings be taken in order to minimize biological local site variation and selection of a less appropriate echo. However, the best way sofar discovered of measuring skin thickness by ultrasound is to outline the contour of a block of skin by the use of the ROI (region of interest) function of the Dermascan C. With this scanner, an average thickness based on 224 A-mode scans and a 22.3 mm piece of skin can be measured quickly.

A group of Danish researchers recently showed that the diameter and wall thickness of subcutaneous arteries can be measured accurately with ultrasound, and the effects of vasoactive drugs in migraine monitored [33, 34]. Arteries with diameters of 1–3 mm and their reactions and diseases are surprisingly little studied, and the ultrasound scanners developed for the examination of skin have obvious applications in this field.

An ongoing study in Copenhagen shows that ultrasound scanners are also useful for the determination of skin and subcutaneous fat thickness in newborn babies and to determine nutritional state and effects of different nutritional regimens (S. Petersen, J.R. Petersen, J. Serup, unpublished data).

Ultrasound B-mode and C-mode is of use whenever cross-sectional imaging provides special information, which is, typically, not directly quantitative. The natural field is skin tumors. Malignancies are generally of low reflectancy [20]. Tumor echo pattern, contour, thickness and depth of invasion can be

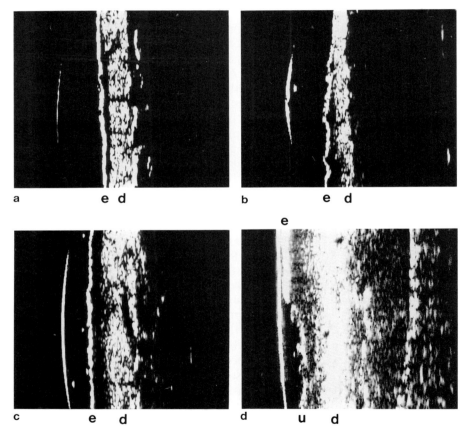

Fig. 5a–d. Different subepidermal band formations: *a* psoriasis vulgaris with band extending into hair follicle (upper part of picture) and with shadows from scales, perpendicular to the surface. *b* Pustular psoriasis. *c* Gravitational syndrome with stasis dermatitis of the legs. (A band in the papillary dermis is seen; the dermis is thickened by edema, with a dilated vein.) *d* Venous leg ulcer with band formation in the papillary dermis extending into the ulcer (lower part of picture); the dermis is thickened; toward the fascia the subcutaneous space is free. *e*, epidermis; *d*, dermis; *u*, ulcer

determined. For this purpose a systematic way of scanning, such as the C-scanning introduced in the Danish equipment, is essential. In basal cell carcinoma it is important for the surgeon to know whether the cancer has already eroded into the subcutaneous space. In Kaposi sarcoma the cancer invades the skin in a discontinuous and irregular way. In malignant melanoma, C-mode scanning is critically needed. However, ultrasound has not yet been sufficiently evaluated with respect to its predictive value in these malignancies. Relations to survival data have to be ascertained and compared to those of histology. However, tumor volume, determined noninvasively and preoperatively, should, from the tumor biologist's point of view, be a better predictor than tumor invasion, defined by the one malignant cell which invades the dermis to the deepest level. Years of research work lie ahead; 20 MHz ultrasound will not have the resolution of histology, but the strategy of treatment may very well be improved.

Inflammatory lesions show characteristic image patterns. In Histamine weals the dermis quickly turns into low reflectancy, and shortly thereafter the profile starts to normalize. Some weals drain to the surrounding papillary dermis, a correlate to pseudopodia. In more persistent inflammation, such as contact dermatitis, patch test reactions, and atopic dermatitis, a *subepidermal edema band* is visible (Fig. 5 and 6). This band is a common feature of cutaneous edema. The background is probably that the papillary dermis is more loose in structure and easier to distend. This is obvious in gravitational syndrome, stasis dermatitis of the legs, and leg ulcer, where a broad subepidermal edema band is very prominent. In ischemic ulcer the skin is thinned. In psoriasis, subepidermal band formation is also typical [35], related to thickening and activity. The background is probably both acanthosis and inflammation of the papillary dermis. As mentioned previously, subepidermal band formation can also be a result of aging [10].

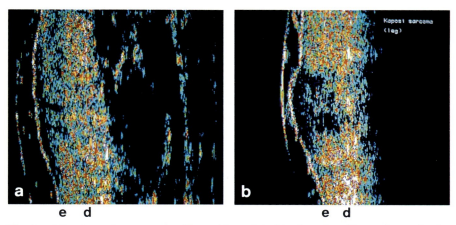

Fig. 6a. Allergic patch test reaction (2+, rubber mix) with edema band formation under the epidermis. *b* Kaposi's sarcoma in an AIDS patient. The tumor is eroding deeper parts of the dermis. *e*, epidermis; *d*, dermis

There are numerous dermatological diagnoses, where ultrasound B- and C-mode scanning is of potential use. For example, in trichoepithelioma, sebaceous-gland-like structures at all levels of the dermis can be visualized by ultrasound. There is scope for much scientific work.

In scleroderma, the skin and septa are thickened, and the subcutaneous fat may be echogenic. In chronic graft-versus-host disease the dermis/subcutaneous interface may be irregular and serrate with thickened attachments of retinacula explaining the dimpling sign. In fasciitis, the thickening of the fascia is easily seen.

In the imaging of skin lesions at various levels it is of major importance that the gain level, slope, and profile can all be adjusted on the live picture to satisfy the special requirements of that particular lesion. This can be called the *live image gain adjusted method*, with which an optimum of information about a specific lesion is obtained; in contrast, the *standard gain method* may be better for interindividual comparison. The beginner will often prefer to use a standard gain. Gain adjustment facility is, generally, more important than different color scales.

In every ultrasound examination it is important that parallel and systematic images are taken to evaluate what is typical and what is atypical for the lesion. Thus, for the purpose of skin imaging, the C-mode principle is superior. However, in certain body regions, the surface anatomy makes scanning with the big C-mode probe impractical, and better scans are obtained with special B-mode probes with which lesions may also be scanned in different sections.

It has to be remembered that selection and processing based on the examiner's choice from an image has a special risk of *observer bias*, and randomization and blinding ought be used whenever possible. As previously mentioned, A-mode scanning has advantages in this respect.

Thus, ultrasound B- and C-mode scanning is directly applicable to a great number of skin conditions. The method must be used critically and combined with sound judgement, or supported by a comparative technique.

Starting up with Ultrasound

The aim of the study should be clear and realistic, and equipment used should permit a favorable cost/benefit relationship. Color images are spectacular and expensive, and they provide special but qualitative information. However, advanced C-scanners have in-built software with facilities for image analysis and quantifications. If analysis of a study design concludes that the information needed is quantitative, if interfaces can be identified reliably, and if data is analyzed statistically, A-mode scanning by a smaller equipment may be preferable. It appears quite easy to operate an ultrasound scanner, but knowledge, training and critical evaluation of results are always needed to perform good ultrasound studies. The examiner needs to have background knowledge of the normal and pathological structure of skin.

Acknowledgements. Development of prototype equipments was supported by the Gerda and Aage Haensch Foundation and by the Danish Medical and Technical Research Councils. Development took place in close cooperation with technicians of the Danish Institute of Medical Engineering, Academy of Technical Sciences, Copenhagen, Denmark, and later in cooperation with technicians of Cortex Technology Aps, Hadsund, Denmark.

References

1. Alexander H, Miller DL (1979) Determining skin thickness with pulsed ultra sound. J Invest Dermatol 72: 17–19
2. Tan CY, Roberts E, Statham B, Marks R (1981) Reproducibility, validation and variability of dermal thickness measurement by pulsed ultrasound. Br J Dermatol 105: 25–26
3. Tan CY, Marks R, Payne P (1981) Comparison of Xeroradiographic and ultrasound detection of corticosteroid induced dermal thinning. J Invest Dermatol 76: 126–128
4. Miyauchi S, Miki Y (1983) Normal human skin echogram. Arch Dermatol Res 275: 345–349
5. Søndergaard J, Serup J, Tikjøb G (1985) Ultrasound A- and B-scanning in clinical and experimental dermatology. Acta Derm Venereol (Stockh) 65 [Suppl 120]: 76–82
6. Fornage BD, Deshayes J-L (1986) Ultrasound of normal skin. J Clin Ultrasound 14: 619–622
7. Payne PA (1989) Skin thickness measurement and cross-sectional imaging. In: Leveque J-L (ed) Cutaneous investigation in health and disease. Noninvasive methods and instrumentation. Dekker, New York, pp 183–213
8. Pugliese PT (1989) Use of ultrasound in evaluation of skin care products. Cosmet Toil 104: 61–75
9. Jemec GBE, Serup J (1989) Ultrasound structure of the human nailplate. Arch Dermatol 125: 643–646
10. de Rigal J, Escoffier, C, Querleux B, Faivre B, Agache P, Leveque J-L (1989) Assessment of aging of the human skin in vivo. Ultrasound imaging. J Invest Dermatol 93: 621–625
11. Kobayasi T, Willeberg A, Serup J, Ullman S (1990) Morphea with blisters. Acta Derm Venereol (Stockh) 70: 454–456
12. Serup J (1985) Punch biopsy of the skin by electric power drill: effect of speed. Dan Med Bull 32: 189–191
13. Edwards C, Payne PA (1984) Ultrasound velocities in skin components. International Society for Bioengineering and the Skin: ultrasound in dermatology. Symposium, Liege, November 9th, 1984
14. Escoffier C, Querleux B, de Rigal J, Leveque J-L (1986) In vitro study of the velocity of ultrasound in the skin. Bioeng Skin 2: 87–94
15. Serup J (1984) Non-invasive quantification of psoriasis plaques – measurement of skin thickness with 15 MHz pulsed ultrasound. Clin Exp Dermatol 9: 502–508
16. Serup J (1984) Localized scleroderma (morphoea): thickness of sclerotic plaques as measured by 15 MHz pulsed ultrasound. Acta Derm Venereol (Stockh) 64: 214–219
17. Serup J (1986) Localized scleroderma (morphoea). Clinical, physiological, biochemical and ultrastructural studies with particular reference to quantification of scleroderma. Acta Derm Venereol (Stockh) 65 [Suppl 122]: 1–61
18. Serup J (1984) Decreased skin thickness of pigmented spots appearing in localized scleroderma (morphoea). Measurement of skin thickness by 15 MHz pulsed ultrasound. Arch Dermatol Res 276: 135–137

19. Serup J (1984) Quantification of acrosclerosis: measurement of skin thickness and skin-phalanx distance in females with 15 MHz pulsed ultrasound. Acta Derm Venereol (Stockh) 64: 35–40
20. Serup J, Drzewiecki KT, Hou-Jensen K (1988) Ultrasound for tissue characterization of skin tumours and nevi. International Society for Bioengineering and the Skin: 7th International symposium on bioengineering and the skin. June 16–18 1988, Milwaukee
21. Jemec GBE, Agner T, Serup J (1989) Transonychial water loss: relation to sex, age and nail-plate thickness. Br J Dermatol 121: 443–446
22. Serup J, Staberg B, Klemp P (1984) Quantification of cutaneous oedema in patch test reactions by measurement of skin thickness with high-frequency pulsed ultrasound. Contact Dermatitits 10: 88–93
23. Serup J, Staberg B (1987) Ultrasound for assessment of allergic and irritant patch test reactions. Contact Dermatitis 17: 80–84
24. Serup J (1984) Diameter, thickness, area, and volume of skinprick histamine weals. Allergy 39: 359–364
25. Agner T, Serup J (1989) Quantification of the DMSO-response – a test for assessment of sensitive skin. Clin Exp Dermatol 14: 214–217
26. Agner, T, Serup J, Handlos V, Batsberg W (1989) Different skin irritation abilities of different qualities of sodium lauryl sulphate. Contact Dermatitis 21: 184–188
27. Agner T, Serup J (1989) Skin reactions to irritants assessed by non-invasive bioengineering methods. Contact Dermatitis 20: 352–359
28. Agner T, Serup J (1990) Individual and instrumental variations in irritant patch-test reactions – clinical evaluation and quantification by bioengineering methods. Clin Exp Dermatol 15: 29–33
29. Agner T, Serup J (1990) A dose-response study of SLS irritation evaluated by different bioengineering methods. J Invest Dermatol 95: 543–547
30. Agner T, Serup J (1989) Seasonal variation of skin resistance to irritants. Br J Dermatol 121: 323–328
31. Serup J, Holm P, Stender IM, Pichard J (1987) Skin atrophy and telangiectasia after topical corticosteroids as measured non-invasively with high frequency ultrasound, evaporimetry and laser Doppler flowmetry. Methodological aspects including evaluations of regional differences. Bioeng Skin 3: 43–58
32. Broby-Johansen U, Karlsmark T, Peterson LJ, Serup J (1990) Ranking of the antipsoriatic effect of various topical corticosteroids applied under a hydrocolloid dressing: skin thickness, blood flow and colour measurements compared to clinical assessments. Clin Exp Dermatol 15: 343–348
33. Nielsen T, Iversen H, Tfelt-Hansen P (1989) Dermascan A, a high-frequency acoustic scanner for non-invasive studies of the luminal diameter of superficially situated, medium-sized arteries. Cephalalgia 9 [Suppl 10]: 72–73
34. Iversen H, Nielsen T, Tfelt-Hansen P, Olesen J (1989) Headache and changes in the diameter of the radial artery during 7 hours intravenous nitroglycerin infusuion. Cephalalgia 9 [Suppl 10]: 82–83
35. Querleux B, Leveque J-L, de Rigal J (1987) In vivo imaging of the skin by ultrasonic technique. American Academy of Dermatology: 46th meeting, San Antonio, December 5–10th

General Phenomena of Ultrasound in Dermatology

P. ALTMEYER, K. HOFFMANN, M. STÜCKER, S. GOERTZ, and S. EL-GAMMAL

Introduction

Zoologists have known about the existence of ultrasound for almost 200 years now. In 1794 the Italians Spallanzani and Lazarro described the ultrasonic sense of orientation in bats. A short while later it was indeed proved that bats do not lose their sense of orientation with loss of sight but on mechanical closure of the auditory canals. Some of their prey such as night-flying moths are, however, also able to perceive ultrasound signals, a fact which has doubtless improved their chances of survival. The discovery of the piezoelectric effect by the Curie brothers in 1881 [10] laid the physical foundations for modern ultrasonography.

Ultrasound scanners did not enter into widespread use in medicine until the 1950s. Today, however, they have become routine in practically all disciplines, with the exception of a few fields which include dermatology.

There are several reasons for this:
1. By using scanners in the range of 3.5–7.5 MHz, the echogenic reflection on the skin surface was too strong and overlapped the underlying superficial details of the skin, including the epidermis and the papillary dermis [17, 18, 20]. This meant that diagnosis of pathological processes limited to the corium was inadequate or impossible. This is, however, an indispensable prerequisite for efficient diagnostic ultrasound in dermatology [7, 28–30].
2. The image resolution of the 3.5- to 10-MHz scanners hitherto available was far from satisfactory when compared with that of routine microscopic sections.
3. The size of the ultrasound transducers is still such that it is difficult or impossible to use them in certain locations such as the nose and eye regions. As these regions are of particular importance from the oncological point of view, the cumbersome nature of the transducers also prevents them from being used efficiently. Unfortunately the demand for higher resolution at present runs contrary to the desire for smaller transducers.
4. For various reasons, the ultrasound scanners generally used in dermatology operate with a water path (see below). This leads to marked disadvantages in operating convenience. Use of the more convenient

commercially available ultrasound gels for coupling the signal to the skin unfortunately produces strong interference echoes in the high-frequency scanners so that we mostly refrain from using them [14].

Ultrasound Scanners in Dermatology

The high-frequency scanners available today operate at frequencies between 20 MHz and 1–2 GHz. The optimal frequency range for dermatological questions is probably between 20 and 150 MHz for scanners used in vivo.

The generation and detection of ultrasound is based on the pulse-echo principle using piezoelectric crystals which are able to convert electrical vibrations to mechanical vibrations and vice versa.

The DUB 20 (Taberna pro medicum, Lüneburg, FRG) is a 20-MHz scanner which can operate in both A and B mode. This pulse-motor driven scanner permits an axial resolution of about 80 µm and a lateral resolution of 200 µm. The image depicts a skin area 12.8 mm wide (8-fold magnification) and about 7 mm deep (24-fold magnification). When computing the dimensions of a structure the computer bases its calculation on a mean velocity of sound of 1580 m/s for all tissues. This leads to imaging inaccuracies as the velocity of sound differs from tissue to tissue; it is considerably higher in tumour tissue and adipose tissue, for example, than in cutaneous connective tissue.

According to its amplitude each echo signal is depicted in a false colour code consisting of 256 colours, the colour black standing for echolucent structures and white for highly echogenic structures. Between the two, in order of increasing echogenicity, lie the colours green, blue, red and yellow. The colour coding permits better differentiation of tissue structures and thus faster comprehension of the sonograms.

In order to understand the structure of the image, it is important to know that the computer builds up the scan on the basis of the interval between transmission and echo return. The echoes which the transducer receives first appear at the top of the image. Echoes received later are added in the appropriate position below. In certain cases this computational operation, which assumes a uniform velocity of sound for all echoes (not in fact found in the individual tissues), leads to imaging artefacts such as the shortening phenomenon (see below).

The degree of echogenicity of a structure can be quantified by densitometry. The respective acoustic density is given a number between 1 and 256 which corresponds to a colour in the false colour representation. In order to standardise the measurement the densitometry value of a region of interest (ROI) is subtracted from the densitometry value of the water path. The densitometry number is dimensionless.

With the Dermascan C produced by the Danish company Cortex it is possible to work in real-time mode, i.e. the sonogram is available immediately. This eliminates the bothersome necessity of having to wait for the scan to be computed. The main advantage of real-time ultrasound, however, is in scanning larger areas of skin. This means that the marginal portions of an area suspicious of malignancy can be examined very meticulously. In additon, alteration of the skin tension can alter its echogenicity while the acoustic characteristics of the tumour remain unchanged. This is an examination techique where the real-time mode has a distinct advantage over other procedures. We should also mention that the patient can follow the examination procedure on the screen.

Ultrasound scanners which operate above the 20-MHz range are at present only available as prototypes. Their advantage lies in their better resolution. Even these scanners are far from fulfilling the dermatologist's need for scanners which are able to provide sufficient resolution of pathological processes in the region of the epidermis.

Acoustic microscopes (Scanning Acoustic Microscope – SAM – Leitz or Olympus) operate in the gigahertz range and permit imaging of microscopic quality. Examination of histological sections or individual cells can be performed with up to 2000-fold magnification. Acoustic microscopes are thus the ideal supplement to the in vivo scanners and permit the solution of detail problems which arise during in vivo diagnosis [8].

Frequency and Depth of Penetration of the Ultrasound Signal

A general principle of ultrasound is that the depth of penetration of the ultrasound waves is dependent on its frequency. Ultrasouund scanners operating in the 20-MHz range reach a depth of signal penetration of about 7 mm. This means that the zones of diagnostic interest in dermatology are covered, i.e. epidermis, corium, and subcutaneous fatty tissue.

Particularly if the subcutis is not very well developed, evaluation of the muscle fasciae is also possible (Fig. 1). In 50-MHz scanners, which have a considerably higher resolution and thus also a better imaging quality, the depth of penetration of the ultrasound signal is about 4 mm. This means that a diagnostic region is covered which is sufficient for most dermatological questions [1, 3, 9, 12, 15, 33]. Noninvasive diagnosis of the subcutaneous fatty tissue can be said to open up a new dimension for the dermatologist as, due to the fact that for technical reasons the subcutaneous fatty tissue often escapes closer examination, knowledge of this region is rather sparse.

General Physical Principles of Ultrasound

The Sound Field

The region lying in the path of the sound beam is known as the sound field, which is divided into near field and far field. In the near field plane waves from the centre of the oscillating crystal overlap with spherical waves emitted by the edge of the crystal. On account of the variations in sound pressure the

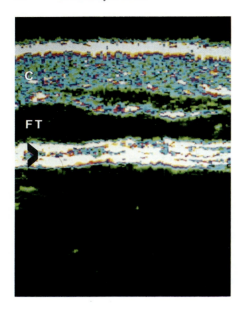

Fig. 1. Ultrasound scan of the forearm of a 45-year-old healthy man. Beneath the band-like entry echo is a moderately echogenic corium (*C*). This is followed by the echolucent subcutaneous fatty tissue (*FT*), the highly reflective muscle fascia (arrow), and the echolucednt musculature.

near field cannot be used for medical purposes. Therefore an optimum distance must be maintained between the transducer and the object to be examined. This can, for example, be achieved by an adequate water path [35] such as is integrated in all scanners used in dermatology today.

Resolution

A distinction is made between lateral resolution (perpendicular to the direction of propagation) and axial resolution, also known as depth resolution. The axial resolution, i.e. the ability to discriminate between two adjacent points, is directly dependent on the frequency. The lateral resolution is a function of the focussing of the acoustic cylinder and the scan spacing in a lateral direction. The term high resolution is frequently used in connection with diagnostic ultrasound in medicine. As this is a relative term it is usual to take standard medical scanners (e.g. 7.5-MHz sonographs), which have a resolution of about 3–5 mm, as the point of reference. From the dermatological point of view we are therefore only justified in using the term high resolution if both the axial and the lateral resolution are below 1 mm.

In order to obtain as high a resolution as possible a high frequency must be selected. At high frequencies, however, the ability of the ultrasound to penetrate tissue diminishes. Hence, we can derive definite physical standards for specific dermatological questions [3, 6]:
– 7.5–10 MHz transducers with a diagnostic depth of penetration of 2–3 cm for evaluation of the subcutaneous lymph nodes

- 20-MHz scanners with depths of penetration of 7 mm for the intermediate region down to the muscle fascia
- Extremely high-resolution sonographs in the 50- to 150-MHz range for evaluation of the epidermis and upper corium alone.

At present the term "high frequency" is used to refer to ultrasound scanners operating at frequencies above 15 MHz.

Ultrasound in Biological Tissues

During propagation of ultrasound in biological tissues ultrasound waves are influenced by various physical effects, the most important of which are reflection, refraction, scattering, and attenuation or absorption. These phenomena together contribute to the formation and influencing of the ultrasonic image.

Only if we understand the interactions between ultrasound waves and tissue can we correctly interpret the characteristic parameters of the ultrasound image and draw diagnostic conclusions. The most important parameters which describe the interactions between the ultrasound field and the tissue through which the waves are transmitted are attenuation, velocity and impedance. The attenuation and velocity of the ultrasound in a tissue increase in proportion to the relative amounts of protein and collagen contained in the tissue. On the other hand they decrease in proportion to the increasing water content [25]. Collagen fibres have a greater modulus of elasticity than other tissues. This leads to a higher velocity and higher impedance [26]. For this reason collagen is one of the main sources of a tissue's echogenicity. Processes which involve changees in the contour-forming connective tissue structures can be recorded particularly well by ultrasound. This is the case in scleroderma [21], for example, where the corial connective tissue increases at the expense of the subcutaneous fatty tissue (Fig. 2). Increases in collagen in the corium itself cannot be detected as clearly on the B scan. Such distinctions are only possible by means of comparative densitometry. In view of these facts it becomes clear that all processes which lead to reduced echogenicity or even to loss of reflection in the corium will appear as negative images within the highly reflective connective tissue (Fig. 3). The high echogenicity of connective tissue can thus be regarded as a sonographic "stroke of luck" for dermatology.

Reflection

The physical phenomenon of reflection is crucial for the creation of an image. A certain amount of the ultrasound beam is reflected at the interface between two media with different acoustic resistances. If the beam strikes the interface at right angles, its reflection is determined mainly by the difference

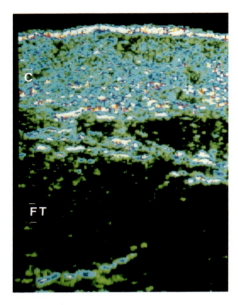

Fig. 2. Scleroderma of the morphea type. High reflective corial connective tissue (*C*) being increased at the expense of the fatty tissue (*FT*)

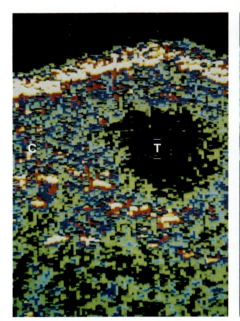

Fig. 3. Small melanoma metastasis in the upper corium (*C*). The almost cmpletely echolucent tumour parenchyma (*T*) is characteristic

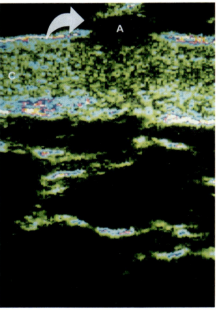

Fig. 4. Lateral scattering of the echo signal by the oblique surfaces of an exophytic tumour (capillary angioma, *A*). Entry echo absent here (*arrow*)

between the impedance of the medium in front of the interface and the impedance behind.

The proportion of the sound waves reflected at right angles and received by the transducer can be measured and forms part of the information used to create the image. The strongest echo is thus obtained at interfaces which lie exactly perpendicular to the direction of propagation of sound.

In reality the acoustic beam usually does not strike an interface at right angles, as assumed above, but obliquely. Here the principle also applicable in optics holds: angle of incidence = angle of reflection. In other words, the ultrasound signal is reflected to the side and can thus not be received by the transducer. The structure concerned is not imaged.

This situation is illustrated particularly clearly in the case of exophytic tumours. The signals from the ascending and descending surfaces of a tumour are reflected sidewards. The echoes do not reach the transducer (Fig. 4). The region appears hypoechoic or echolucent.

The physical principles described above lead to some statements of practical relevance for dermatology:
– At the interface between air and soft tissue the extreme difference in impedance leads to reflection of 99 % of the applied acoustic energy, i.e. practically total reflection [16]. This can be avoided by coupling the transducer to the skin via a contact medium.
– At the interface between water and skin reflection of the applied sound waves is only minimal (0.23 %) so that water represents an optimum coupling medium [16].
– Within soft tissue the reflection at interfaces can be very small ($r = 0.10$ for the fat-muscle interface) [16]. This means that evaluation in this region is difficult. At the corium-subcutis boundary we have a different situation. As a result of the high echogenicity of the corium and the almost entire absence of echogenicity in the subcutaneous fatty tissue this border is well defined.

Refraction

If an ultrasound beam strikes the boundary between two tissues with different acoustic conductivities at an oblique angle it is refracted, i.e. deflected from its original direction. According to Snell's law the ratio of the angle of incidence and the angle of refraction is equal to the ratio of the velocities of the incident beam and the refracted beam.

Scattering

Scattering of the signal can also lead to the absence of echoes in a tissue. Each cell represents an interface for the ultrasound wave but as this interface is smaller than the wavelength of the sound wave the latter is able to spread practically unimpeded.

However, if aggregates of cells occur with an overall size in the region of the wavelength, this results in diffuse reflection or scattering of the signal. The consequence is that a small amount of energy is removed from the incident sound wave and scattered in various directions while the entire wave is able to spread with only minimal interference.

Absorption

Absorption is the transformation of the ordered, sound-bearing oscillations of the particles in a medium into random, undirected thermal vibrations or intramolecular energy, or simply: the transformation of movement to heat. When an ultrasound wave passes through an absorbing medium its amplitude, and thus its energy, decreases exponentially as a function of an absorption coefficient. This absorption coefficient is determined by the properties of the medium and the sound frequency. As the absorption also increases with increasing frequency, the depth of penetration of the ultrasound signal decreases with increasing frequency. Thus energy is removed from the ultrasound wave with increasing depth of tissue penetration. The problem of absorption or attenuation is very familiar in dermatology, e.g. in the ultrasound examination of very thick skin such as thes kin of the back (see Fig. 16).

Here the attenuation of the signal in the upper and middle portions of the very compact and broad corium is so great that the deep portions of the corium are frequently depicted only weakly or not at all. The basal structures of the corium thus fade into the background on the ultrasound image. A further morphological phenomenon which arises in certain topographic situations is the so-called shortening phenomenon. This results from the fact that the computer builds up the image on the basis of a certain interval between transmission and echo return. If the velocity of sound in a region of interest (ROI, e.g. in a melanoma) is increased the echoes from dorsally or basally situated structures will reach the transducer sooner than those from neighbouring regions. The consequence is a computer artefact. The base of the tumour appears higher than in reality.

Morphological Analysis and Description of a Sonographic Structure

A sonographic ROI is described schematically, beginning with characterisation of the structure's shape and surroundings. Then the interior of the structure, i.e. its echogenicity, is defined.

The following schematic categories are used to describe the shape:
– Circle: circle and semicircle

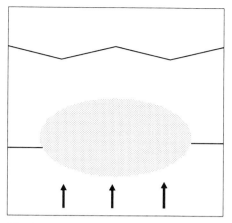
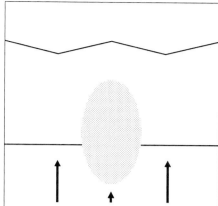

Fig. 5. Logitudinal ellipse   **Fig. 6.** Transverse ellipse

- Longitudinal ellipse: the axis of the ellipse lies in the direction of the sound beam (Fig. 5)
- Transverse ellipse: the axis of the ellipse lies perpendicular to the sound beam (Fig. 6)
- Band-like: narrow echo-poor or echo-rich band-like formations
- Others: nongeometric structures

Delimitation of the ROI

Here the configuration of the boundaries of a sonographic structure is described. Broadly speaking a distinction is made between regular or smooth boundaries and irregular boundaries (Fig. 7). A smooth boundary can have a echo-rich or echo-poor border (Fig. 8). A structure with irregular boundaries displays either hyporeflective or hyperreflective, variously shaped (squat, arciform, finger-like etc.) projections.

The transition between the structure and its surroundings may be abrupt (sharp, well-defined) or gradual (blurred, indistinct; Fig. 9).

Internal Structure of the ROI

The internal structure of the ROI is described in terms of the intensity, structure and distribution of the echoes.

Intensity. The description of the degree of echogenicity of the ROI is relative as it is made by comparison with the surroundings. The appearance of the internal echoes can be as follows:

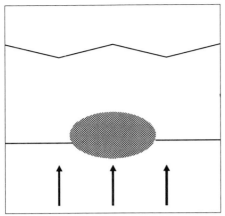

Fig. 7. Regular boundary

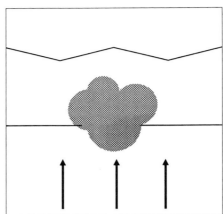

Fig. 8. Irregular boundary

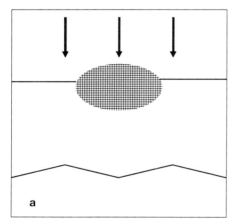

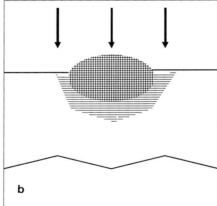

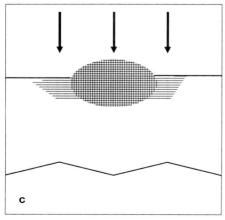

Fig. 9 a–c. Transition between the structure and its surroundings:
a abrupt;
b indistinct;
c partly abrupt, partly indistinct

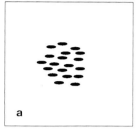 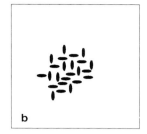 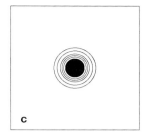

Fig. 10 a–c. Structure of individual internal echoes:
a regular;
b irregular;
c weak

- More intense than in the surrounding tissue – echo-rich
- Of equal intensity
- Less intense than in the surrounding tissue – echo-poor to echolucent

Structure. Each individual internal echo has a certain structure. The internal echo can be regularly or irregularly structured. Weak internal echoes do not display a sharply defined structure but merge diffusely with their surroundings (Fig. 10).

Distribution. The internal echoes of an ROI form varying patterns of distribution which are usually described as even or homogeneous, or uneven or inhomogeneous or mottled (Fig. 11).

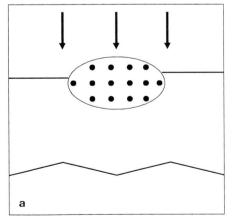 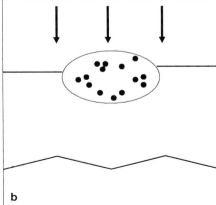

Fig. 11 a, b. Distribution of internal echoes:
a homogeneous; **b** inhomogeneous

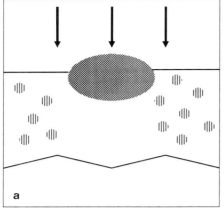
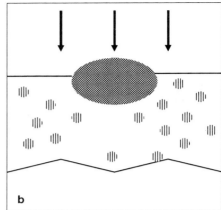
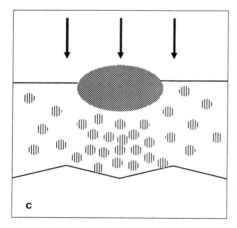
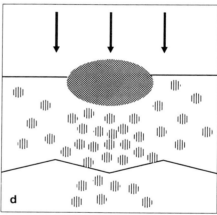
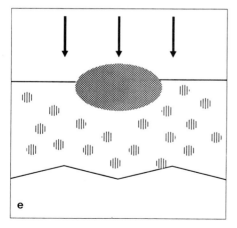

Fig. 12 a–e. Alteration of the echoes beyond or beneath the region of interest:
a dorsal acoustic shadow;
b dorsal acoustic attenuation;
c dorsal acoustic intensification;
d strong dorsal acoustic intensification;
e dorsal acoustic pattern unchanged

Acoustic Behaviour Beyond a Structure

The dorsal or distal acoustic behaviour describes the properties of the echoes beyond or beneath the ROI. They are compared with the echoes in the surrounding tissue.

The pattern of dorsal echoes can be altered behind the entire structure or only behind certain portions (Fig. 12).
- Dorsal acoustic shadow – extinction of the echoes
- Dorsal acoustic attenuation – attenuation of the echoes
- Dorsal acoustic intensification – intensificatin of the echoes
- Dorsal acoustic pattern unchanged

Lateral Shadows

While dorsal acoustic shadows or attenuated dorsal echoes lie behind a highly reflective zone; lateral shadows lie behind the lateral reflex boundary. Lateral shadows can be unilateral or bilateral, symmetrical or asymmetrical (Fig. 13). As the scanners generally used in dermatology operate with perpendicular, linear movement of the transducer lateral shadows are rare.

Special Phenomena of Ultrasound in Dermatology

After this introduction to the relevant ultrasound phenomena we will now look in detail at the individual layers of the skin.

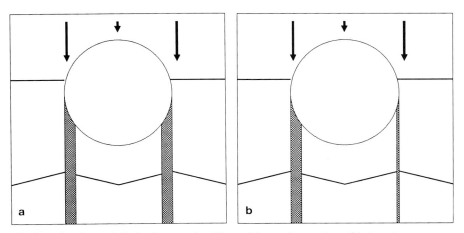

Fig. 13 a, b. Acoustic behaviour at the side and beneath a region of interest:
a lateral shadow, symmetrical;
b lateral shadow, asymmetrical

The Entry Echo

When evaluating an ultrasound scan of the skin a strong band-like echo is seen at the boundary between the waterpath and the skin, the so-called entry echo. Some authors equate this with the epidermis [11, 22–24]. This was not, however, confirmed by our more recent results.

In our opinion the highly reflective entry echo originates from the uppermost portions of the epidermis, probably as a result of the change in impedance from the coupling medium to the stratum corneum. The width of the entry echo is not identical with that of the epidermis.

Skin regions with a broad stratum corneum, e.g. on the sole of the foot, induce a highly reflective entry echo. The strong reflection of the ultrasound signal leads to attenuation of the dorsal echoes or to formation of a complete acoustic shadow. The consequence is that the underlying portions of the corium are imaged either incompletely or not at all. This phenomenon can, for example, be demonstrated as a broad acoustic shadow in seborrhoeic keratosis.

A similar phenomenon can be elicited by sticking a strip of cellotape to the skin. The strong band of reflection induced by the cellotape is not, as may have been expected, superimposed upon the original entry echo but appears as a broad (by far exceeding the thickness of the cellotape) echo-rich pseudo-entry echo. Structures of the papillary layer lying immediately below are eclipsed. Attenuation of dorsal echoes is also found (Fig. 14).

The entry echo undergoes a remarkable change in response to alteration of skin tension. An artificial increase in tension leads to a marked increase in the reflectivity of the entry echo. A reduction in tension reduces the intensity of the entry echo or even eliminates it completely (see Fig. 20).

The entry echo itself is not unstructured. This can be illustrated by sonograms of skin from the palms or soles or of acanthotic epidermis, e.g. in chronic atopic dermatitis. On the palms and the soles (Fig. 15) 50-MHz scanners indicate the presence of three layers, a phenomenon already described by Japanese authors [20]. This phenomenon, which is highly important for an understanding of the entry echo, can be further analysed with higher-frequency scanners.

Here we see a highly reflective linear initial signal followed by a echo-poor layer and finally, towards the corium, a linear exit echo. According to these investigations the entry echo arises in the uppermost portions of the stratum corneum. The echolucent intermediate layer probably corresponds to the cellular portion of the epidermis.

In acanthotic epidermis we find a broad entry echo with an irregularly structured superficial relief. We can deduce from this that it is global contourforming alterations of the gross relief of the epidermis and not alterations of its microscopic structure which contribute to the entry echo.

Highly parakeratotic horny plaques with their numerous interfaces cause total reflection with a focal dorsal acoustic shadow. The same phenomenon can be found under fibrin-impregnated crusts (e.g. under an encrusted

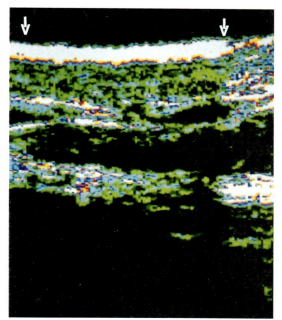

Fig. 14. Pseudo-entry echo induced by a strip of cellotype stuck to the skin (*arrows*). Distinct attenuation of dorsal echoes

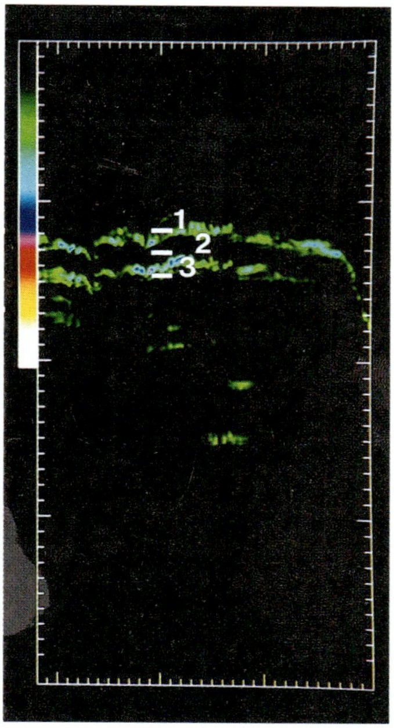

Fig. 15. Sonogram of the soles (50-MHz scanner). There are three layers in the entry echo. High reflective linear initial signal (*1*), followed by a echo-lucent to echo-poor layer (*2*), and a linear exit echo (*3*)

erosion). A further feature which illuminates the phenomenon of the entry echo can be found in junction naevi. Here, from the physical point of view, we find close interweaving between the epidermis and the nests of naevus cells.

The 20-MHz scanner does not discriminate between the epidermis and the naevus cell nests but computes from both a weakish compound entry echo. Horn pearls enclosed in the epithelium appear as bright spots.

Corium

Apart from the entry echo it is the corium, and within it the collagenous fibres, which is the main echogenic structure of the skin. Depending on the plane of section the bundles of collagenous fibres appear as plaque-like or band-like, moderately or highly reflective structures.

In general the border with the highly reflective entry echo is well defined and smooth. In acanthotic epidermis there can be an irregularly wavy border

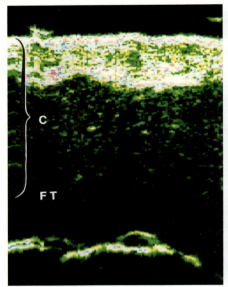 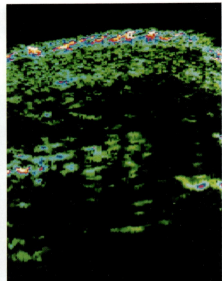

Fig. 16. Ultrasound scan of back skin of a 44-year-old man. The deep portions of the corium (*c*) are depicted only weakly. *FT*, fatty tissue

Fig. 17. Sonogram of the extensor surface of the thigh (24-year-old woman)

zone. In fact, depending on the location, the sonographical demonstrated structure of the corium displays considerable morphological differences which we will present below on the basis of illustrations Figure 16 shows the ultrasound scan of back skin of a 44-year-old man. The highly reflective corium can be seen beneath the entry echo as an irregularly structured zone which is not sharply demarcated from the subcutaneous fatty tissue. The lower layers of the corium are depicted only weakly.

On the extensor surface of the thigh (Fig. 17) the boundary between the corium and the subcutaneous fatty tissue is for the most part well defined.

In addition to follicular structures (hair follicles appear as longish, echo-poor areas traversing the corium), the ultrasound texture of the corium is also characterised by sections of larger vessels (Fig. 18). In contrast to the follicles, blood vessels are round and bordered on all sides. The lumen is completely free of internal echoes. Note the broad echo-poor zone beneath the entry echo as the expression of the presence of a severe actinic elastosis.

The palm of the hand of a 30-year-old man (Fig. 19) shows in the 20-MHz scan an inhomogeneous entry echo. The corium itself contains only weak echoes; the border with the subcutaneous tissue is not clearly identifiable.

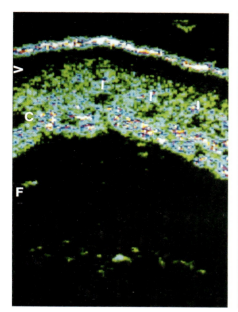

Fig. 18. Sonogram of the upper lip of a 77-year-old woman with three blood vessels (whitze bars). Severe actinic elastosis (*arrow*). F, subcutaneous fat tissue

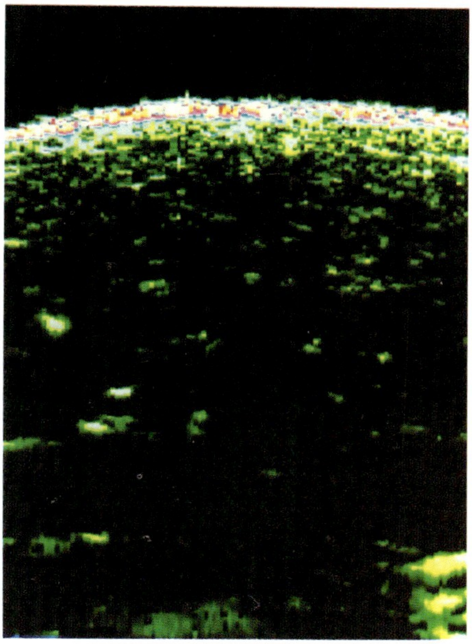

Fig. 19. Typical sonogram of the palm of the hand of a 25-year-old man. The corium contains only weak echoes

Influence of Skin Tension on the Ultrasound Image

An important finding in our investigations has been that the degree of skin tension considerably influences the entry signal and the echoes within the corium. The lax skin of an old person produces a relatively weak entry echo although the epidermis is only insignificantly thinner than that of a young person. If the senile atrophic skin is drawn taut to all sides, there is marked enhancement of the entry echo. In other words the degree of tension of the epidermis is of eminent importance for its acoustic behaviour. The extreme is total loss of the entry echo when there is complete loss of skin tension. This can be demonstrated in ultrasound scans of excised and thus tensionless skin (Fig. 20).

But it is not only the entry echo which alters its echogenicity with varying degress of tension but also the corium. Tautening of the skin leads to a marked increase in echoes. There are probably two reasons for the increase in echogenicity of the corial connective tissue under tension: on the one hand the tension on the bundles of collagen fibres, on the other hand the flattening of the previously steep lattice-like arrangement of the collagen. This means

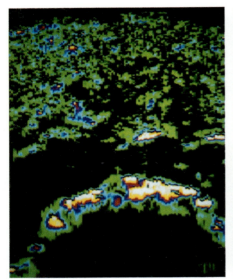 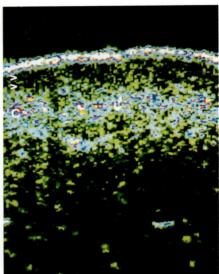

Fig. 20. Total loss of the entry echo in excised skin. Hyporeflective corium

Fig. 21. Actinic elastosis (*arrows*). Cheek of a 77-year-old woman. Beneath the entry echo a broad echo-poor band with irregularly distributed internal echoes. *C*, corium

that not only the tension but also the angle of reflection of the applied ultrasound signal is altered.

Actinic Elastosis

A commonly found change in the ultrasound properties of the cutaneous connective tissue which is important from the differential diagnostic point of view is that caused by actinic elastosis. This is an actinically induced alteration of the collagenous connective tissue. The altered collagen stains in the same manner as elastic tissue, hence the name elastosis.

This actinically altered tissue is deposited subepidermally in bands. Depending on its severity, the elastosis is shown by ultrasound scanners operating in the 20-MHz range as echo-poor or echolucent band with sawtooth-like, usually marginally situated internal echoes (Fig. 21). In the case of the basal cell carcinomas often occurring in actinic skin, severe actinic elastosis presents particular problems of sonographic differentiation as both tumour and elastosis are echo-poor in appearance (Fig. 22). In such cases comparison of the region in question with the contralateral nontumorous skin can be of help. In addition, tautening of the skin increases its echogenicity while the tumour parenchyma itself remains unchanged. This facilitates

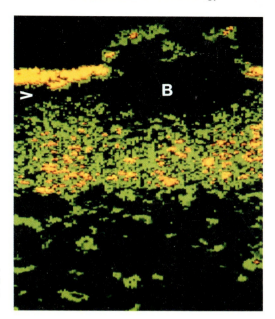

Fig. 22. Basal cell carcinoma (*B*) in severe actinic elastosis (*arrow*). No differentiation between parenchyma of the tumour and actinic elastosis

differentiation. On the other hand, as elastotic connective tissue can be clearly distinguished morphologically from the deeper layers of unchanged connective tissue, ultrasound examination provides quantifiable information on the actinic damage in skin subjected to chronic actinic exposure. Densitometry also opens up further possibilities of specification of the elastosis.

Rosacea

The echo-poor or echolucent processes which occur in advanced rosacea also present problems of differentiation. The loosely arranged oedematous-gelatinous corium appears below the entry echo as a broad, band-like zone, usually with an indistinct distal boundary. As with actinic elastosis, demarcation of tumour parenchyma is sometimes not possible.

Fine-Fibrillary Connective Tissue

An unexpected problem is found in fine-fibrillary connective tissue, for example in a fresh scar, in the neurogenic connective tissue of naevus cell naevi or neurofibromas or in the stroma of a basal cell carcinoma, for example. We would normally expect to find strong reflection of the echo signal in connective tissue. This is after all the case in the regional connective tissue of the corium.

However, a change in the texture of the connective tissue, e.g. the development of fine-fibrillary connective tissue, leads to attenuation or even to complete loss of its echogenicity. The signal is reflected diffusely by the irregularly arranged fine fibrillary fibres and can thus no longer be picked up.

Conclusions. It becomes clear from these examples that the anatomical texture of the corium is of crucial significance for the ultrasound imaging of the entire skin. To begin with the degree of echogenicity of the corium depends on the amount of collagen fibre material per unit volume (mass/unit volume). Any change in this ratio leads to a change in the acoustic properties. Increased tension leads to compression of the connective tissue and thus increases this ratio. Relaxation has the opposite effect. This is illustrated by the weak corial echoes of the lax skin found in senile involution.

Development of loosely arranged, oedematous corium also reduces the number of echogenic structures per unit volume (e.g. wheal). Since all tumorous and inflammatory processes in the corium, unless they are accompanied by increased production of collagenous fibres or other echogenic structures (horn pearls, calcium), are echo-poor compared with the corium, they appear as negative images within the corial connective tissue. They thus alter the physiological echogenic structure of the cutaneous connective tissue in a more or less characteristic manner. This leads to the following fundamental statement with respect to ultrasound imaging in dermatology.

In contrast to histological diagnosis, an ultrasonic diagnosis of a physiological or pathological process in the corium cannot be made on the basis of a particular internal texture. The process must be evaluated on the basis of its topography, its outline characteristics and the specific ultrasonic phenomena which it induces in the surrounding tissue.

Subcutaneous fatty tissue

The subcutaneous fatty tissue appears echolucent on the ultrasound scan. Only the fibrous septa traversing the fatty tissue are echo-rich. Inflammatory processes in the subcutaneous fatty tissue are not detected by the 20-MHz scanners either as they, too, are echolucent.

All fibrosing processes are, however, of great interest. This applies to older scars and also, for example, to circumscribed or progressive systemic scleroderma (see Fig. 2).

Muscle Fascia and Muscle

The muscle fasciae are detected by 20-MHz scanners in all regions where there is only a thin layer of subcutaneous fatty tissue (e.g. flexor aspect of the forearm, neck, various parts of the face). They appear highly reflective, either as a homogeneous band or split into several bands by echo-poor zones. The musculature itself is echolucent (see Fig. 1).

Cartilage

Cartilage, like fatty tissue, is completely echolucent. Figure 23 shows a cross section through the entire auricle of a 30-year-old man. We see a strong entry echo and the somewhat irregularly structured ventral corium. Next follows the completely echolucent cartilage, followed by the dorsal corium and the epithelial echo. The cartilage is sharply demarcated on both sides.

Application in Tumour Diagnosis

One of the main indications for ultrasound scanning in dermatology is preoperative tumour diagnosis [14, 19, 27]. Here we are interested less in a diagnosis in the histological sense, i.e. tissue differentiation, than in information which will facilitate or confirm the preoperative diagnosis.

In most cases, for example, the characteristic acoustic behaviour of the seborrhoeic verruca permits us to rule out a malignant melanoma. On account of their internal structures angiomas also present a typical ultrasound pattern. The tumour parenchyma can usually be delimited clearly on all sides with the modern 20- or 50-MHz scanners.

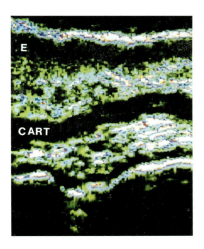

Fig. 23. Cross section through the entire auricle of a 30-year-old man. Sharply demarcated complete echolucent cartilage (*CART*); *E*, elastosis

Apart from the two-dimensional measurement of the tumour, computerized processing of serial ultrasound sections permits us to enter the "third dimension". Using the computer program ANAT 3D (Dr. el-Gammal) specially developed for this purpose, a three-dimensional representation of the tumour can be constructed without difficulty. The computer makes it possible to rotate the tumour in all planes and thus gives us a good insight into the topographic situation. It provides exact information on the surface and volume of the computed structure [31, 32]. The parameter invasive tumour mass (i.e. the proportion of the malignant melanoma shown to be invasive tumour parenchyma) might in future come to supplement the currently used tumour indices of Clark or Breslow.

In lateral and basal delimitation of a tumour 20-MHz ultrasound scanning is of great help. This important clinical question arises in the diagnosis of basal cell carcinomas, particularly in the case of the sclerodermiform basal cell carcinoma. In the sclerodermiform basal cell carcinoma exact lateral delimitation is often not possible with conventional noninvasive clinical methods so that several punch biopsies have to be made preoperatively in the marginal region of the tumour. Specific use of high-resolution dermatological ultrasound would render this superfluous (Fig. 4).

Delimitation of a tumorous process in actinically damaged skin, however, confronts the ultrasound examiner with the problem that both the tumour and the elastosis are echo-poor. Here ultrasound examination of the contralateral healthy skin can be of help. In addition firm tautening of the skin increases the echogenicity of the actinic elastosis but not that of the tumour.

Subtumoral Inflammatory Infiltrate

At present most examiners [7, 13] point out that unequivocal differentiation between the inflammatory infiltrate at the base of the tumour and the actual tumour parenchyma is not possible. Both appear echo-poor to echolucent.

In ultrasound measurement of tumour thickness (Breslow index), an indispensable parameter for the surgical regime, this physical phenomenon leads to higher values. The error is greater the thinner the tumour, as in the case of thinner tumours the subtumoral band of inflammatory infiltrate is relatively wider than in very thick melanomas.

Experimental Approaches

A further very interesting possibility of diagnostic ultrasound are noninvasive longitudinal studies, for example observation of the time course of an inflammatory or atrophying process. Here the development of an experimentally induced inflammation (e.g. after intracutaneous administration of a

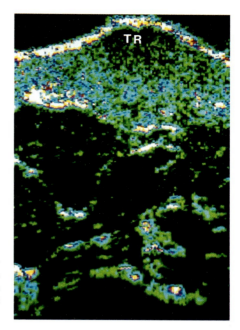

Fig. 24. Tuberculin reaction (*TR*) 48 h after intracutaneous administration of the allergen. Exo- and endophytic expansion of the corium. Irregular echo pattern within the lesion

defined amount of allergen, e.g. tuberculin) is a suitable object of study [4].

The progressive inflammatory reaction is shown by the expansion of the corium both above the level of the epidermis and in the direction of the subcutaneous fatty tissue (Fig. 24). The corial echo is broken up. The originally highly echogenic texture becomes very irregularly interspersed with echolucent zones. All the above parameters can be exactly quantified. Both the length and the breadth of the inflammatory zone can be measured. The quality of the inflammation can also be evaluated by densitometric procedures.

A further example of ultrasound quantification of an inflammatory reaction is in psoriasis. The untreated psoriatic plaque shows a strong entry echo often combined with focal dorsal acoustic shadowing. Histologically these acoustic shadows are shown to be zones of parakeratosis. The underling echo-poor to echolucent band is composed of acanthotic epithelium and inflammatory infiltration.

An eczematous reaction can also be evaluated on the basis sonographic parameters in respect of both the extent and, via densitometry, the quality of infiltration. It can thus be seen that dermatological ultrasound permits us to examine and measure inflammatory processes in the skin more exactly than is possible on the basis of the clinical parameters already available. The possibility of noninvasive longitudinal investigations provides objectifiable information on the dynamics of a process. In this context it should be emphasized that ultrasound examination is completely harmless for the patient and can thus be repeated as often as desired.

Steroid effects on the skin can also be examined noninvasively by ultrasound scanning [34]. Both anti-inflammatory analysis and continuous observation of the atrophogenic effect of an external steroid are possible.

References

1. Alexander H, Miller DL (1979) Determining skin thickness with pulsed ultrasound. J Invest Dermatol 72:17–19
2. Altmeyer P (1989) Dermatologische Ultraschalldiagnostik. Gegenwärtiger Stand und Perspektiven. Z Hautkr 61:727–728
3. Altmeyer P, el-Gammal S, Hoffmann K (1990) Blick in die Haut-ohne Schnitt und Biopsie. MMW 132:14–22
4. Beck JS, Spence VA, Lowe JG (1986) Measurement of skin swelling in the tuberculin test by ultrasonography. J Immunol Methods 86:125–129
5. Breitbart EW, Rehpenning W (1983) Möglichkeit und Grenzen der Ultraschalldiagnostik zur in vivo Bestimmung der Invasionstiefe des malignen Melanoms. Z Hautkr 58:975–987
6. Breitbart EW, Hicks R, Rehpeninng W (1985) Möglichkeiten der Ultraschalldiagnostik in der Dermatologie. Z Hautkr 61:522–526
7. Breitbart EW, Müller CE, Hicks R, RehpenningW, Vieluf D (1989) Neue Entwicklungen der Ultraschalldiagnostik in der Dermatologie. Akt Dermatol 15:57–61
8. Buhles N, Altmeyer P (1988) Ultraschallmikroskopie an Hautschnitten. Z Hautkr 63:926–934
9. Cole GW, Handler SJ, Burnett K (1981) The ultrasonic evaluation of skin thickness in scleroderma. JCU 9:501–503
10. Curie J, Curie P (1881) Développement par pression de l'électricité polaire dans lees cristaux hemièdres à faces incliees. CR Acad Sci 91:294–295
11. Dines KA, Sheets PW, Brink JA, Hanke CW, Condra KA, Clendenon JL, Goss SA, Smith DJ, Franklin TD (1984) High frequency ultrasonic imaging of skin: experimental results. Ultrason Imaging 6:408–434
12. Fornage BD, Deshayes JL (1986) Ultrasound of normal skin. JCU 14:619–622
13. Gassenmaier G, Schell H (1989) Wertigkeit und Grenzen des Ultraschallverfahrens bei Diagnostik und Differentialdiagnostik von Pigmenttumoren. Zentralbl Haut Geschlechtskr 156:558
14. Hoffmann K, el-Gammal S, Matthes U, Altmeyer P (1989) Digitale 20-MHz-Sonographie der Haut in der präoperativen Diagnostik. Z Hautkr 64:851–858
15. Kraus W, Nake-Elias A, Schramm P (1985) Diagnostische Fortschritte bei malignen Melanomen durch die hochauflösende Real-Time-Sonographie. Hautarzt 36:386–392
16. McDicken WN (1976) Diagnostic ultrasonics: principles and use of instruments. Crosby Lockwood Staples, London
17. Miyauchi S, Miki Y (1983) Normal human skin echogram. Arch Dermatol Res 275:345–348
18. Miyauchi S, Masanori T, Miki Y (1983) Echographic evaluation of nodular lesions of the skin. J Dermatol 10:221–227
19. Müller C, Breitbart EW, Hicks R, Schulte I (1989) Ultraschalldiagnose maligner Tumoren der Haut, speziell des malignen Melanoms. Hautarzt 40:382–383
20. Murakami S, Yoshiharu M (1989) Human skin histology using high-resolution echocardiography. JCU 17:77–82
21. Myers SL, Cohen JS, Sheet PW, Bies JR (1986) B-mode ultrasound evaluation of skin thickness in progressive saysstemic sclerosis. J Rheumatol 13:577–580

22. Payne P (1985) Medical and industrial applicationas of high resolution ultrasound. J Phys E Sci Instrum 18:465–472
23. Payne P (1985) Ultrasound in dermatology-non-invasive skin measurement by ultrasound. RNM 13:24–26
24. Payne P, Grove GL, Alexander H, Quilliam RM, Miller DL (1982) Cross sectional ultrasonic scanning of skin using plastic film transducers. Bioeng Skin 3:241–246
25. Price RR, Jones TB, Goddard J, James AE (1980) Basic concepts of ultrasonic tissue characterisation. Radiol Clin North Am 18:21–30
26. Quereleux B, Leveque JL, de Rigal J (1988) In vivo cross sectional ultrasonic imaging of human skin. Dermatologica 177:332–337
27. Schwaighofer B, Pohl-Markl H, Frühwald F, Stiglbauer R, Kokoschka EM (1987) Der diagnostische Stellenwert des Ultraschalls beim malignen Melanom. Fortschr Geb Röntgenstr 146:409–411
28. Serup J (1984) Non-invasive quantification of psoriasis plaques. Measurement of skin thickness with 15 MHz pulsed ultrasound. Clin Exp Dermatol 9:502–505
29. Serup J (1984) Quantification of acrosclerosis: measurement of skin thickness and skin-phalanx distance in females with 15 MHz pulsed ultrasound. Acta Derm Venereol (Stockh) 64:35–40
30. Serup J, Staberg B, Klemp P (1984) Quantification of cutaneous oedema in patch test reaction by measurement of skin thickness with high-frequency pulsed ultrasound. Contact Dermatitis 10:88–93
31. Sohn C, Grotepaß J, Schneider W, et al. (1988) Erste Untersuchungen zur dreidimensionalen Darstellung mittels Ultraschall. Z Geburtshilfe Perinatol 192:241–248
32. Sohn C, Grotepaß J, Swobodnik W (1989) Möglichkeit der 3dimensionalen Ultraschalldarstellung. Ultraschall 10:307–313
33. Strasser W, Vanscheidt W, Hagedorn M, Wokalek H (1986) B-Scan-Ultraschall in der Dermatologie. Fortschr Med 104:495–498
34. Tan CY, Marks R, Payne P (1981) Comparison of xeroradiographie and ultrasound detection of corticosteroid induced dermal thinning. J Invest Dermatol 76:126–129
35. Weinraub Z, Brenner S, Krakowski A, Caspi E (1982) The water cushion in dermatological diagnostic ultrasound. Dermatologica 164:357–359
36. Weiss LW, Clark FC (1987) Three protocols for measuring subcutaneous fat thickness on the upper extremities. Eur J Appl Physiol 56:217–221

Automatic Measurement of Skin Thickness

A. Pech, E.-G. Loch, and W. v. Seelen

Introduction

Skin thickness measurement is an important instrument in diagnosis, therapy control, and the testing of medicaments. Changes in the structure of human skin indicate processes inside the human body [3] as well as external influences. Nowadays, the measurement of human skin thickness in vivo is carried out by high frequency ultrasound. During this kind of measurement some problems occur concerning the character of the signal and the anatomic structure of the investigated organ. Therefore, the ultrasonic measurement of skin thickness should be standardized and automated to gain accuracy and velocity in clinical routine.

Methods

The boundaries between the different skin layers are not smooth, so there is not a single echo caused by the different impedances of the materials but a group of echoes with internal phase shifts. This results from the fact that the ultrasonic field is, extending over a region of tissue where the boundaries vary (Fig. 1), and therefore the echo is not a clear sharp pulse. Although this kind of integration is useful while determining the mean value of skin thickness, a broader ultrasonic field would not be helpful because the average boundaries would be undetectable.

In order to obtain exact measurements of skin thickness, the sonography has to be applied to more than a single point. The mean value of several measurements within a small region provides a good estimate for the mean skin thickness if more than ten samples are collected and the average thickness is computed. A computer removes the time-consuming element from registration.

Some properties of high frequency images should be mentioned. First of all, the radio frequency (RF) signal should be used for feature extraction because the phase information is important at the boundaries of tissue types. Secondly, B-Scan images should be presented only with linear gray or color scales if the full information is to be obtained. Other (nonlinear) color scales can produce artifacts resulting in pattern without histological correspondence.

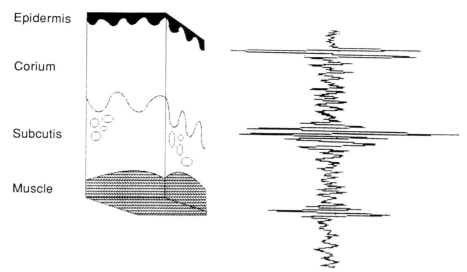

Fig. 1. Cross section of human skin and corresponding echo pattern

Using a Minhorst Donoson 2 (Fig. 2) with a probe having an upper frequency level of 25 MHz, skin measurements were made, digitized and stored in a computer system.

Mathematical models based on the theory of autoregressive moving average (ARMA) processes [1] are formed in the z-domain. If $u(z)$ is the input signal and $y(z)$ represents the output of the system, the equation

$$\frac{y(z)}{u(z)} = \frac{b_0 + b_1 z^{-1} + \ldots + b_m z^{-m}}{1 + a_1 z^{-1} + \ldots + a_n z^{-n}}$$

describes the behavior of the tissue. The constants a_i (i = 1, 2, 3...) and b_j (j = 0, 1, 2 ...) are dependent on the tissue type and have to be estimated by a least squares algorithm.

A second class of models works on first order Markov chains. A Markov chain can be described by its transition matrix containing all transition probabilities and including, therefore the properties of the chain [2]. Both models were designed in order to describe the behavior of the ultrasound pulse inside the tissue [4].

Characterizing the skin tissue by features extracted from the above models, the different types of skin tissue are detected by a maximum likelihood classifier [4].

The knowledge base of the system is found by extracting the features in a preclassified set of training data and estimating the joint probability distributions of the feature vectors. This is done recursively, so new feature

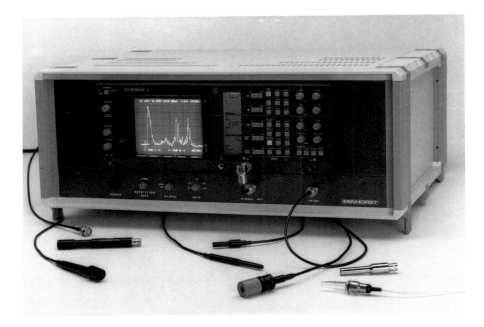

Fig. 2. Ultrasound equipment: Minhorst Donoson 2

vectors may be added to the knowledge base at any time. After repeating the classification process on every single A-line within the B-scan image, the skin thickness is found easily by counting the pixels of each skin class and multiplying the sum by a factor determined from the sound velocity and sample rate. The mean value and standard deviation of the skin thickness within the insonified region are computed from 100 A-lines.

Results

Figure 3 shows a B-scan image of normal human skin presented by a linear color scale. The original data corresponding to that image have been classified by the procedure described earlier. The result of the classification can be seen in fig. 4. The skin layers (epidermis, corium, and subcutaneous fat) are marked by different colors. From this classified image the average skin thickness is computed.

The average skin thickness becomes a quite good and reliable estimate due to the high number of measurements taken. Automatic evaluation and classification prevents this method from being time consuming.

The knowledge base may be altered by the user at any time, and therefore the measurement system is very flexible in use.

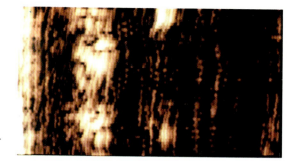

Fig. 3. Ultrasound image of human skin with linear color scale

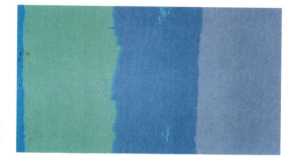

Fig. 4. Result of the application of the classification process to the data corresponding to Fig. 3

Conclusions

The system we have described for automatic measurement of skin thickness improves both velocity and accuracy of measurement and is therefore, a powerful tool in dermatology. Fast computer-aided evaluation of high frequency RF signals completes skin measurement system.

References

1. Isermann R (1977) Digitale Regelsysteme. Springer, Berlin Heidelberg New York
2. Langrock P, Jahn W (1979) Einführung in die Theorie der Markovschen Ketten und ihre Anwendungen. Teubner, Leipzig
3. Loch E-G, Pech A, Kluge A, Wasmayr M (1990) Ultraschall-Hautmessung: Zusammenhang von Hautdicke und Knochendichte als diagnostischem Kriterium der Osteoporose. In: Gebhardt J, Hackelöer BJ, v. Klinggräff G, Seitz K (Eds) Ultraschalldiagnostik 89. Springer, Berlin Heidelberg New York (in press)
4. Pech A, Loch EG, von Seelen W (1990) Pattern recognition on human skin tissue. In: Wade G, Lee H (eds) Acoustical imaging 18. Plenum, New York (in press)

Lymphnodes in 5- to 7.5-MHz Ultrasound

B-Scan Ultrasound of Regional Lymph Nodes in Different Dermatological Diseases

B. Riedl, D. Hiller, and N. Stosiek

Introduction

In recent years the examination of lymph nodes by ultrasound has become an important diagnostic method in otorhinolaryngology [3, 9, 13, 18], internal medicine [1, 5, 6, 15], and gynecology [4]. In dermatology, ultrasound is used for detection of lymph node macrometastases and for evaluation of tumor thickness in malignant melanomas [2, 8, 12, 14, 19]. Here, the sonographical findings of the regional lymph nodes in different dermatological diseases are shown. Applications for this noninvasive method are also given.

Patients and methods

A total of 83 patients with different dermatological diseases were examined by sonography (Table 1). For the examination of lymph node regions a signal depth penetration of about 6–7 cm is required. Furthermore, for satisfactory discrimination of 3 mm large lymph node structures, an axial and lateral

Table 1. Distribution of the diagnoses of the examined patients ($n = 83$)

Diagnosis	Number of patients
Malignant melanoma	52
Non-Hodgkin's lymphoma	7
Carcinoma	4
Mycosis fungoides (T_2, N_1, M_0, B_0)	3
Psoriasis	3
Erysipelas	2
Atopic eczema	2
Eczema (otherwise classified)	2
Large plaque parapsoriasis	2
AIDS (WR II)	1
Epidermal nevus syndrome	1
Classic Kaposi's sarcoma	1
Paraneoplastic erythroderma	1
Persistent light reaction	1
Eosinophilic pustular folliculitis	1

WR, Walter Reed Classification

resolution of 0.4 mm and 0.9 mm, respectively, is needed. A 7.5 MHz linear scanner (Sonoline SL 1, Siemens Co.) complies with both conditions [11].

Results

The Normal Lymph Node

The shape of a normal lymph node either resembles that of a bean or is spherical [10]. The size ranges between a few millimeters and 3 cm [10, 17]. Inflammation causes an enlargement of the regional lymph nodes.

The sonographical aspects of normal lymph nodes are judged differently in the literature. Marchal found somewhat flattened hypodense masses [16]. According to Beyer and Bruneton, normal lymph nodes of healthy individuals cannot be separated from surrounding tissue, because their acoustic impedance is identical [1, 5]. In normals, we also saw the typical echo pattern of fatty tissue, but no circumscribed masses.

Lymph Nodes in Inflammatory Dermatological Diseases

Noninfectious (e.g., psoriasis, eczema) and contagious inflammatory diseases show the same sonographical pattern. Oval or spherical masses, different in size, with marginal hypodensities and increased center reflexions are found (Fig. 1). Rarely inflammatory lymph nodes present as totally hypodense masses, resembling the alterations in neoplastic lymph nodes [2,

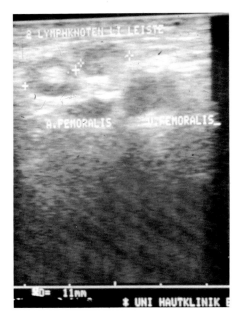

Fig. 1. Lymph node changes in inflammatory diseases: hyperechoic center reflexion and hypoechoic margin

5]. In these cases the sonographical follow-up is used for differentiation between tumorous lymph node involvement and inflammatory changes. A gradually more intense echo pattern, finally not distinguishable from surrounding tissue, is found in inflammation following antibiotic therapy [1, 2]. Histologically, this change corresponds to a disappearance of the initial edema and inflammatory cellular hyperplasia [1].

Malignant Lymphomas

Involvement of the regional lymph nodes in malignant lymphomas is sonographically nonuniform. In agreement with the literature [1, 2, 5], we found echo-poor, palpable, enlarged lymph nodes. A patient suffering from chronic lymphoblastic leukemia had multiple palpable lymph nodes with a sonographic picture similar to the changes described for inflammation: a cockade-like structure with a echo-rich center and echo-poor circumference, as already reported by Beyer [1]. In a patient with a low grade non-Hodgkin's lymphoma of B cell type, we found both totally echo-poor and cockade-like patterns.

Sonography shows a gradual increase in echogenicity in involved lymph nodes, with finally the same echo pattern as the surrounding tissue when the lymphoma is treated by chemotherapy or radiotherapy. Therefore, at this point sonographical imaging is no longer possible [1, 2]. Patients suffering from mycosis fungoides had palpable lymph node enlargement with a cockade-like echo pattern (increased center reflexion with marginal hypodensity), resembling the changes described in inflammatory lymph nodes. According to the findings of Brockmann [2], circumscribed echo-poor areas in lymph nodes represent T cell growth.

Malignant Melanoma

Several groups have used B-scan ultrasound for staging malignant melanoma [2, 12, 14, 19]. Our group investigated the regional lymph nodes of patients with malignant melanoma when tumor thickness, as measured by high frequency (20 MHz) ultrasound, was more than 1.5 mm [8]. These patients were treated by local tumor excision and a simultaneously performed lymph node dissection. Well-marked, echo-poor masses with spherical or irregular shapes were classified as suspect. This corresponds to the sonographic criteria of malignancy with respect to the findings of Stutte and Kraus ([12, 19]; Fig. 2). So far, we have not missed any metastatic involvement of regional lymph nodes, as confined by the histological findings; however, a final result will be given when a greater number of patients has been examined by this method.

We feel that masses smaller than 3-4 mm in diameter cannot be detected by the 7.5 MHz ultrasound imaging system with sufficient accuracy, if no

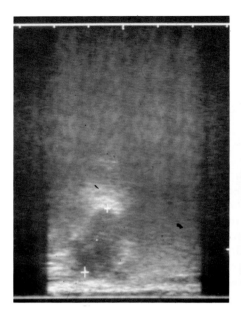 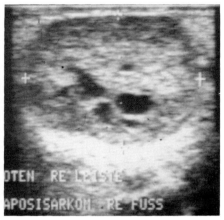

Fig. 2. Lymph node metastasis of a malignant melanoma: nearly spherical, sharp edged inhomogenous echo-poor mass

Fig. 3. Lymph node metastasis in Kaposi's sarcoma. In the center pronounced hyperechoic mass with echolucent cleft-like spaces corresponding to sections of vessels

additional inflammatory infiltration is present. In the assessment of questionable lymph node relapses in the postoperative course of patients with malignant melanoma who underwent lymph node dissection, one has to keep in mind that postoperative seromas, hematomas, abscesses, and lymphogenous liquid masses present themselves as sharply defined, homogenous, echo-poor or anechoic masses [19].

Case Report of a Patient with Classic Kaposi's Sarcoma

An 81-year-old male patient, suffering from Kaposi's sarcoma in the right foot and lower leg for 17 years, presented with signs of superinfection combined with lymph node swelling of the right groin a few weeks before hospital admission. The sonographically found enlarged lymph node showed a few echo-poor, sharply defined areas that corresponded to vessel sections, as found by the histological workup. This confirmed the ultrasonic diagnosis "lymph node metastasis" of Kaposi's sarcoma (Fig. 3). In such lymph node metastases there are pathological vessels, analogous to the structure of the primary tumor [7]. This might be an unusual observation; Mende described metastases in HIV associated Kaposi's sarcoma as homogenous masses (lecture at international congress on ultrasound in dermatology, Bochum, FRG, 1990).

Conclusions

According to both the literature [2, 12, 14, 19] and our own experience, applications of B-scan ultrasound in examining regional lymph nodes in dermatology include the following:
1. Identification of suspicious palpable masses in the area of the regional lymph nodes.
2. Discrimination of inflammatory or tumorous lymph nodes; however, sometimes an exact differentiation is not possible, thus requiring further histological exploration or sonographical follow-up.
3. Real size measurement of lymph nodes.
4. Follow-up on size and echo pattern of lymph nodes in the therapy of inflammatory and lymphoreticular dermatological diseases.
5. Early detection of lymph node metastases as part of tumor after-care.

In our opinion this noninvasive, inexpensive, and reproducible technique should be established in dermatology as a routine method. The criteria for the discrimination of benign lymph node changes from metastatic involvement obviously cannot be absolute, since this method can miss micrometastases. Therefore, diagnostic B-scan sonography of peripheral lymph nodes should be considered as a supplementary but valuable diagnostic tool, particularly in dermatological oncology.

References

1. Beyer D, Peters PE, Friedmann G (1982) Leistungsbreite der Real-time-Sonographie bei Lymphknotenerkrankungen. Röntgenpraxis 35: 393–402
2. Brockmann WP, Maas R, Voigt H, Thoma G, Schweer S (1985) Veränderungen peripherer Lymphknoten im Ultraschall. Ultraschall 6: 164–169
3. Bruneton JN, Roux P, Caramella E, Demard F, Vallicioni J, Chauvel P (1984) Ear, nose, and throat cancer: ultrasound diagnosis of metastasis to cervical lymph nodes. Radiology 152: 771–773
4. Bruneton JN, Caramella A, Hery M, Aubanel D, Manzino JJ, Picard JL (1986) Axillary lymph node metastases in breast cancer: preoperative detection with US. Radiology 158: 325–326
5. Bruneton JN, Normand F, Balu-Maestro C, Kerboul P, Santini N, Thyss A, Schneider M (1987) Lymphomatous superficial lymph nodes: US detection. Radiology 165: 233–235
6. Elke M, Livers M, Tan KG, Faust H (1986) Wandel der bildgebenden Diagnostik bei Non-Hodgkin-Lymphomen in den letzten Jahren. Radiologe 26: 109–117
7. Finkbeiner WE, Egbert BM, Groundwater R, Sagebiel RW (1982) Kaposi's sarcoma in young homosexual men. Arch Pathol Lab Med 106: 261–264
8. Gassenmeier G, Kiesewetter F, Schell H, Hornstein OP (1989) Wertigkeit der hochauflösenden Sonographie in der präoperativen Diagnostik des malignen Mela-

noms. Symposium on malignant melanoma, Deutsche Dermatologische Gesellschaft, Klinikum Steglitz der Freien Universität, 16–17 June 1989, Berlin
9. Gritzmann N, Czembirek H, Hajek P, Karnel F, Türk R, Frühwald F (1987) Sonographie bei cervicalen Lymphknotenmetastasen. Radiologe 27: 118–122
10. Knoche H (1979) Lehrbuch der Histologie. Springer, Berlin Heidelberg New York, pp 203–206
11. Knoche J, Schmitt KJ, Hebel RM (1989) Möglichkeiten und Grenzen der Hochfrequenzsonographie aus technischer Sicht. Workshop on ultrasound in dermatology, 119th meeting Vereinigung Südwestdeutscher Dermatologen, 6–8 Oct 1989, Erlangen
12. Kraus W, Nake-Elias A, Schramm P (1985) Diagnostische Fortschritte bei malignen Melanomen durch die hochauflösende Real-time-Sonographie. Hautarzt 36: 386–392
13. Kuhn FP, Mika M, Schild H, Klose K (1983) Spektrum der Sonographie von lateralen Kopf- und Halsweichteilen. Fortschr Röntgenstr 138: 435–439
14. Löhnert JD, Bongartz G, Wernecke K, Peters PE, Macher E, Bröcker EB (1988) Sensitivität und Spezifität der sonographischen Lymphknotendiagnostik beim malignen Melanom. Radiologe 28: 317–319
15. Magnusson A, Hagberg H, Hemmingsson A, Lindgren PG (1981) Computed tomography, ultrasound and lymphography in the diagnosis of malignant lymphoma. Acta Radiol [Diagn] (Stockh) 23: 29–35
16. Marchal G, Oyen R, Verschakelen J, Gelin J, Baert AL, Stessens RC (1985) Sonographic appearance of normal lymph nodes. J Ultrasound Med 4: 417–419
17. Peters PE, Beyer K (1985) Querdurchmesser normaler Lymphknoten in verschiedenen anatomischen Regionen und ihre Bedeutung für die computertomographische Diagnostik. Radiologe 25: 193–198
18. Schmelzeisen R, Milbradt H, Reimer P (1988) Sonographie im Kopf-Halsbereich, die Einsatzmöglichkeiten sind vielfältig. Klinikarzt 17: 591–599
19. Stutte H, Erbe S, Rassner G (1989) Lymphknotensonographie in der Nachsorge des malignen Melanoms. Hautarzt 40: 344–349

Comparison of Ultrasound with Clinical Findings in the Early Detection of Regional Metastatic Lymph Nodes in Patients with Malignant Melanoma

R. LOOSE, J. WEISS, W. KÜHN, R. SIMON, J. TEUBNER, and M. GEORGI

Introduction

The continuous development of new ultrasound techniques offers a wide range of medium- and high-resolution ultrasound scanners, enabling the detection and differentiation of lesions in the cutaneous and subcutaneous tissue. Hence, in addition to a careful clinical examination, ultrasound plays an important role in detection of metastatic lymph nodes and local recurrences [1–3, 5, 7, 9].

Patients and Methods

In a prospective clinical study, in cooperation with our dermatology department, we tried to determine the value of postsurgical ultrasound screening in patients with malignant melanoma. We examined the cervical, axillary, and inguinal lymph nodes and compared our results with the clinical findings. Over a period of 3.5 years we performed follow-up examinations in 282 patients who underwent surgical removal of a malignant melanoma. For 2273 lymphatic outflow areas we were able to compare our ultrasound results and the clinical findings with the final diagnoses, which are explained below.

Examinations were performed with a 5 MHz real time linear scanner (Picker LS 3000) with a resolution < 1.3 mm at 17 mm depth in the near focus range. We used standard settings for gain (30 dB), near gain (−15 dB), and far gain (6.0 dB) to be able to compare the echo patterns of different examinations [8].

Clinical findings were divided into three groups: normal findings, inflammatory changes, and metastasis. Ultrasound findings were divided into four groups: normal findings, inflammatory changes, ambiguous metastasis, and metastasis.

All 2273 ultrasound findings and clinical examinations were compared with the final diagnoses. Metastatic disease was assumed when:
– A surgically removed lymph node demonstrated a positive histology (tumor cells)
– A fine needle aspiration demonstrated a positive cytology (tumor cells)

- A patient died with obvious metastatic disease (bulks of lymph nodes affected)

No metastatic disease was assumed when:
- A surgically removed lymph node demonstrated a negative histology.
- A clinical and/or ultrasound follow-up at 6 months demonstrated normal findings.

Fine needle aspirations with negative cytology were classified as nondiagnostic because of the high risk of false-negative results.

Results

Figure 1 shows a typical metastatic lymph node of the right groin. A transformation from an elliptical to a nearly spherical shape with low homogeneous echo density is seen. Most of these lymph nodes are not flexible. Figure 2 shows the exact position of the needle tip during fine needle aspiration in the same lymph node. The aspirated material contained tumor cells of a melanoma and the patient underwent lymph node dissection a few days later. It is easy to verify the exact position of a needle tip during aspiration of lesions down to 5 mm diameter [4].

Figure 3 is a sonogram of a patient's right axillary region after lymph node dissection. A melanoma of the right arm and one metastatic axillary lymph node had been removed. It shows scar tissue and a seroma without any echo

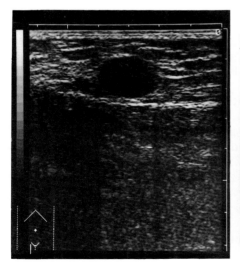
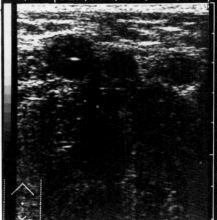

Fig. 1. Typical lymph node metastasis of the right groin with low homogeneous echo density

Fig. 2. Metastatic lymph node during fine needle aspiration (white spot corresponds to needle tip)

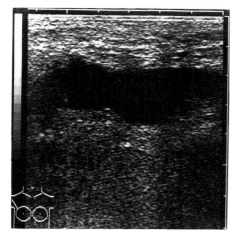 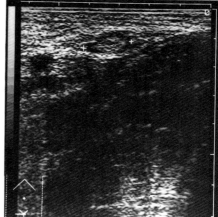

Fig. 3. Axillary region with seroma after preceding lymph node dissection

Fig. 4. Typical inflammatory lymph node

structure. Some 5 month later we found a 3 cm irregular mass with low echo density. Because of the scar tissue, this mass was missed during the clinical examination. The fine needle aspiration yielded tumor cells and the mass was removed surgically. The patient has been free of any recurrence for 3.5 years now.

Most palpable lymph nodes demonstrated inflammatory sonographic changes. Figure 4 shows a typical sonographic finding, with a sharply outlined elliptical lesion, a peripheral rim of low echo density, and a center with high echo density. This is due to inflammation in the borderline area and fatty degeneration in the center. A ratio of longitudinal to transverse diameter above 1.5 has been reported to be typical for inflammatory changes [6]. Most of these lymph nodes are flexible and can be found bilaterally.

Tables 1 and 2 show our results comparing clinical and ultrasound findings. The data contain all lymph node findings; local recurrences are excluded.

Table 1. Ultrasound vs clinical examination in the final diagnosis of metastatic disease ($n = 89$)

	Clinical		
	Normal findings	Inflammatory changes	Metastatic disease
Ultrasound			
Normal findings	0	0	0
Inflammatory changes	0	0	0
Ambiguous	10	5	0
Metastatic disease	6	11	57

In Table 1, 89 outflow areas with the final diagnosis of metastatic disease are listed. None of the proven lymph mode metastases was missed by ultrasound. There were 15 outflow areas with proven lymph node metastases demonstrating uncertain metastatic disease in ultrasound and requiring further exploration with dissection, fine needle aspiration, or a short range follow-up examination. In 32 outflow areas, lymph node metastases were detected only by ultrasound with normal clinical findings or inflammatory changes.

Table 2 summarizes 2184 outflow areas with the final diagnosis no metastasis. In this group ultrasound prevented unnecessary biopsies in 38 patients in whom clinical examinations had suggested metastatic disease. False-positive diagnoses were made by ultrasound in six patients. In 42 outflow areas, ultrasound demonstrated ambiguous findings requiring further exploration.

Table 2. Ultrasound vs clinical examination in the final diagnosis of no metastasis ($n = 2184$)

	Clinical		
	Normal findings	Inflammatory changes	Metastatic disease
Ultrasound			
Normal findings	1634	140	21
Inflammatory changes	233	91	17
Ambiguous	36	4	2
Metastatic disease	1	3	2

Sensitivity and specificity of clinical examinations were 64% and 98%, respectively. The reason for the rather low sensitivity and high specificity of clinical findings may be explained as follows: Clinical examination reveals many palpable lymph nodes with inflammatory changes and, therefore, only obvious metastases are classified as pathologic. The sensitivity and specificity of ultrasound depends on the classification of "ambiguous findings" and yields results between 83% and 98%.

If sensitivities of ultrasound and clinical examination are compared as a function of lymph node size, a decreasing sensitivity of palpation from 100% for lymph nodes >3 cm down to 29% for lymph nodes ≤1 cm is found (Fig. 5). Furthermore, 61% of all groin metastases were palpable but only 45% in the axillary region (Fig. 6) We found no loss of sensitivity of ultrasound in patients with preceding surgical intervention, whereas palpation demonstrated 70% of metastases in patients without lymph node dissection but only 33% after surgical treatment (Fig. 7).

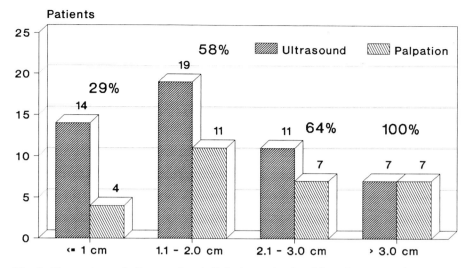

Fig. 5. Comparison of ultrasound and clinical examination (size of metastases)

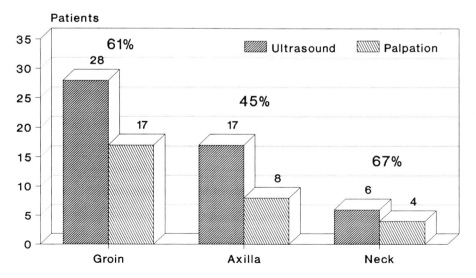

Fig. 6. Comparison of ultrasound and clinical examination (localization of metastases)

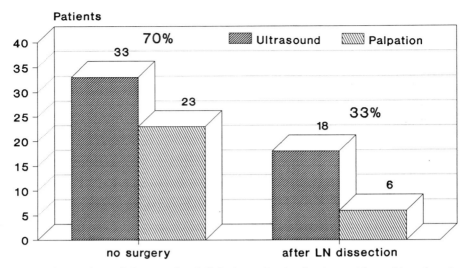

Fig. 7. Comparison of ultrasound and clinical examination (patients with or without lymph node dissection)

Summary

Ultrasound of regional lymphatic outflow areas is an efficient method for postsurgical screening of patients with malignant melanoma.

It is mandatory for high-risk patients with Clark's level IV and V to repeat the follow-up examinations every 3 month for at least 5 years.

Ultrasound can detect small lymph node metastases not demonstrated by clinical examination and thus enable early surgical removal. In addition, it can prevent unnecessary biopsies in patients with ambiguous clinical findings. This fact is very important in patients with scar tissue after prior surgical interventions, especially in the axillary region where the sensitivity of clinical examination is rather low.

References

1. Brockmann WP, Maas R, Voigt H, Schweer S (1985) Veränderungen peripherer Lymphknoten im Ultraschall. Ultraschall 6: 164–169
2. Erbe S (1989) Der Stellenwert der Lymph- u. Hautknotensonographie in der Nachsorge des Malignen Melanoms der Haut. University of Tübingen
3. Kraus W, Nake-Elias A, Schramm P (1986) Hochauflösende Real-Time-Sonographie in der Beurteilung regionaler lymphogener Metastasen von malignen Melanomen. Z Hautkr 61: 9–14

4. Perry MD, Seigler HF, Johnston WW (1986) Diagnosis of metastatic malignant melanoma by fine needle aspiration biopsy: a clinical and pathologic correlation of 298 cases. JNCI 77: 1013–1019
5. Schmidt D (1988) Diagnostische Wertigkeit der Real-time Sonographie bei Lymphknoten- u. Transitmetastasen des malignen Melanoms der Haut. University of Köln
6. Solbiati L, Rizzatto G, Bellotti E, Montali G, Cioffi V, Croce F (1988) High-resolution sonography of cervical lymph nodes in head and neck cancer: criteria for differentiation of reactive versus malignant nodes. 74th scientific assembly and annual meeting of the Radiological Society of North America, Chicago 1988
7. Stutte H, Erbe S, Rassner G (1989) Lymphknotensonographie in der Nachsorge des malignen Melanoms. Hautarzt 40: 344–349
8. Teubner J, van Kaick G, Junkermann H (1985) 5 MHz Realtime-Sonographie der Brustdrüse, part 1: gerätetechnische Untersuchungen. Radiologe 25: 449–456
9. Weiss H, Weiss A (1985) Ultraschallatlas: internistische Ultraschalldiagnostik mit schnellen B-Bild-Geräten. Edition Medizin, Weinheim, pp 231–242

The Value of Sonography in Diagnosis and Follow-Up of Lymph Nodes in HIV-Patients

U. MENDE, W. TILGEN, U. PEKAR, and M. HARTMANN

Introduction

With 1538 new reports of patients with AIDS and an estimated 50 000 persons with HIV-infection in the old FRG and West Berlin, the health statistics for 1989 (Bundesgesundheitsamt, BGA) emphasize the growing importance of this complex of diseases for epidemiology and public health [3]. Besides a number of diseases with diagnostic value [2], a visible or palpable involvement of the lymph nodes is often the first sign of an HIV infection. In addition to clinical examination, for effective staging and analysis of these pathologic nodal changes quantification by imaging methods is mandatory. Among these, sonography as a noninvasive, inexpensive, available, and efficient procedure should not only be applied to the investigation of abdominal structures [1, 5, 6], but also to the peripheral (cervical to inguinal) lymph nodes as a valuable adjunct to diagnosis, therapy planning, and follow-up in this group of patients.

Patients and Methods

From November 1985 until December 1989 a group of 57 patients with known HIV infection, who were under the diagnostic and therapeutic care of the Departments of Dermatology and Radiology at the University of Heidelberg, underwent up to three sonographic examinations of the (peripheral) lymph nodes in addition to clinical and laboratory findings. The sex distribution was 40 male and 17 female patients. The mean age was 32.1 ± 7.7 years; the range was 17–51 years. Based on the Center for Disease Control (CDC) classification 2 patients (3.5%) were in stage IIa, 1 (1.8%) in IIB, 15 (26.3%) in IIIA, 21 (36.8%) in IIIB, 3 (5.3%) in IVA, 4 (7.0%) in IVB, 2 (3.5%) in IVC1, 3 (5.3%) in IVC2, and 6 patients (10.5%) in IVD/E.

The modes of infection and the risk groups are shown in Table 1. These data indicate that probably due to the differences in the availability of drugs in Heidelberg, the proportion of IV drug users (IVDU), which rose from 33.3% to 51.9% for new patients in 1989, is about three times higher in our group than in the AIDS statistics of the BGA [2] (an increase from 12.7% to 15.6% in 1989).

Table 1. Mode of infection resp. risk groups

	1985–1989		1989 only	
Homosexual male	26	45.6%	9	33.3%
Bisexual male	3	5.3%	1	3.7%
Heterosexual	7	12.3%	3	11.1%
IV drug use	19	33.3%	14	51.9%
Endemic (Central Africa)	1	1.8%	–	–
Unknown	1	1.8%	–	–
Total	57	100.0%	27	100.0%

The examinations were performed on a Picker LSC 7000 machine with 5 MHz linear and curved array transducers using water soluble gel as coupling agent. A silicon block (3M) or a water filled pad (Picker GmbH) were used only for cutaneous and subcutaneous infiltrations to avoid near field artifacts or for very irregular surfaces with insufficient coupling by the contact gel.

A description of the nodal (cervical to inguinal) status included an evaluation of affected regions and multiplicity, and was used for diagnosis and especially follow-up. In addition, the echogenicity of representative pathologic lymph nodes was quantified by greyscale histograms; the nodal volumes were calculated in good approximation on the basis of rotational bodies using measured areas and perpendicular diameters [7].

In case of symptoms or pathologic cervical lymph nodes, the structures of the oral cavity and the pharynx were also examined [8].

The volume and structure (greyscale histogram) of representative cutaneous and soft-tissue infiltrations in Kaposi's sarcoma patients were measured for therapy planning, monitoring, and follow-up.

To obtain reproducible control data for both the group and the individual patient, the setting of the machine was kept constant. The planes of the corresponding sonographic sections were identical.

Results

The extent of sonographic alterations of the examined lymph nodes depending on the CDC stage is listed in Table 2. For the clinical examination, nodes with a diameter of more than 10 mm, corresponding to a volume of .5 ml and more, were considered to be pathologic [11]. The largest lymph nodes found in this study had a volume of 17 ml in patients with infections or lymphadenopathy (Figs. 1, 2) and 20 ml in patients with nodes showing malignant changes (Kaposi's sarcoma; Fig. 3, top left). Further criteria for sonographic evaluation were shape, contours and multiplicity of the nodes, affected regions, and, most importantly, the lack of echogenicity, especially in patients with acute infections and malignant diseases.

Table 2. Sonographic changes of the lymph nodes (size and/or echogenicity)

CDC stage	+ (n=13)	++ (n=19)	+++ (n=25)	Total number of patients (n=57)
I A	2	–	–	2
I B	1	–	–	1
III A	2	7	6	15
III B	3	7	11	21
IV A	2	1	–	3
IIV B	1	2	1	4
IV C1	–	–	2	2
IV C2	–	2	1	3
IV D/E	2	–	4	6

+, minor changes; ++, expressed changes; +++, massive changes

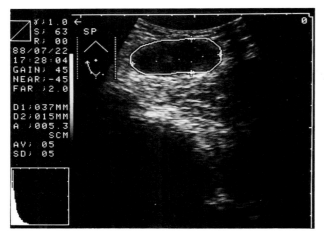

Fig. 1. 26-year-old homosexual male; CDC III A. Enlarged echolucent inguinal lymph nodes maximum diameter 37 mm, volume 8.6 ml

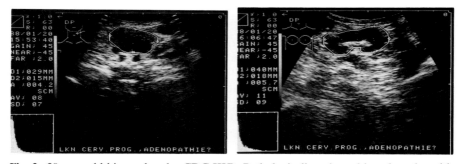

Fig. 2. 29-year-old bisexual male; CDC III B. Pathologically enlarged lymph nodes with reduced echogenicity. *Left*, cervical, volume 11.0 ml; *right*, axilla, volume 17.1 ml

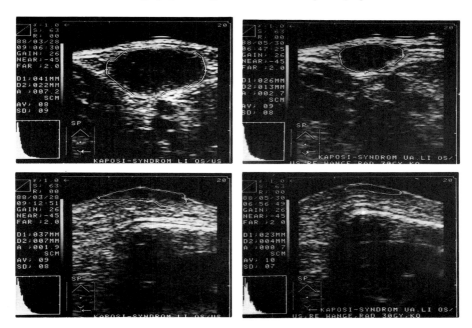

Fig. 3. 49-year-old bisexual male; CDC IV D; Kaposi's sarcoma; therapy monitoring. Inguinal lymphnodes (*top*) and cutaneous infiltrations (*bottom*). *Left*, before radiotherapy; *right*, good response after 30 Gy. Residual tumour volumes 17.8% and 13.2%, respectively

Corresponding to clinical and laboratory data, the most marked nodal changes with respect to size and structure, were found in patients with advanced stages of disease: 87.8% in CDC III and 72.2% in CDC IV, but 100% in patients with opportunistic and general infections (CDC IV C1 and IV C2).

Discussion

Prognosis and quality of life of HIV patients ultimately depend on the control of opportunistic and general infections as well as the malignant diseases [9]. Successful treatment requires an exact diagnosis with besser chances of survival as a result of **early detection.** This is especially true for the multimorbid patient with reduced tolerance to (aggressive) therapeutic approaches.

Due to the altered immunological situation the clinical appearance is often uncharacteristic; reactions and laboratory data may be atypical and nonspecific resulting in the enhanced importance of imaging methods to secure the

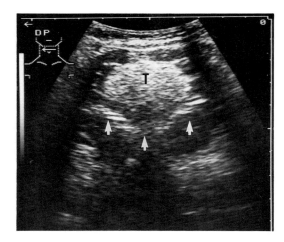

Fig. 4. 17-year-old female (partner with HIV infection); CDC III A. Besides massively enlarged lymph nodes, echolucent pharyngeal structures with echogenic contours (*arrows*); *T*, tongue. Transverse submental section

diagnosis. In this context, the evaluation of the nodal status, with its indicative function, is of special significance. However, whereas in clinical examination the diagnosis of pathologic lymph nodes is mainly based on the palpable size, sonography as a sensitive and effective procedure, not only quantities the diameter and volume, but also provides additional important diagnostic criteria, such as structural changes (loss of echogenicity, e.g.) and shape and contours of the affected nodes, thereby allowing an earlier diagnosis [7].

Symptoms or enlarged cervical lymph nodes point to **oral infections** (viral, bacterial, mycotic). Structural changes, such as loss of echogenicity of the pharyngeal tissues (especially tonsils, pillar of fauces, and palate) and echogenic contours of tongue and palate, as further sensitive diagnostic criteria are easily quantified and documented by sonography (Fig. 4).

A marked low echogenicity of enlarged lymph nodes in combination with echolucent oropharyngeal structures should therefore always trigger a differential diagnosis that includes HIV infection for all patients, not only those in the known risk groups.

Staging of the lymph nodes, with the criteria multiplicity, size, volume, and structure, on the safer C2 level indicates a **follow-up,** either just to "wait and see" (Fig. 5), or to monitor a systemic or local therapeutic schedule (Figs. 3, 6). This is especially important for those patients with malignant diseases.

The therapeutic strategies for Kaposi's sarcoma include systemic and local measures such as radiotherapy. Here, the discussion about single and total dose and fractionation schemes is still open [4, 10]. Sonography provides the necessary data for effective diagnosis, therapy planning, and monitoring with the opportunity to calculate response rates for both lymph nodes and cutaneous and soft-tissue infiltrations (Fig. 3).

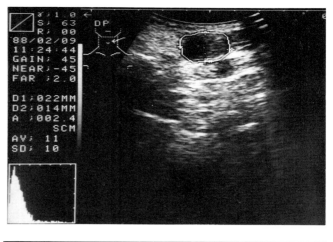
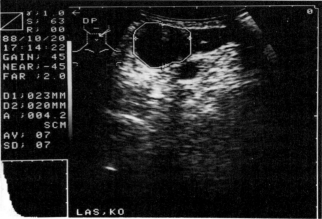

Fig. 5. 48-year-old homosexual male; CDC III B; sonographic follow-up. *Left*, pathologic cervical lymph nodes; *right*, 8 months later increase in volume (350%) and decrease in echogenicity

The high risk of transformation into malignant lymphomas (non-Hodgkin's lymphoma, Hodgkin's disease) is well-known [12]. Sonography is an essential part of the diagnostic methods used for staging, follow-up, and posttherapeutic care in this category of diseases. It is even more important in HIV patients, who have limited tolerance to more or less aggressive therapy modalities due to the immunological depression. Sonography can help to optimize therapy, avoid over- as well as undertreatment, and reduce side effects (Fig. 6).

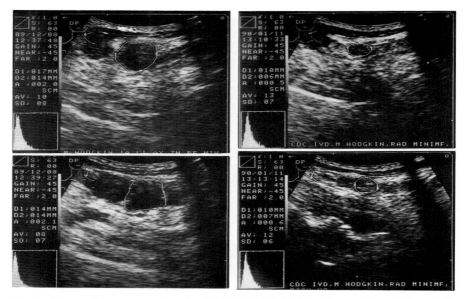

Fig. 6. 51-year-old homosexual male; CDC IV E; Hodgkin's disease CS IA (left axilla); sonographic staging IIA (cervical and left axilla). Cervical lymph nodes; therapy monitoring. *Left*, before radiotherapy; *right*, after 36 Gy, excellent response (residual nodal volume 17.3%, increase in echogenicity)

Conclusion and Summary

Based on the analyses of 57 patients with known HIV infection (CDC II–IV), sonography of the lymph nodes and, in special cases, of the pharyngeal structures has proven to be a valuable method for safer and more objective staging, follow-up, therapy monitoring, and post-therapeutic care.

As a noninvasive, inexpensive, available, and efficient method, it is the ideal adjunct to clinical and laboratory examinations.

References

1. Abiri MM, Kirpekar M, Abiri S (1985) The role of ultrasonography in the detection of extrapulmonary tuberkulosis in patients with acquired immunodeficiency syndrome (AIDS). J Ultrasound Med 4: 471–473
2. AIDS-Zentrum im Bundesgesundheitsamt (1988) AIDS: Neufassung der CDC-Falldefinition zur einheitlichen epidemiologischen Erfassung. Dtsch Arztebl 85: 845–853
3. AIDS-Zentrum im Bundesgesundheitsamt (1990) AIDS-Statistik 31. Dezember 1989. Dtsch Artzebl 87: 294–296
4. Cooper JS, Fried PR (1987) Defining the role of radiation therapy in the management of epidemic Kaposi's Sarcoma. Int J Radiat Oncol Biol Phys 13: 35–39

5. Langer M (1989) Bildgebende Diagnostik bei AIDS. Springer, Berlin Heidelberg New York
6. Langer R, Langer M, Schütze B, Zwicker C, Wakat JP, Felix R (1989) Abdominelle Sonographiebefunde bei Patienten mit AIDS. Röntgenblätter 42: 121–125
7. Mende U, Flentje M, Haels J, Zöller J (1987) Sonographische Lymphknotendiagnostik bei Malignomen im Kopf- Hals-Bereich. Picker Aktuell 5: 15–18
8. Mende U, Flentje M, Weischedel U, Zöller J, Lenarz T (1989) Sonographische Diagnostik von Kopf- Hals-Tumoren im therapeutischen Umfeld. Röntgenblätter 42: 19–23
9. Neumann G (1990) AIDS und Tuberkulose. ÄBW 45: 20–23
10. Nobler MP, Leddy ME, Huh SH (1987) The impact of palliative irradiation on the management of patients with acquired immune deficiency syndrome. J Clin Oncol 5: 107–112
11. Schäublin C (1989) AIDS-Kompendium Hoechst 1989. Hoffmann, Berlin
12. Tirelli U, Vaccher E, Rezza G, Barbui T, Bernasconi C, Cajazzo A, Cargnel A, de Lalla F, Dessalvi P, Fassio PG, Gobbi M, Lambertenghi Deliliers FMG, Lazzarin A, Luzi G, Luzzati R, Mandelli F, Maserati R, Piersantelle N, Puppo F, Raise G, Rossi E, Salvia G, Scanni A, Sinicco A, Foà R, Gavosto F, Monfardini S for the Gruppo Italiano Cooperativo AIDS and Tumori (1989) Hodgkin's disease in association with acquired immunodeficiency syndrome (AIDS). Acta Oncol 28: 637–639

Tumors in 5- to 7.5-MHz Ultrasound

Efficacy of Sonography in Differential Diagnosis of Soft-Tissue Tumors

H. Merk, D. Esser, G. Merk, and L. Langen

Introduction

Rapid development of imaging techniques has opened up completely new outlets for the diagnosis of soft-tissue tumors of unknown etiology [2, 7, 10, 14]. In particular, reliable differentiation between soft-tissue tumors and tumor simulating diseases, primarily inflammatory diseases and vascular alterations, are of substantial interdisciplinary interest. In addition to computed tomography (CT) and magnetic resonance imaging (MRI), high-resolution, real time sonography, which is free from side effects, easy to use, and provides meaningful information, has gained increasing importance [1, 4–6, 12]. The features of sonography relevant to the diagnosis of soft-tissue alterations are based on the differentiated visualization of soft-tissue structures and bony margins. Sonography of tumors can be adapted to provide information on [3, 9]:
1. Tumor quality: solid, cystic, complex
2. Inner structure of the tumor: homogeneous, inhomogeneous, calcification foci, necroses, foreign body/air inclusions
3. Localization and initially affected tumor tissues
4. Size (three-dimensional) and location relative to neighboring organs and vessels: displacement, infiltration

Sonography is not suitable to assess the malignancy of tumors [8, 16]. The information quality provided by real time sonography mainly depends on both the examiner's experience and the way the sonographic finding is incorporated into the overall clinical picture.

Reviewing 4 years of experience gathered by our group, the present work was undertaken to critically report on the ability of sonography to assess soft-tissue tumors.

Patients and Methods

The findings obtained from a total of 379 patients from the Orthopedic Clinic (284), the ENT Clinic (45), the Dermatological Clinic (45) and the Clinic for Urology (5) of the Magdeburg Medical Academy were evaluated. In a prospective study conducted from May 1984 to February 1988, all 379 patients, who had soft-tissue swellings of unknown etiology, were examined by sonography. In this approach, it was considered essential that the previous clinical findings had not clearly established the diagnosis. A Toshiba SSA 90 A linear scanner with a 7.5 MHz high-resolution transducer was used for the investigation. A gel pad was employed to eliminate radiation interference

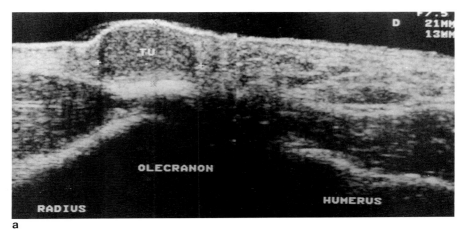

a

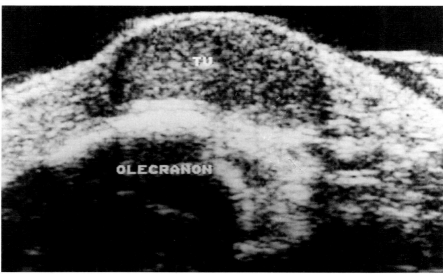

b

Fig. 1a, b. 48-year-old patient with a lipoma (histologically verified) above the left elbow joint. **a** Sonographic longitudinal section: well-defined oval tumor (*TU*) in subcutaneous tissue, producing uniformly distributed inner echoes and clearly differentiated from muscles. **b** Expanded scan: sonographic transverse section above the olecranon, visualizing the homogeneous structure of the lipoma with regular alterations of low-echo and high-echo fractions; clearly differentiated from the joint capsule

Efficacy of Sonography in Differential Diagnosis of Soft-Tissue Tumors   113

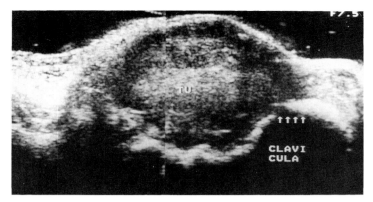

Fig. 2. 77-year-old patient with a fusocellular sarcoma above the sternoclavicular joint (histologically demonstrated). Sonographic longitudinal section: longitudinal oval tumor (*TU*) growing in an infiltrative way; no reliable classification of tissue; inhomogeneous structure, cone shaped penetration medially and laterally; additional osteolysis of the clavicle. The sternoclavicular joint was destroyed and, hence, not visualized

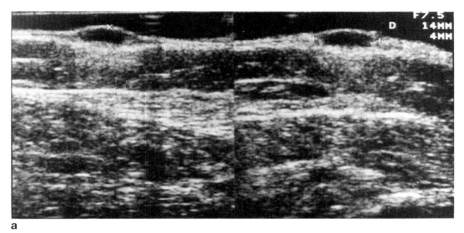

a

Fig. 3a, b. 64-year-old patient with a nodular malignant melanoma with in-transit metastasis on the lower left leg (histologically demonstrated). **a** Sonographic visualization of melanoma in longitudinal section (*right*) and transversal section (*left*). Typical image of melanoma in the sonographic scan: well-defined cone shaped tumor in the cutis; echo-free structure with high-reflection border; depth 4 mm; melanoma well-differentiated from subcutis and muscles. **b** Sonographic visualization of in-transit metastasis (*MET*) in longitudinal section; well-defined low echo tumor in the subcutis; fascia of gastrochemius muscle clearly displaced. Tumor size: 14 × 14 × 10 mm

b

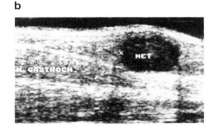

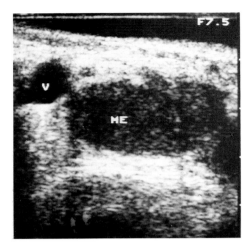

Fig. 4. 48-year-old patient with lymph node metastasis (*ME*) from a melanoma in the left axilla (histologically verified), low-echo longitudinal oval tumor with adjacent axillary vein (*V*)

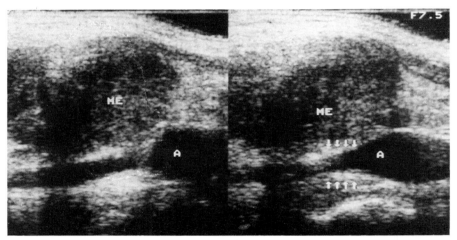

Fig. 5. 43-year-old patient with metastasis (*ME*) of a carcinoma of the larynx on the left side of the neck (histologically demonstrated). Sonographic longitudinal section: low-echo tumor nonuniformly defined and growing infiltratively; carotid artery (*A*) compressed by the metastasis, with beginning infiltration into the vascular wall

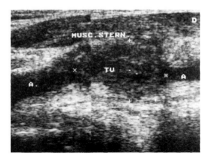

Fig. 6. 52-year-old patient with metastasis of a carcinoma of the larynx on the left side of the neck (histologically demonstrated). Sonographic longitudinal section: inhomogeneous, nonuniformly defined low echo tumor (*TU*); the metastatic tissue has infiltrated into the vascular wall of the carotid artery (*A*); above the latter, the sternocleidomastoid muscle

and improve coupling. No special preparation of the patients was required. Positioning of patients and the examination technique were varied as a function of the tumor site. Our interest was focused on localizing the tumor relative to adjacent vessels and analyzing the ensuing surgical consequences. Intraoperative and histological findings were evaluated comparatively to confirm the sonographic diagnosis. The soft-tissue tumors were classified using WHO 1969 recommendations, except that epithelial tumors were also included in the classification.

Results

Using a prospective ultrasound examination, we classified by differential diagnosis 379 soft-tissue alterations of undetermined origin. The overall sensitivity of sonography was 88%. Table 1 presents the sonographic results vs intraoperative or histologic findings. Sonographic diagnosis of tumor simulating diseases was correct in 96% of the patients; thus, these diseases could be differentiated with the highest degree of reliability. In contrast, 82% of the true soft-tissue tumors were identified by ultrasound. With increasing experience, evidence of malignancy was gathered for some of the tumors. Typically, for soft-tissue tumors of the locomotor system, demonstration of cortical defects was suggestive of infiltrative growth and penetration into the bone. Melanomas were well-discerned as low-echo oval foci in the cutis and subcutis. Similarly, vascular infiltration of tumors was considered as a sign of malignancy. Table 2 shows the correspondence between preoperative sonographic classification of tissues and the histologic diagnosis for the 112 soft-tissue tumors. The sensitivity was very high (91%), demonstrating that tissues can be well-differentiated in the sonographic scan when high-resolution transducers are used. In particular, soft tissue tumors near the surface can be clearly classified.

Table 1. Comparison between preoperative sonographic diagnosis and histologic or intraoperative (as applicable) findings, with sensitivity of sonography indicated ($n = 379$)

Type of soft-tissue alteration	Incidence among our patients	Correct sonographic diagnosis	Sensitivity (%)
True soft-tissue tumors	112	92	82
Metastases	42	36	86
Lymph node metastases	34	32	94
Tumor simulating diseases	106	98	96
Inflammatory diseases	56	48	86
Vascular alterations	29	27	93
Total	379	333	88

Table 2. Differentiation of true soft-tissue tumors, in view of histological findings vs preoperative sonographic tissue classification ($n = 122$)

Type of tumor	Incidence among our patients	Correct sonographic tissue classification (no malignancy assessment)
Lipoma	38	37
Fibroma	14	12
Myoma	8	6
Hemangioma	18	16
Lymphangioma	4	3
Benign synovioma	1	1
Neurofibroma	6	5
Malignant fibrous histiocytoma	2	2
Fibrosarcoma	1	0
Myosarcoma	1	1
Fusocellular sarcoma	1	1
Melanomas	16	16
Basilomas	2	2
Total	112	102

Sensitivity: 91 %

There is a wide range of other soft-tissue diseases which show the clinical picture of a soft-tissue tumor. Among the tumor simulating diseases, those affecting the ganglia predominated (89 patients). Of the 56 patients with inflammatory diseases, we differentiated 10 cases of osteomyelitis, 16 of arthritis, and 28 of solitary soft-tissue abscesses. Differentiation of vascular alterations was of particular relevance.

Discussion

Clinically, many soft-tissue tumors are easily revealed by inspection and palpation due to their location near to the skin surface [8]. Still, the use of imaging techniques is essential for the differential diagnosis of circumscribed tumors [6, 13, 15]. To this end, high-resolution real time sonography has gained increasing importance. Besides providing relevant information, the ultrasound method is the only approach that can be easily applied and does not entail side effects. Hence, a prospective interdisciplinary study involving 379 patients with soft-tissue alterations was conducted to assess the efficacy of sonography. The only methods considered suitable as reference regarding the current clinical picture were histologic examination and intraoperative findings. By analysing and classifying the different sonographic features of soft-tissue masses, pathological processes can be well differentiated due to tissue differences in reflectance [10, 11]. The sensitivity of sonography in classifying soft-tissue lesions by differential diagnosis, 88 %, is considered very good. This is also true of the percentage of correct tissue classifications (91%).

To date, there have been no comparable reports in the literature studied. Furthermore, the approach presented in this work is advantageous in that the size of a tumor can be determined and its location relative to adjacent soft-tissues visualized [3, 16]. Also for surgical removal of soft-tissue tumors, assessing the relation to neighboring vessels is of substantial importance. Typically, sonography can be used to define the location relative to a vessel or verify vascular wall infiltration of a tumor [8, 9]. With increasing experience, we noted typical sonographic patterns suggestive of the malignancy of individual tumors.

In summary, while unable to provide malignancy specific information, sonography is nonetheless capable of revealing the three-dimensional size of a tumor and its relation to adjacent vessels. Therefore, in stepwise application of imaging techniques, sonography should be considered the method of choice: (a) for the diagnosis of soft-tissue tumors, (b) in the evaluation of recurrence, and (c) in ruling out soft-tissue metastases.

The sonographic approach is particularly suitable for interdisciplinary tumor examination during the follow-ups of patients undergoing chemotherapy or radiotherapy. Hence, it is possible to fill a diagnostic gap using an imaging method, which can be documented especially in outpatient practice.

References

1. Breitbart EW, Hicks R, Rehpenning W (1986) Möglichkeiten der Ultraschalldiagnostik in der Dermatologie. Z Hautkr 61:522–526
2. Bücheler E, Friedmann G, Thelen M (1983) Real-time-Sonographie des Körpers. Thieme, Stuttgart
3. Eichhorn Th, Schroeder H-J, Glanz H, Schwark WB (1987) Histologisch konsolitärer Vergleich von Palpation und Sonographie bei der Diagnose von Halslymphknotenmetastasen. Laryingol Rhinol Otol (Stuttg) 66:266–274
4. Glasier CM (1987) High resolution ultrasound characterization of soft tissue masses in children. Pediatr Radiol 17:233–237
5. Gritzmann N et al. (1987) Sonographie bei cervicalen Lymphknotenmetastasen. Radiologe 27:118–122
6. Harland U (1987) Darstellung von Tumoren des Bewegungsapparates im Ultraschall. In: Stuhler Th, Feige A (Hrsg) Ultraschalldiagnostik des Bewegungsapparates. Springer, Berlin Heidelberg New York, pp 107–111
7. Kinnas PA, Woddham CH, MacLarnon JC (1984) Ultrasonic measurements of haematomata of joints and soft tissues in the haemophiliac. Scand J Haematol [Suppl] 40 (33):225–235
8. Kratochwil A, Zweymüller K (1975) Ultraschalldiagnostik bei Knochen- und Weichteiltumoren. Wien Klin Wochenschr 87:397–407
9. Krause W, Nake-Elias A, Schramm P (1986) Hochauflösende Real-time-Sonographie in der Beurteilung lymphogener Metastasen von malignen Melanomen. Z Hautkr 61:9–14
10. Kremer H, Dobrinski W (1987) Sonographische Diagnostik. Urban and Schwarzenberg, Munich

11. Mann WJ (1984) Ultraschall im Hals-Kopf-Bereich. Springer, Berlin Heidelberg New York
12. Merk H, von Roden L (1988) Bewegungsapparat. In: Hofmann V (ed) Ultraschalldiagnostik in der Pädiatrie und Kinderchirurgie. Thieme, Leipzig
13. Papavasiliou V, Beslikas Th, Manolikakis G (1985) Akute hämatogene Neugeborenenosteomyelitis – eine Analyse von 105 Fällen. Beitr Orthop Traumatol 32:463–469
14. Weber U, Müller K (1983) Periphere Weichteiltumoren. Thieme, Stuttgart
15. Weitzel D, Dinkel E, Dittrich M (1984) Pädiatrische Ultraschalldiagnostik. Springer, Berlin Heidelberg New York
16. Westhofen M, Hagemann J, Schröder S, Herberhold C (1985) B-Mode Sonographie des Halses. Laryngol Rhinol Otol 64:409–417

Sonography: The Ideal Imaging Method for Staging and Follow-Up of Malignant Melanoma

U. Mende, W. Petzoldt, W. Tilgen, and P. Schraube

Introduction

The incidence of malignant melanoma is increasing worldwide [2, 3]. Improvement of the prognosis requires safe and early detection not only of the primary tumor, but also of possible metastatic spread [5–7, 9, 10]. Exact therapy planning must therefore be based on both clinical staging and imaging methods [4, 11]. This is especially true for the lymph nodes, where up to 39% of involved nodes are not discovered by clinical examination alone [1]. To reduce this rate of false-negative results sonography, which is an efficient, inexpensive, and noninvasive method, has become an integral part of staging, follow-up, and post-therapeutic care of lymph nodes as well as cutaneous and soft-tissue infiltrations.

Patients and Methods

From March 1985 to December 1989 205 patients (113 male, 92 female; mean age 51.9 ± 15.3 years, range 16–84 years) with malignant melanoma underwent up to eight sonographic examinations of lymph nodes, cutaneous infiltrations, soft-tissue areas, and bones in up to 12 regions for diagnostic staging, therapy monitoring and post-therapeutic care.

The sonographic examinations were performed using 5 and 7.5 MHz linear and 3.5 (abdomen) and 5 MHz curved array transducers with a Picker LSC 7000 device. Examinations were performed on the day of or within a very few days of clinical evaluation. Water soluble gel was used as a coupling agent. A silicon elastomer block or a water filled pad were only applied to patients with cutaneous and low lying subcutaneous infiltrations (near field artifacts).

Clinically representative and/or sonographically suspect or pathologic processes were documented and analyzed for volume (calculated from measured areas and diameters) and structure (gray scale histograms), as described elsewhere [8], and compared to the clinical findings.

Markedly echolucent lymph nodes and soft-tissue processes were considered positive for metastatic involvement. If the findings were only questionably suspect, due to a short postoperative interval or were not likely metastatic, short-term follow-up controls were done. A node was considered to be sonographically negative when oval shaped with an echogenic cortex, an even more echogenic center, and a definable hilum. Constant findings in repeated controls were considered to be free from metastases.

Patients with sonographically positive processes underwent surgery. In patients in whom surgery was not performed (local or general inoperability, advanced stages with ubiquitous metastases, etc.), the sonographic data were used to plan local radiotherapy or systemic therapy and thus provided information for follow-up controls.

Results

The smallest lymph node metastasis seen in sonography had a diameter of 3 mm, corresponding to a volume of 0.014 ml, the largest node had a volume of 149 ml with a maximum diameter of more than 80 mm.

The comparison between clinical palpation and sonographic examination of 801 evaluated regions showed coincidently negative results in 537 patients (67.0%) and coincidently positive results in 128 patients (16.0%). A metastatic involvement was unlikely or ruled out by sonography in 79 (9.9%) patients with suspect clinical findings. In addition, ultrasound revealed 57 (7.1%) metastatic processes which were not disclosed by clinical examination.

There were three false-positive results. In one patient with malignant melanoma a progressive right cervical tumor was mistaken for a lymph node metastasis due to the echolucent structure. The intraoperative and histological diagnosis disclosed a branchiogenic cyst (Fig. 1 left). In another patient with malignant melanoma and progressive cervical lymph nodes discovered during post-therapeutic care, sonography did not rule out the clinical suspicion of metastatic invasion. Histology of the echolucent nodes, however, showed that the sonographic changes in the structure were due to a toxoplasmosis infection and not to metastatic disease (Fig. 2). Another moderately echolucent lymph node in the supraclavicular region of a patient with malignant melanoma was considered to be sonographically pathologic, though with an atypical structure for malignant melanoma. Histology revealed the metastasis of an until then undetected carcinoma of the thymus as a second tumor. In another patient with malignant melanoma and a palpable node in the left breast, sonography correctly diagnosed a T1 carcinoma of the breast (maximum diameter 14 mm) as a second tumor, confirmed by operation and histology.

Discussion

The diagnosis of pathologic changes and subsequent evaluation for therapy planning is based on the patient's history, clinical examination, biopsy with pathohistological analysis, and radiological imaging techniques. In particu-

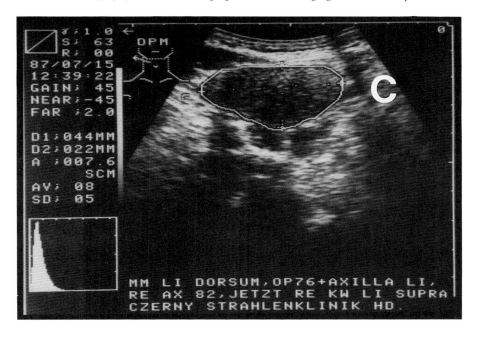

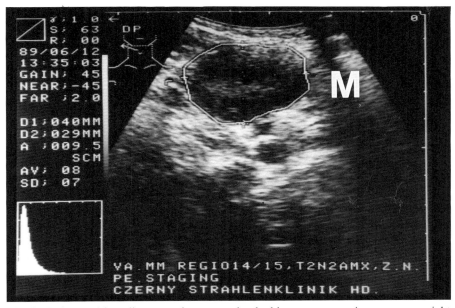

Fig. 1. Patients with malignant melanoma and palpable space-occupying processes, right cervical region. Sonography: echolucent processes, almost identical gray scale histograms. *Top*, branchiogenic cyst (*C*), confirmed intraoperatively and by histology; *bottom*, metastasis (*M*), confirmed by histology

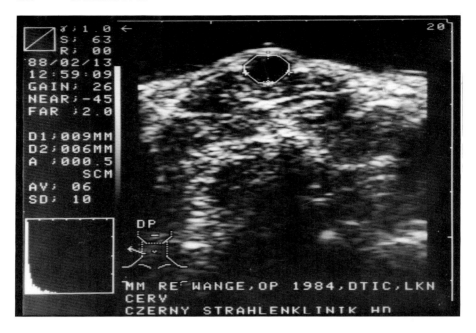
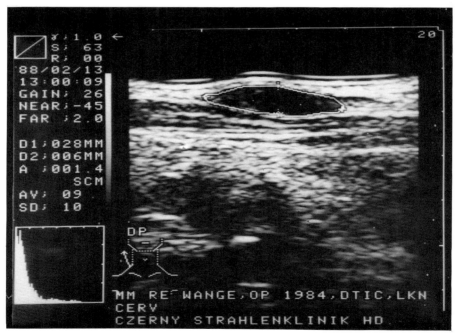

Fig. 2. Patient with malignant melanoma; palpable cervical lymph nodes (*circled area*). Sonography: very echolucent node, suspicion of metastatic involvement. Histology: toxoplasmosis

lar, for tumors such as malignant melanoma, with a marked tendency to metastatic spread, excellent prognosis in case of early detection, but rapid progression in advanced stages, sonography provides a nonaggressive, noninvasive, and repeatable method. Moreover, sonography is efficient and inexpensive for the therapy oriented diagnostic schedule [5, 7, 9, 11]. This is especially true for metastatic disease in lymph nodes and subcutaneous structures which, according to autopsy findings, are rather frequent localizations (65% and 75%, respectively) [1].

Even in patients with clinically apparent metastatic cancers, clinical examination alone will often not provide the objective criteria as to multiplicity of the pathologic processes, their three dimensional spread, and the possible invasion of therapy relevant structures (large vessels, bones, etc.), which are the basis for adequate treatment planning. The rate of 15%–39% histologically positive lymph nodes not detected by palpation obviously shows the limits of staging based on clinical examination alone [1, 11]. To reduce this high number of false-negative results, early detection must be the first aim of an imaging method such as sonography.

Therapy planning, follow-up, detection of recurrent disease and the unknown primary metastatic tumors, and exclusion of a malignant tumor in cases of suspect clinical evidence are further indications for this procedure.

To provide objective criteria for this purpose, sonographic analysis must include data about the affected regions, multiplicity, dimensions, structure, contours, and vascularization of the tumor as well as its relation to neighboring structures.

The general opinion, that malignant changes of lymph nodes or soft-tissue tumors are always echolucent in relation to neighboring structures, has to be qualified for a number of primary tumors such as carcinomas of the breast (Fig. 3), the head and neck region, and others [8], but *not* for malignant melanoma. The generally low level of echogenicity of malignant melanoma metastases is mainly due to pathologic vessels and hypervascular tumors and not to necrotic areas, which can also be demonstrated by angiographic methods (Fig. 4).

Low echogenicity means good contrast with the more echogenic surrounding tissues, resulting in a high degree of sensitivity with an actual detection limit of about 3 mm for pathologic nodes under favorable conditions. As the amount of time required by the experienced examiner is reasonable, sonography will be the preferred imaging method to check even unsuspected regions in a risk-adapted screening in addition to clinical findings.

Sonographic follow-up under standardized conditions allows determination of tumor volume, calculation of the kinetics of tumorous processes, analysis of the treatment results, and, in case of therapeutic failure, early adjustment of the therapy. This is especially important in patients with aggressive tumors such as malignant melanoma, where we found tumor doubling times as low as 8 days (in Fig. 5, 18 days). In these patients, even "no change" situations must be considered as a therapeutic success. For good

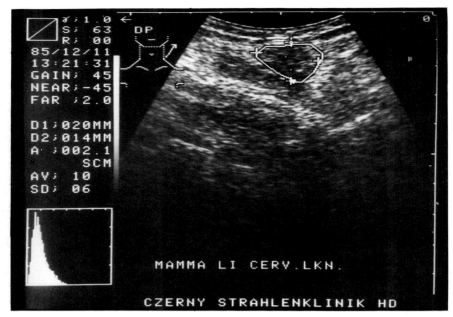

Fig. 3. Left cervical lymph node with only moderately reduced echogenicity in a patient with breast cancer

response rates, objectified on the safer level of the imaging methods (Fig. 4). To optimize therapy, monitoring should not only be applied to local measures such as radiotherapy (Fig. 6), but also to other schedules e.g., dacar bazine (DTIC), monoclonal antibodies, interferon, lymphocyte-activated killer cells, etc. Controls have to be performed at short-term intervals in high-risk patients with the first examination about 2 weeks postoperative.

Few differential diagnostic problems with palpable processes are encountered in echogenic lymph nodes with characteristics of chronic changes (Fig. 7) [9] or in patients with lipoma, calcified hematoma, or a Baker's cyst.

The problematic findings are subacute infections (toxoplasmosis, tuberculosis, etc.) (Fig. 2), branchiogenic cysts (Fig. 1), and metastases of an unknown second primary tumor. In case of the diagnosis "metastases of an unknown primary origin", the combination of echolucent lymph nodes and echolucent soft-tissue metastases may be an indication for a possibly amelanotic malignant melanoma.

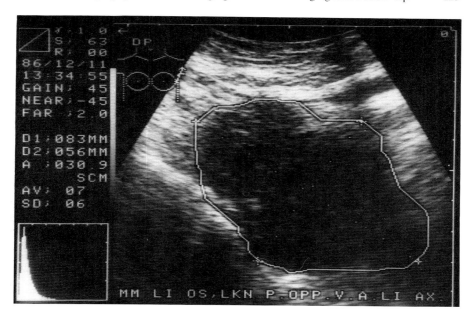

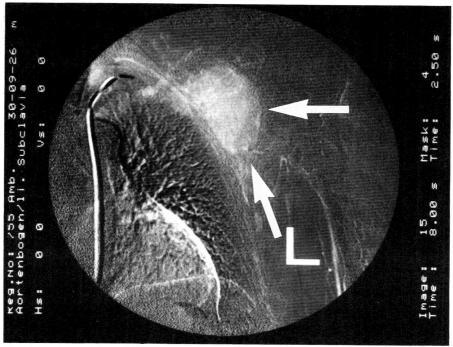

Fig. 4. Patient with malignant melanoma; large metastatic lymph node left axilla. *Top*, sonography: echolucent tumor with pathologic vessels; *bottom*, pathologic vessels, hypervascularized tumor (*arrows*)

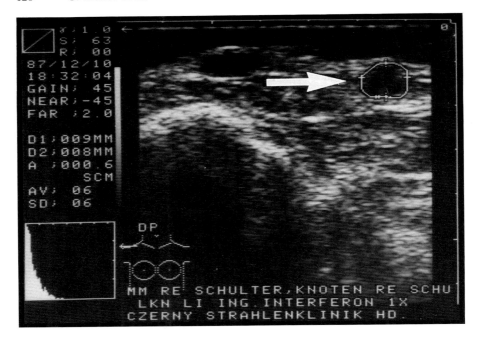

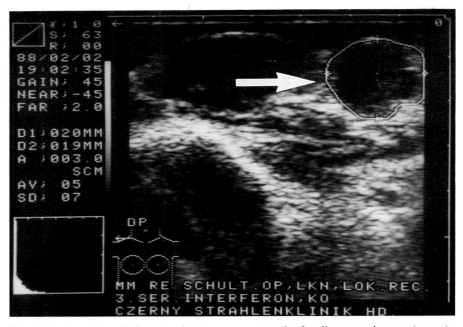

Fig. 5. Fast growing echolucent, subcutaneous metastasis of malignant melanoma (*arrow*). *Top*, sonography Dec. 1987; *bottom* control February 1988. Tumor doubling time 18 days

Sonography: The Ideal Imaging Method for Staging and Follow-Up

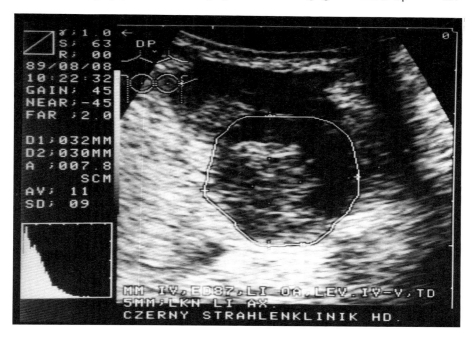

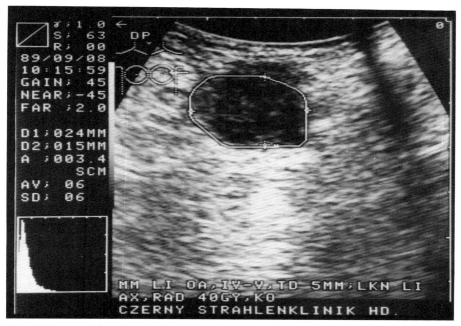

Fig. 6. Metastatic lymph node (*circled area*) left axilla before therapy (*top*) and after 40 Gy (*bottom*); a response rate of 70%

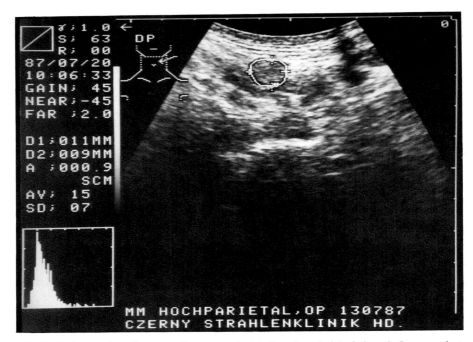

Fig. 7. Patient with malignant melanoma; palpable lymph node (*circled area*). Sonography: very echogenic structure; chronic inflammation, no indication of malignancy

Conclusion and Summary

In support of the findings of other authors [5, 7, 9, 10] our results with 205 patients with malignant melanoma demonstrate the excellent sensitivity and very good specificity of sonography in the diagnosis of metastatic processes of the lymph nodes as well as soft-tissue tumors. Discrepant low rates of sensitivity [6] may be to equipment problems.

Sonographic monitoring of the response of the tumorous processes to different therapy modalities allows an objective verification and quick adjustment of the treatment plan if necessary. As the sonographic result had a direct influence on the therapeutic procedure in 50% of our patients, we consider the risk-adapted application of sonography with sophisticated analysis as a noninvasive, efficient and inexpensive method to be used as an integral part of the diagnosis, monitoring, and follow-up schedule in patients undergoing therapy for malignant melanoma.

References

1. Altmeyer P, Nödl F, Merkel H (1980) Lymphogene Metastasierungsbereitschaft des malignen Melanoms. Dtsch Med Wochenschr 105: 1769–1772

2. Blois MS, Sagebiel RW, Abarbanel RM (1983) Malignant melanoma of the skin. Cancer 52: 1330–1341
3. Braun-Falco O, Landthaler M (1990) Das maligne Melanom der Haut. Dtsch Arztebl 87: 689–691
4. Garbe C, Stadler R, Orfanos CE (1986) Prognose-orientierte Therapie bei malignem Melanom. Hautarzt 37: 365–372
5. Kraus W, Nake-Elias A, Schramm P (1986) Hochauflösende Real-Time-Sonographie in der Beurteilung regionaler lymphogener Metastasen von malignen Melanomen. Z Hautkr 61: 9–12
6. Krüger I, Ghussen F, Groth W (1989) Maligne Melanome der Extremitäten. Ein Vergleich der verschiedenen Stadieneinteilungen. Tumor Diagn Ther 10: 54–59
7. Löhnert JD, Bongartz G, Wernecke K, Peters PE, Macher E, Bröcker E-B (1988) Sensitivität und Spezifität der sonographischen Lymphknotendiagnostik beim malignen Melanom. Radiologe 28: 317–319
8. Mende U, Flentje M, Haels J, Zöller J (1987) Sonographische Lymphknotendiagnostik bei Malignomen im Kopf-Hals-Bereich. Picker Aktuell 5: 15–18
9. Prayer L, Winkelbauer F, Gritzmann N, Weislein H, Helmer M, Pehamberger H (1989) Untersuchung der primären Lymphknotenstationen beim malignen Melanom mittels hochauflösender Realtime-Sonographie – Stellenwert und Indikation. Fortschr Rontgenstr 151: 294–297
10. Schwaighofer B, Pohl-Markl H, Frühwald F, Stiglbauer R, Kokoschka EM (1987) Der diagnostische Stellenwert des Ultraschalls beim malignen Melanom. Fortschr Rontgenstr 146: 409–411
11. Voigt H, Kleeberg UR (eds) (1986) Malignes melanom. Springer, Berlin Heidelberg New York

Observations and Experiences in Sonographic Grading and Staging of Malignant Melanomas

G. MERK, H. MERK, J. ULRICH, K.-H. KÜHNE, and C. WILLGEROTH

Introduction

This work presents some results using ultrasound at the Department of Dermatology at Medizinische Akademie Magdeburg.

Using the SSA 90 scanner (Toshiba) we obtained images of skin tumors which could be further analysed. This instrument is equipped with a high-resolution 7.5 MHz transducer, well-suited for the clinical problems we encounter.

Sonography is suitable for the following indications:
1. Preoperative measurement of tumor thickness
2. Evaluation of the size and location of subcutaneous tumors
3. Differentiation of tumor structures
4. Exclusion of regional subcutaneous lymph node metastases

Additional benefits of sonography are listed in Table 1.

Results

Since 1987, we have investigated 318 patients. Of a total of 388 examinations, 206 sonographic findings were examined. Among these were 82 patients with malignant melanomas, 52 with lymph node metastases, 37 with subcutaneous melanotic metastases, and 18 with benign skin tumors. Sonographically, malignant melanoma can usually be shown as a spindle shaped, echo-poor focus within the highly reflective cutis band (Figs. 1–3).

Within the loosely structured subcutis, pervaded by irregular streaky reflections, sonography allows definition of subcutaneous melanotic metastases; these appear as round foci the echogenicity of which ranges from echo-poor to echolucent. Topographical details, such as the relation of tumor location to vessels or an infiltration of the muscle, may yield essential indications for surgical planning (Fig. 4). The sonographic technique also enables superficial lymph node metastases to be easily visualized and differentiated from non-specific lymph node swellings. The structure of lymph node metastases sonographically coincides with that of subcutaneous melanotic metastases. Nonspecific lymph nodes show the regular structure of

Observations and Experiences in Sonographic Grading and Staging 131

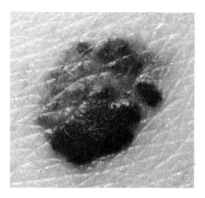

Fig. 1. Left upper arm of a 67-year-old female patient

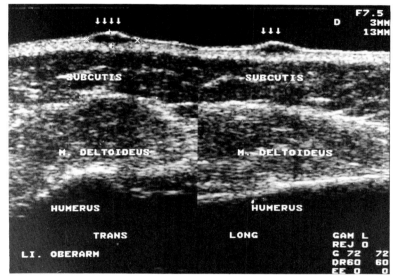

Fig. 2. Sonogram of the tumor shown in Fig. 1; *arrows*, melanoma

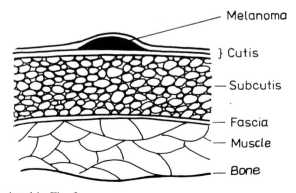

Fig. 3. Scheme of sonogram depicted in Fig. 2

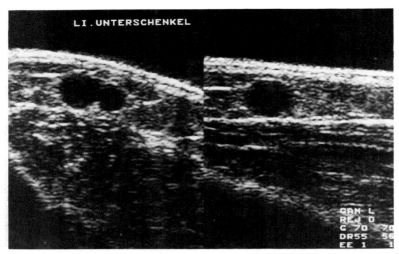

Fig. 4. Sonogram of a subcutaneous melanotic metastasis in the left lower leg of a 56-year-old female patient

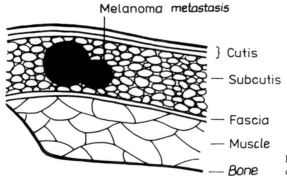

Fig. 5. Scheme of the sonogram depicted in Fig. 4

capsule (echo-rich), cortex (echo-poor), and center (echo-rich) (Figs. 6–8).

A correlation between sonographic findings and histological diagnosis of the clinical course yielded the following results: Of the 82 melanomas, we detected 65 with a tumor thickness of >1 mm sonographically, 55 of which could be confirmed histologically. The sensitivity was thus 84%. The main sources of errors were acro-lentiginous melanomas, which are echo-rich and blue nevi which are sonographically identical to melanomas (Fig. 9). Specificity of lymph node examinations was about 96% (Figs. 9, 10). Comparable results have been obtained by Kraus et al. [2, 3]. A correlation of the sonographically determined tumor thickness values with histology

Observations and Experiences in Sonographic Grading and Staging 133

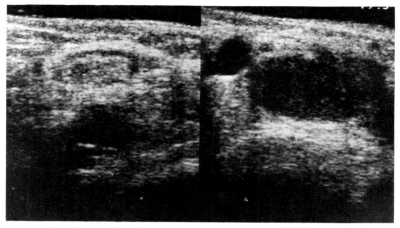

Fig. 6. Sonogram of an inguinal lymph node metastasis (*right*) and of a normal inguinal lymph node (*left*) in a 58-year-old female patient

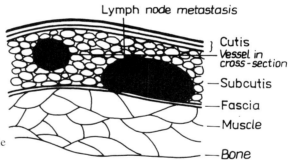

Fig. 7. Scheme of the right side sonogram depicted in Fig. 6

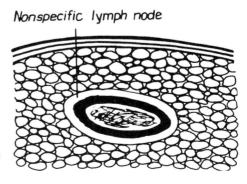

Fig. 8. Scheme the left side sonogram depicted in Fig. 6

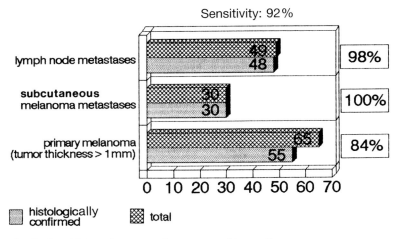

Fig. 9. Sensitivity of preoperative sonographic results

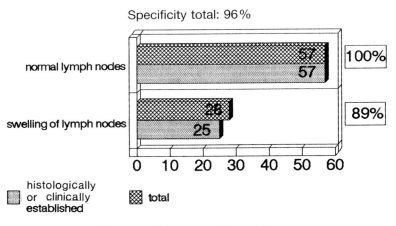

Fig. 10. Specifity of preoperative sonographic results

showed that the sonographically measured tumor thickness values were higher. Moreover, with respect to differences between single melanomas, note the "no deviation" line in Fig. 11. Above this value, sonographically thicker tumors are depicted and below, thinner ones.

In general there is good agreement between sonographically and histologically determined tumor thickness values. Similar results were presented by Breitbart and Rehpennig 1983 [1].

In summary, our findings strongly suggest the following:
1. The sonogram does not yield clear hints to diagnose a melanoma.

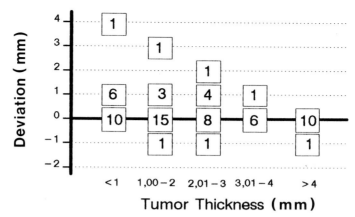

Fig. 11. Comparison of sonographically and histologically determined tumor thickness (malignant melanomas)

2. In our view, difficulties result from the fact that the tumor is echo-poor and spindle shaped. Another problem is the jagged border and the lack of dorsal echo enhancement. However, ultrasound provides further support in finding the correct diagnosis (Table 1).

Table 1. Advantages of sonography

Dynamic depiction of tumors
Tumour puncture under ultrasonic control
Intraoperational application
Bedside application
Course of therapy control, location of metastases, assessment of recidivism
On-the-spot documentation
No exposure to radiation
A noninvasive method, no side effects

A disadvantage of ultrasound is that visualization of tumors which are less than 1 mm thick is not possible at 7.5 MHz. In addition, the quality of the diagnosis depends on the type of ultrasound instrument used and the skill of the examiner.

Conclusions

Sonography is an exact and reproducible tool to gain additional diagnostic information. This method is particularly interesting for dermatological oncology.

References

1. Breitbart EW, Rehpenning W (1983) Möglichkeiten und Grenzen der Ultraschalldiagnostik zur in vivo-Bestimmung der Invasionstiefe des malignen Melanoms. Z Hautkr 58: 975–987
2. Kraus W, Nake-Elias A, Schramm P (1985) Diagnostische Fortschritte bei malignen Melanomen durch die hochauflösende Real-Time-Sonographie. Hautarzt 36: 386–392
3. Kraus W, Nake-Elias A, Schramm P (1986) High resolution real-time sonography for the assessment of regional lymph node metastases of malignant melanoma. Z Hautkr 61: 9–14

Doppler Ultrasound and Ultrasound Duplex

Basis and Clinical Applications of Ultrasound Doppler Systems

P. A. Payne, A. Ayatollahi, and R. Y. Faddoul

Introduction

Clinical applications of Doppler ultrasound go back almost 30 years. However, this history is much shorter than that of the use of ultrasound in a more conventional imaging modality. The reasons for the slow acceptance of Doppler ultrasound techniques are many and complex, but they are almost certainly principally due to the very difficult physical concepts that must be understood in order to maximise the benefit that can be obtained from the technique. Such an understanding has clearly begun to emerge and today there are many ultrasound Doppler systems in use, ranging from very simple battery operated devices that employ a small loudspeaker to indicate the patency of a blood vessel through to the Duplex systems that combine Doppler flow measurements with cross-sectional imaging and the even more complex systems that produce colour flow images.

The Doppler effect, in conjunction with ultrasound, is also used extensively as a means of, for example, monitoring the foetal heart rate in utero. This is just one example of the use of ultrasound Doppler to obtain data derived from movement and then to further analyse it, in this case to obtain timing information. Applications such as this are outside the scope of this present paper and we will concentrate on ultrasound Doppler systems that may be used for the measurement of blood velocity and volume flow.

Acoustic Scattering by Red Corpuscles

The majority of the scatterers in human blood comprise red blood cells or corpuscles. These are biconcave discs about 7 μm in diameter and some 2 μm thick. If we assume that the wavelength of ultrasound is much greater than the dimensions of the red blood cell, then certain simplifications can be used in any analysis of the physical effects. This simplifying assumption is certainly true for frequencies in common clinical use, i.e. between 2 and 20 MHz. If we use a factor of ten as representing the condition referred to above, then the maximum frequency at which the simplifications will work is a little over 20 MHz.

It was shown by Rschevkin [8] that the amplitude of a back scattered acoustic wave resulting from interaction with a red blood cell is independent of the shape of the cell and depends only on its volume and the mismatch in acoustic impedance with respect to the plasma.

Atkinson and Woodcock [1] also present a useful analysis in terms of statistical diffraction theory, which can form the basis for an understanding of the type of interaction that ultrasound has with blood. In particular, they describe the axial and radial fading phenomena which are linked to the effect obtained from bandpass filtering of white noise.

The Doppler Equation

The relationship between the Doppler frequency f_D and the transmitted frequency is given by:

$$f_D = \frac{2v}{c} f_T \qquad (1)$$

in which v is the velocity of a scatterer, c is the velocity of sound in the plasma and f_T is the transmit frequency. This equation assumes that the scatterer is moving normally with respect to the transmitter/receiver. If this is not the case, a term $\cos\theta$ must be introduced where θ is the angle between the axis of the ultrasound beam and the direction of travel of the scatterer.

Continuous Wave and Pulsed Doppler Systems

There are two fundamental ways in which ultrasound Doppler systems operate. The first and most simple is that based on a continuous wave (CW) approach. Here the transmitted signal is "sent" continuously and a separate receive transducer collects the back scattered energy and this is then further processed.

In the alternative pulsed Doppler system a single transducer can be employed and this is used to send out a "toneburst" which is a signal that is brief in time, but that has a characteristic centre frequency. By processing the back scattered version of the toneburst, the shift in the characteristic frequency can be obtained, giving rise to Doppler information. The difference compared with CW, however, is that by timing the transmission and reception of the acoustic energy, it is possible to define a so-called sample volume out in front of the transducer from which the back scattered data are obtained. Any acoustic signals outside the sample volume are rejected and thus it becomes possible to select points within the body from which Doppler signals are accepted. This removes the confusing interaction of signals present in the continuous wave systems when many blood vessels are interrogated simultaneously.

Current Instrumentation

The simplest instruments merely use the Doppler difference frequency, suitably amplified, to drive a loudspeaker or headphones. Analysis of these signals, which fortunately usually lie in the audio range, is left to the user. The next stage in complexity tends to be associated with CW instruments that use low cost techniques for providing spectral analysis of the Doppler signals. These are usually three-dimensional figures plotting Doppler shift frequency against time and giving an indication of the intensity of the spectrum at any point. A further degree of complexity gives rise to the pulsed Doppler systems which can be employed to accurately locate the sample volume in the position across an artery, for example, of interest to the clinician. Such systems have been combined with sophisticated B-scanning ultrasound instruments to produce the so-called Duplex systems, in which a cross-sectional image of the soft tissue surrounding a blood vessel is obtained and a pulsed Doppler channel is added to this, enabling an additional display of flow velocities to be given. By combining these two modalities, it becomes possible to measure the diameter of a blood vessel, measure the velocities across the lumen, and hence, calculate volume flow. In a recent review of arterial blood flow as measured by Doppler ultrasound, Hoskins [6] surveyed a number of reports on the accuracy of ultrasound Doppler volume flow based mostly on the Duplex instrument principle and has found a wide range of root mean square (RMS) errors, from 9% to 101%. Much better results are associated with the measurement of cardiac volume flow, where the average RMS error was some 19%.

To date, the most complex (and hence most costly!) ultrasound Doppler instrumentation is that associated with colour flow imaging. In this technique a real time colour image represents the flow of blood; shades of red and blue usually represent blood velocities away from and towards the transducer. In addition, turbulence is often displayed, sometimes separately, very often using shades of green. In almost all cases, the Duplex systems and the colour flow imaging systems use multielement phased or linear array transducers. The requirements for simultaneous measurement of Doppler signals, together with imaging, make the use of mechanical scanners almost impossible.

Considerable work has been done on techniques of waveform analysis associated with Doppler ultrasound signals and a number of these are reviewed by Hoskins [6].

Clinical Applications

Studies of Arterial Flow

A lot of work, on measurements of lower limb blood flow using ultrasound Doppler, has been reported, many of these studies being based on the use of fairly simple instrumentation, together with relatively complex signal analysis. Most of these techniques, however, are still research tools and have not found their way into general clinical use, despite the fact that the earliest work dates back to the mid 1960s.

Another major area of interest is in measuring blood flow in the carotid arteries and quite accurate diagnosis of stenosis in these arteries is now being obtained.

Ultrasound Doppler blood flow measurements are also employed in the area of obstetrics, neonatal studies and studies of blood flow in tumours. The paper by Hoskins [6] contains good reviews of these and a number of other areas of application.

Ultrasound Doppler for Dermatology

The measurement of blood flow in the skin would, at first sight, appear to be a much simpler problem than that of measuring blood flow in some deeply sited artery. This turns out not to be the case and principally this is due to the complexity of the microcirculation in the skin and of the physiological interactions with blood flow that can readily occur. Numerous methods have been used in the past for measuring blood flow and these have been reviewed by Payne [7]. In addition, the use of skin thermal conductivity as an index of blood flow has been described by Dittmar [3]. Stüttgen et al. [9] have described techniques based on optical plethysmography among a number of other techniques.

There is little work reported to date on the use of ultrasound to measure skin blood flow.

We might conveniently group the blood in skin into three regions: the capillary flow, flow in the dermal plexus and flow in the subdermal plexus. An instrument devised to enable these three components of skin blood flow to be independently measured has been described recently by Ayatollahi [2], based on earlier work by Faddoul [4], which gave rise to a single channel pulsed Doppler ultrasound blood flowmeter.

Payne [7] has shown how the single channel instrument can be calibrated to enable an estimate of volume flow to be obtained for a given volume of tissue. The instrument described has a calibration constant of 0.0055 µl per second and the instrument sensitivity is sufficient to detect changes in skin blood flow due to cigarette smoking or small thermal stimuli applied to the skin.

Using just one channel of the three channel instrument referred to previously, the effect of raising and lowering the arm on the capillary flow in the thumb pad was measured; the results are shown in Fig. 1. In Fig. 2 two channels of this same flowmeter have been used to monitor the blood flow in the thumb pad whilst the hand was held at the level of the heart. In one case the timing settings of the instrument were chosen so that channel one responded only to the capillary flow, whilst channel two was adjusted to measure dermal plexus blood flow.

Basis and Clinical Applications of Ultrasound Doppler Systems 143

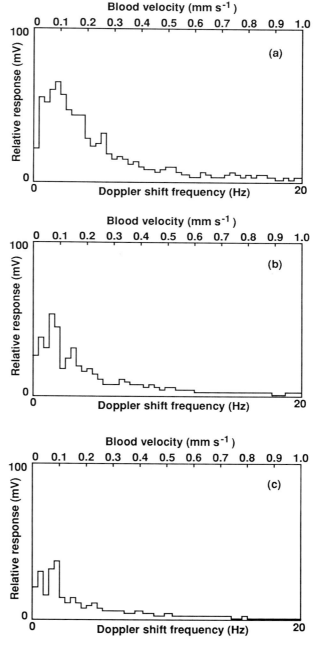

Fig. 1a–c. Skin blood flow results obtained from a single channel of the three-channel blood flowmeter on the inner forearm of a normal volunteer with **a** the hand positioned below the heart, **b** level with the heart and **c** above the heart

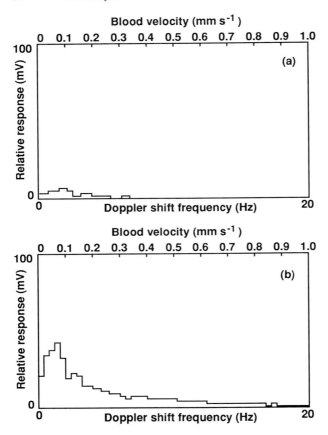

Fig. 2a, b. Simultaneous Doppler shift measurements from **a** capillary bed and **b** dermal plexus

The instruments described above were both capable of operating over a wide range of centre frequencies and the data in Figs. 1 and 2 were obtained at a centre frequency of 20 MHz. Clearly, as the frequency is raised so the effect of attenuation in the skin increases. However, the intensity of the back scattered signal from red blood cells alters with frequency raised to the power four. The combination of these two effects was investigated by Frew and Giblin [5] and they showed that, for an observation distance of 100 μm, the optimum frequency at which to operate a skin blood flowmeter was 120 MHz. However, if our interest is in measuring at a number of depths within the skin, then this optimum frequency is changed considerably. In Fig. 3 a graph is shown of pulsed Doppler centre frequency against total power loss in the system and for three different depths within the skin. As can be seen, a frequency of around 20–30 MHz is about optimum for depths of 2–3 mm.

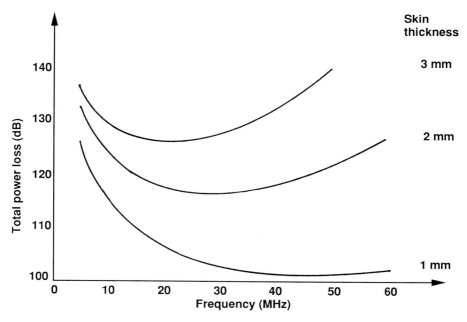

Fig. 3. Relationship between total power loss (dB) and frequency of operation for a Doppler blood flow measurement at three depths within the skin

However, the total power loss involved makes the design of a blood flowmeter extremely difficult. If we restrict ourselves to depths of around 1 mm, then the optimum frequency appears to be around 40–50 MHz. The majority of the experiments performed in Manchester have, however, been carried out at frequencies below this.

In addition to the difficulties associated with the power loss involved at greater and greater depths within the skin, there is also the problem of adjusting the timing gates of the instrument so that measurements are made at the appropriate points within the skin's microcirculation. In our work we have found that we must use a high resolution ultrasound A-scan instrument in order to find interfaces within the skin, such as the junction between the epidermis and the dermis and the junction between the dermal tissue and subcutaneous fat. By using these landmarks we can position the gates of the instrument relatively accurately. At present a simultaneous display of both A-scan and blood flow is not possible. However, in some circumstances the toneburst signal can be used as the basis for an A-scan display.

Conclusions

Ultrasound Doppler techniques are now widely used in clinical investigations and the emergence of Duplex and colour flow imaging systems will increase the number of applications by a large factor. The goal of using ultrasound Doppler techniques to detect early onset of vascular disease has yet to be fully achieved, but as better instrumentation systems are developed we are likely to approach this desirable result.

Ultrasound Doppler measurements of skin blood flow are very much in their infancy. However, we can probably learn from the history of Doppler ultrasound applied to other areas of the body. It would appear that the best results will be achieved by an instrument, yet to be designed, that will combine B-scan imaging with Doppler flow measurement.

References

1. Atkinson P, Woodcock JP (1982) Doppler ultrasound and its use in clinical measurement. Academic, London
2. Ayatollahi A (1989) A three channel pulsed Doppler skin blood flowmeter. PhD thesis, University of Manchester (UMIST)
3. Dittmar A (1989) Skin thermal conductivity: a reliable index of skin blood flow and skin hydration. In: Leveque JL (ed) Cutaneous investigation in health and disease. Dekker, New York, pp 323–358
4. Faddoul RY (1985) A high frequency ultrasound pulsed Doppler system for the measurement of skin blood flow. PhD thesis, University of Manchester (UMIST)
5. Frew HS, Giblin RA (1985) The choice of ultrasound frequency for skin blood flow investigation. Bioeng Skin 1:193–205
6. Hoskins PR (1990) Measurement of arterial blood flow by Doppler ultrasound. Clin Phys Physiol Meas 11:1–26
7. Payne PA (1988) Measurement of cutaneous blood flow. In: Marks RM, Barton SP, Edwards C (eds) The physical nature of the skin. MTP Press, Lancaster, pp 115–128
8. Rschevkin SN (1963) A course of lectures on the theory of sound. Pergamon, Oxford
9. Stüttgen G, Ott A, Flesch U (1989) Measurement of skin microcirculation. In: Leveque JL (ed) Cutaneous investigation in health and disease. Dekker, New York, pp 359–384

Duplex Sonography and Color Encoded Blood Flow Imaging

P. SCHLICHTING, D. BRECHTELSBAUER, and L. HEUSER

Both conventional duplex sonography and color encoded blood flow imaging (color flow) combine gray scale ultrasound and the pulsed Doppler technique. According to the Doppler equation, qualitative and quantitative detection and analysis of flow signals presuppose knowledge of the angle of the ultrasound beam in relation to the blood flow.

Amplitude data provide a real time, gray scale image of the vessel, the so-called B-scan. Real time B-scanning can show a relatively large segment of the vessel wall and lumen. Since conventional duplex sonography combines B-scanning and pulsed Doppler in the same object plane, it allows an exact spatial allocation of Doppler flow signals. However, flow information can be obtained only from one small area at a time (the sample volume). A number of areas must be investigated separately to get an adequate impression of flow characteristics. Thus, duplex sonography is a technically demanding and time consuming procedure. Nonetheless, it has a fixed value in perioperative diagnosis of carotid disease, since this area is readily accessible and Duplex sonography is an accurate, noninvasive, and low cost method.

Contrary to Duplex sonography, color flow instruments record both Doppler shift information and echo amplitude for all reflecting points in the field of view. They allow simultanous detection of Doppler information throughout the whole section. Flowing blood is displayed in real time in color superimposed on the gray scale image. Color assignment depends on flow direction with respect to the transducer position. Flow away from the transducer is represented by red and flow toward the transducer by blue. Color code reflects the frequency shift which is dependent on flow velocity and the angle of the sound beam in relation to the blood flow. High frequencies result in greater color saturation towards the lighter shades of red and blue. When there is transverse turbulence, green or yellow is admixed to red and blue. Aliasing is shown as a reversal of color, i.e., a spot of blue within the red stream. In interpreting the color flow signal in pronounced kinking or dilative angiopathy, knowledge of the probe-to-flow angle is of decisive importance in order to avoid misinterpretation of "turbulence signals." These are caused by variable Doppler angle and aliasing. It is important to recognize that color flow information is qualitative, not quantitative, because the color flow image is usually based on average Doppler shift, rather than on spectral frequency analysis, and Doppler information is not corrected for the Doppler angle. Like in conventional Duplex sonography, color flow equipment is capable of performing spectral analysis and providing an audible presentation of the Doppler signal [8].

With more than 4000 conventional Duplex examinations we found that a wide angle between the external and internal carotid arteries causes reversal of flow even during systole at the outer walls of the carotid bifurcation (Fig. 1a). This flow reversal can angiographically be proven by a delayed washout phenomenon in an extended digital subtraction angiography (DSA) series. Multiple studies, including ultrasound, angiography, and intraoperative findings, showed that atherosclerotic plaques tend to be located precisely in this region of flow reversal at the posterolateral wall of the bifurcation [1, 3, 6, 8]. In fact, there are complex secondary flow velocity patterns at the three-dimensional bifurcation consisting of helical flow, flow separation, and

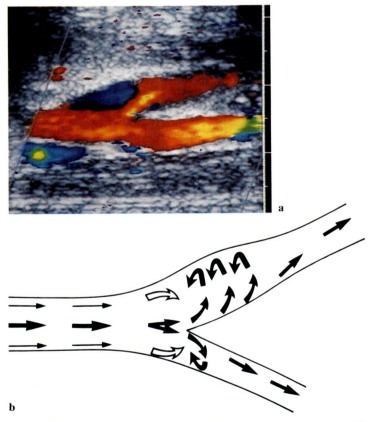

Fig. 1a, b. a Color flow image of the carotid bifurcation during systole. Flow reversal can be seen at the outer wall of the carotid bifurcation assigned by the *blue color*. Antegrade flow is shown in the internal and external carotid arteries near and along the apical divider providing the majority of blood flow. **b** Schematic diagram of the location of complex secondary flow patterns at the carotid bifurcation in one plane

flow reversal (Fig. 1b). Though the precise mechanism of plaque formation in this region is still unknown, it may be due to altered metabolism of the vessel wall or local formation of platelet aggregates [5, 7, 10]. In a study of 88 carotid bifurcations we observed that, with increasing bifurcation, angle flow separation becomes more pronounced and plaques and stenoses occur more frequently (Figs. 2, 3).

In a prospective correlative study between color flow Doppler and conventional Duplex sonography of carotid arteries we examined 45 patients

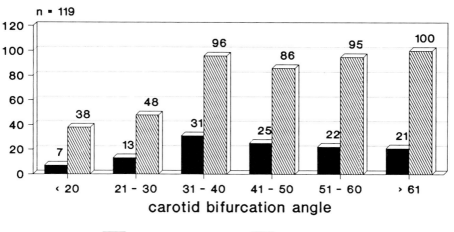

Fig. 2 ■ absolute number ▨ frequency in %

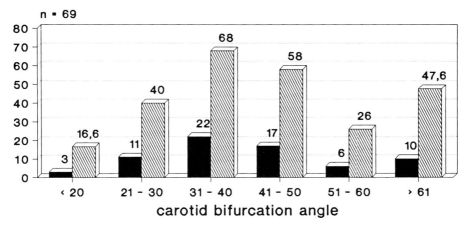

Fig. 3 ■ absolute number ▨ frequency in %

(Table 1). Both qualitative and quantitative data from angle-corrected spectral analysis were compared. Correlation for vessel diameter and blood flow was significant ($p < 0.1\%$) (Table 2). However, the measured absolute blood flow differed by a factor of three to four because in Duplex sonography it was calculated from peak systolic velocity, whereas in color flow the calculation was based on mean systolic velocity (Table 3). The sum of calculated blood flow in the internal and external carotid arteries was twice that found in the common carotid artery. This may be due to the fact that we examined diseased vessels with calcified stenoses, in which the automatically measured diameter of the residual lumen was overestimated. There was no

Table 1. Clinical history of patients examined with color flow. Duplex sonography, and DSA

	Color flow $n = 45$	Duplex sonography $n = 39$	DSA $n = 16$
TIA	16	13	16
Stroke	20	20	–
Asymptomatic	6	6	–

Table 2. Color flow – Duplex sonography correlation for the quantitative criteria vessel diameter, peak systolic velocity, and blood flow (p-values and correlation coefficient r) in the common carotid artery, the carotid bulb, the internal carotid artery, and the external carotid artery

	Vessel diameter			Peak systolic velocity			Blood flow		
	n	p	r	n	p	r	n	p	r
Common carotid artery	50	0.1	0.66	51	–	0.11	50	0.1	0.61
Carotid bulb	49	0.1	0.54	52	–	0.22	45	0.1	0.53
Internal carotid artery	43	0.1	0.67	45	5	0.34	42	0.1	0.55
External carotid artery	55	1.0	0.38	52	–	0.0003	52	1.0	0.37

Table 3. Blood flow in the common, internal and external carotid artery in ml/sec (average value and SD, $n = 50$ vessels) calculated from the area of the vessel lumen and mean systolic velocity in color flow and from peak systolic velocity using Duplex sonography

	Color flow (ml/sec)	Duplex sonography (ml/sec)
Common carotid artery	3.9 ± 2.7	18.5 ± 16.8
Internal carotid artery	3.2 ± 2.0	17.9 ± 8.8
External carotid artery	4.4 ± 3.0	13.6 ± 9.9

Table 4. Diagnostic results using color flow (Duplex sonography) ($n = 78$ vessels)

	Soft plaque	Hard plaque	Stenosis	Occlusion
Common carotid artery	36 (23)	32 (20)	3 (3)	2 (2)
Carotid bulb	29 (19)	33 (20)	11 (11)	1 (1)
Internal carotid artery	26 (17)	29 (28)	9 (9)	4 (4)
External carotid artery	27 (14)	21 (11)	6 (6)	2 (2)

correlation for peak systolic velocities. The results for qualitative criteria showed good agreement. All stenoses and occlusions detected with duplex sonography were corroborated by color flow and vice versa, but color flow was more sensitive in detection of small plaques (Table 4) [9].

Color flow helps to direct the attention to areas of stenosis within a vessel for more detailed spectral analysis. Since high flow and turbulence shine brighter, the areas of stenosis and plaque are easy to identify (Fig. 4). In addition, atherosclerotic plaques are more conspicuous by color flow enhancing them with the color coded lumen. Low-grade echolucent plaques can only be identified by encroachment of the color flow lumen (Fig. 5). The major pitfalls in color flow are calcified plaques, which cause acoustic shadowing extinguishing flow and image signal. When a calcified plaque within a high grade stenosis obscures the residual lumen flow, imaging and measurement is only possible beyond the acoustic shadowing. In these cases conventional Duplex sonography equipment with a 3 MHz Doppler may be helpful.

Comparing color flow and DSA, there is high accuracy using color flow for detection of disease and critical stenosis. Direct measurements to determine the degree of stenosis can be performed with color flow both in multiple longitudinal and transverse planes. Errors occur mainly in severely calcified vessels and in patients with unfavorable body habitus whose bifurcations cannot be examined properly. For minimal disease, color flow is more sensitive than angiography. A major limitation of Duplex sonography in relation to angiography was the difficulty to distinguish very high-grade stenosis with minimal residual flow from occlusion (Table 5). This limitation is not solely instrument dependent, but is related to operative skill and the experience of the interpreter. However, in color flow a trickle of blood flow may be seen more readily.

Color flow is an exciting progress in sonography. Many new applications have been described in pertinent literature reports, e.g., intraoperative assessment of cerebral AV malformations, imaging of thyroid gland adenomas, and detection of flow characteristics in malignant neoplasms and in occlusive disease of femoral and popliteal arteries [4]. The great advantage of color flow is that vessels are visualized even if they are too small to be resolved

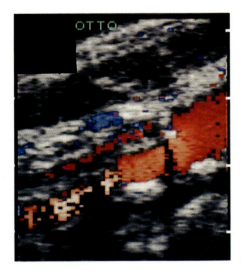

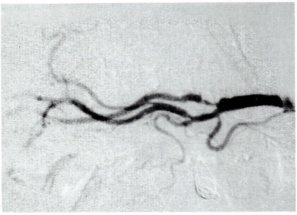

Fig. 4. a Color flow image of a stenosis at the origin of the internal carotid artery due to an inhomogenous, partly calcified, atherosclerotic plaque. Notice the area of increased velocity encoded by the *brighter shades of red*. In addition there is acoustic shadowing beneath the calcified areas of the vessel wall. **b** Corresponding angiogram

Table 5. Color flow – angiography correlation in detection of carotid arteriosclerotic disease in 15 patients with 78 findings

Agreement ($n = 65$)	Disagreement	
	Color flow	DSA
Plaque stenosis	Plaque ($n = 3$)	Ulceration ($n = 1$)
Kinking occlusion	Kinking ($n = 3$)	
	Subtotal stenosis ($n = 3$)	Occlusion ($n = 3$)

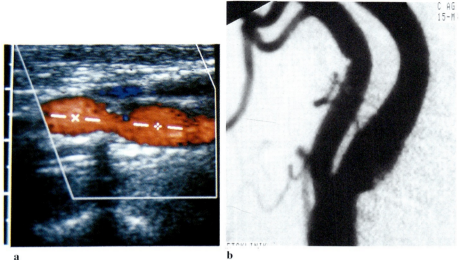

Fig. 5. a Soft plaque in the internal carotid artery with encroachment of the color flow lumen. **b** Corresponding angiogram in which the plaque is less apparent

on a gray scale image. Currently available color flow equipment works with linear or curved array 3.5–7.5 MHz transducers. For sonography of the skin high frequency ultrasound with 20 or even 50 MHz is required. Thus, color flow is limited to visualizing large subcutaneous vessels such as the greater or lesser saphenous veins. A problem encountered with venous color flow imaging is the low velocity range. Special software with slow pulse repetition frequency for the color flow component is needed to enable operators to portray color flow signals from small veins. Research on veins using color flow has concentrated on lower extremity venous disease, in particular lower extremity venous thrombosis. Normal phasic venous flow caused by respiration can be appreciated on a real time color flow image in normal femoral popliteal systems. As with B-mode sonography, there is good agreement between color flow and conventional phlebography in detection of thrombosis in the femoral-popliteal system with exception of the adductor canal (Figs. 6, 7). With the advent of slow flow detecting software, diagnostic accuracy of deep calf vein thrombosis is increased, but is still unsatisfactory. The major advantage of color flow in imaging venous thrombosis appears to be the demonstration of recanalized venous segments that cannot be visualized by common B-scan [2]. The role of color flow imaging in the management of varicosis remains to be precisely defined, a field in which dermatologists will be involved in future.

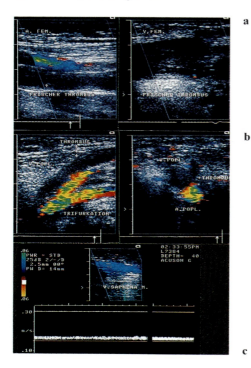

Fig. 6a–c. Venous thrombosis of the **a** common femoral vein and **b** the calf veins at the trifurcation. The lumen of the veins is filled low echoic thrombotic material. The veins are not compressible and there is no flow signal. **c** Blue encoded color flow image of the greater saphenous vein in the same patient. The lack of flow modulation by respiration and Valsalva maneuver indicates extention of the thrombus into the common iliac vein

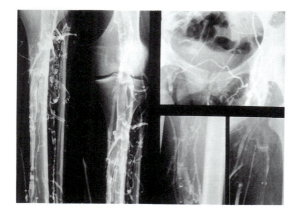

Fig. 7. Conventional venogram corresponding to Fig. 6

References

1. Bürrig K-F, Hort W (1988) Pathogenesis of carotid arteriosclerosis. In: Hennerici MG, Sitzer G, Weger H-D (eds) Carotid artery plaques. Workshop, Gütersloh 1987. Karger, Basel, pp 101–114

2. Foley DW, Middleton WD, Lawson TL, Erickson S, Quiroz FA, Macrander S (1989) Color Doppler ultrasound imaging of lower-extremity venous disease. AJR 162:371–378
3. Gellhaus M (1987) Experimentelle Untersuchung zur Bestimmung des optimalen Verzweigungswinkels der Halsschlagader. Institut für Thermo- und Fluiddynamik, Ruhr-Universität-Bochum, Diplomarbeit
4. Landwehr P, Tschammler A, Höhmann M (1990) Gefäßdiagnostik mit der farbcodierten Duplexsonographie. Dtsch Med Wochenschr 115:343–351
5. Lighthill J (1973) Atherogenesis: initiating factors. Ciba Foundation Symposion 12. Elsevier Excerpta Medica, Amsterdam
6. Nicholls SC, Phillips DJ, Primozich JF, Lawrence RL, Kohler TR, Rudd TG, Strandness DE Jr (1989) Diagnostic significance of flow separation in the carotid bulb. Stroke 20 (2):175–182
7. Reneman RS, van Merode T, Smeets FAM, Hoeks APG (1988) Velocity patterns and wall properties in the carotid bulb in man – their relation to atherogenesis. In: Hennerici MG, Sitzer G, Weger H-D (eds) Carotid artery plaques. Workshop, Gütersloh 1987. Karger, Basel, pp 143–162
8. Schlichting P, Edelmann M (1989) Farbcodierte Duplex-Scan-Untersuchungen der hirnversorgenden Gefäße. In: Schütz R-M, Hohlbach G (eds) Neue diagnostische und therapeutische Verfahren in Angiologie und Gefäßchirurgie. 10. Norddeutsche Angiologentage Lübeck-Travemünde, 1989. Graphische Werkstätten, Lübeck, pp 7–18
9. Schlichting P, v d Gaag C, de Swart P (1988) Erste Erfahrungen mit der Angiodynographie (farbcodierte Duplexsonographie) in der prä- und postoperativen Diagnostik arteriosklerotischer Carotisläsionen. 69. Deutscher Röntgenkongreß, Freiburg, 2–4 June 1988
10. Schmid-Schönbein H, Wurzinger LJ (1988) Vortex transport phenomena of the carotid trifurcation: interaction between fluid-dynamic transport phenomena and hemostatic reactions. In: Hennerici MG, Sitzer G, Weger H-D (eds) Carotid artery plaques. Workshop, Gütersloh 1987. Karger, Basel, pp 64–91

The Value of Duplex Sonography in Diagnosing Phlebologic Diseases

G. Hesse

The value of Duplex sonography (DUS) and color flow Doppler (CFD) has only recently been established for diagnosis of diseases of the superficial venous system of the legs [2, 3, 4]. The advantages of DUS and CFD are that they are noninvasive and reproducible. CFD has the following advantages over DUS:
1. complex anatomical situations can be analyzed better,
2. slow venous flow can be visualized,
3. the correlation of CFD with phlebography (85%) is better than with DUS (67%) and
4. the total investigation time is shorter with CFD [2].

By means of either system, the therapy of phlebological diseases can be planned exactly. Anatomy of the deep and superficial veins, from the pelvis down to the foot, perforating veins, and venous valves, can be shown (Figs. 1–8). The advantage of CFD and DUS compared to phlebography is the possibility of analyzing the function of the veins, as to direction and amount of blood flow, and of visualizing the venous valves. In determining the thickness of the venous wall, visualizing nonperfused veins (thrombosis), and analyzing the structure of a venous thrombus (differentiating between acute and chronic venous thrombosis and visualizing partially thrombosed sapheno-femoral junctions in ascending thrombophlebitis of the greater saphenous vein), both ultrasound systems offer diagnostic facilities which are not possible with phlebography. In the same examination, most arterial diseases, hernia, lymph nodes, some diseases of the joints and muscles, and malignancies can be visualized. Thus, the main structures of the lower extremity which could be affected by or contribute to both phlebological diseases and possible accompanying diseases can be evaluated.

The examinations of L. Bork-Wölwer [3] using DUS showed that the sapheno-femoral or sapheno-popliteal junction can be analyzed equally well as with the invasive method of phlebography. Modern venous surgery should preserve as much as possible from the venous system of the lower extremities, since the veins might be important in arterial surgery some years later. For this kind of venous surgery, exact examination of the so-called points of reflux is essential because surgery at these points seems to be sufficient for the treatment of many varicose veins.

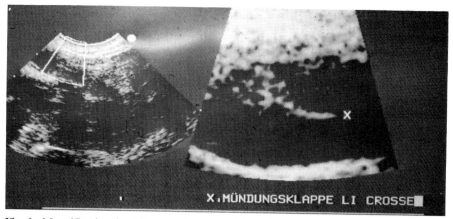

Fig. 1. Magnification (*right*) of the first valve (x) of the vena saphena magna (Sonos 100, HP). Area of the vain which is magnified (*left*)

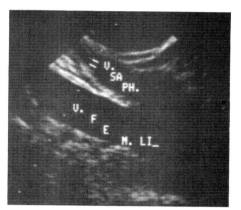

Fig. 2. Insufficient sapheno-femoral junction. (SL 2, Siemens)

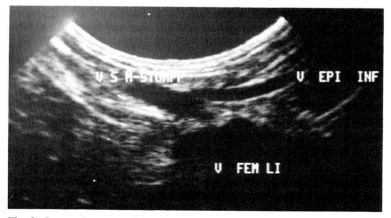

Fig. 3. Incomplete resection of the sapheno-femoral junction. (SL 2, Siemens)

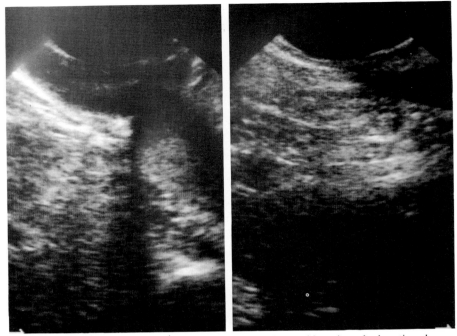

Fig. 4. Sign of complete compression of the sapheno-femoral junction, the junction shown is dilated (*left*, no compression; *right*, complete compression) (SL 2, Siemens)

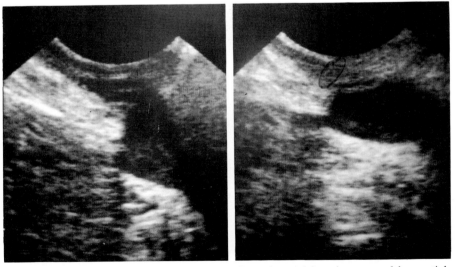

Fig. 5. Incomplete compression (0) of the sapheno-femoral junction, caused by partial thrombosis of the sapheno-femoral junction. (SL 2, Siemens). *Left*, no pressure on the skin by the duplex probe; *right*, the duplex probe is pressed strongly on the skin but due to the thrombus the vein is not completely compressed

The Value of Duplex Sonography in Diagnosing Phlebologic Diseases

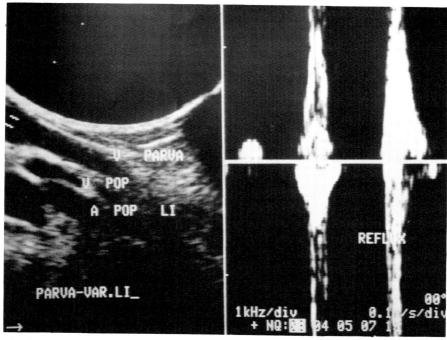

Fig. 6. Reflux into the dilated varicose vena saphena parva provoked by compression from the upper leg. (SL 2, Siemens). *Left*, two-dimensional image of the anatomical situation; *right*, Doppler frequency analysis of the venous blood flow

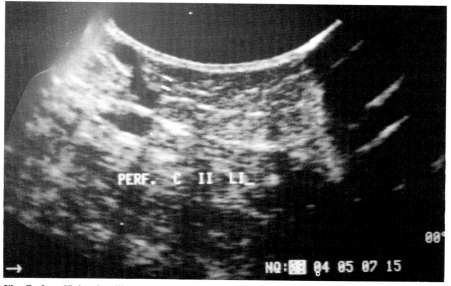

Fig. 7. Insufficiently dilated perforating vein, Cockett II. (Duplex sample not in the perforating vein.) (SL 2, Siemens)

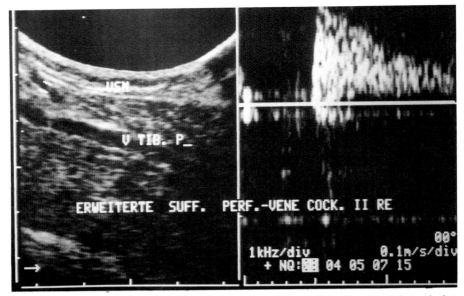

Fig. 8. Slightly dilated perforating vein, Cockett II, without reflux. The signal shown is the flux toward the heart provoked by decompression of the upper lower leg. (SL 2, Siemens). *Left*, two-dimensional image of the anatomical situation; *right*, Doppler frequency analysis of the venous blood flow

In the diagnosis of deep venous thrombosis of the femoral and popliteal veins, sensitivity is 90.5% and specificity 89% for DUS or CFD [1]. These qualities of DUS and CFD change the indications for phlebography, which thus should only be performed if the results of DUS and/or CFD do not concur with clinical results. DUS and CFD are particularly important in evaluating phlebological-dermatological diseases of the extremities, where erythema and swelling often suggest the differential diagnosis of thrombosis which is very important for planning therapy. DUS and CFD are the methods of the future in the noninvasive examination of the venous system and should always be undergone before invasive examinations or treatments are planned.

References

1. Bajardi G, Mastrandrea G, Ricevuto G, Pischedda G (1989) Duplex-scanning in the diagnosis of deep venous thrombosis of lower limbs. Phlebologie 89: 360–362
2. Belcaro G, Laurora G, Cesarone MR (1989) Colour duplex scanning (angiodynography). Evaluation of venous diseases using the slow flow systems. Phlebologie 89: 357–359
3. Bork-Wölwer L, Wuppermann Th (1989) Duplex-Sonographie der primären Varikosis. Vasa [Suppl.] 27: 149
4. Marshall M (1989) The duplex-sonography in phlebology. Phlebologie 89: 342–343

Bi-planar Transesophageal Echocardiography

R. HAMMENTGEN, S. EL-GAMMAL, M. HAUSMANN,
K. HOFFMANN, M. BERGBAUER, and D. RICKEN

Not only the skin but also internal organs can be analyzed with high frequency ultrasound by advancing the transducer into a compartment of the body. The following article describes the echocardiographic examination with an ultrasound probe placed into the esophagus. This method is called transesophageal echocardiography (TEE) [12].

Theory and Method

Modern Two-Dimensional Ultrasound Imaging and Color Flow Mapping

Using a refined technique and fast image processing we are able to perform a two-dimensional examination of the beating heart with 55 frames per second. The size of the heart chambers, its wall thickness and motion, as well as different pathological structures can be observed.

According to the Doppler effect, if reflected from moving erythrocytes, the frequency of ultrasound is shifted proportionally to the velocity, the so-called Doppler shift. Thus, conventional Doppler technique provides noninvasive measurement of flow velocities. Applying different physical formulas, pressure gradients (formula of Bernoulli), the orifice areas of stenotic valves (formula of continuity) and cardiac output can be calculated. The simultaneous pulsed wave measurement in a few thousand points and its visualization using a false-color technique forms the basis of what is known as color flow mapping (CFM) [12]. The vectors of velocity are coded in the following manner:
1. The direction of flow towards the transducer is represented in red. The flow away from the transducer is depicted in blue.
2. The mean flow velocity in a certain sample volume is coded in color brightness. Here, only the relative movement in the direction of the ultrasound beam is measured.
3. Velocity variance (e.g., turbulence) within the flow is coded by the green or yellow. The CFM makes it therefore possible to visualize valvular insufficiencies and intracardial shunts.

Unfortunately the transthoracic ultrasound approach (TTE) to the heart is limited by artifacts due to pulmonary air and a decreased lateral resolution of sector scanners with increasing distance from the transducer. These handicaps are overcome using the TEE approach, which produces quality high resolution images.

Equipment

TEE probes correspond to gastroscopes with an ultrasound transducer mounted to the tip. Today, if available, bi-plane transducers (BI-TEE) [10] are used; they consist of two independent ultrasound crystals which scan two planes oriented perpendicularly to each other (Fig. 1). By angulation and rotation of the tip nearly all conceivable sections of the heart can be registered via the esophagus. The standardized examination uses three points to deduce the scan planes [12]: aortic root, ventricular level, and gastric fund (Fig. 2).

Examination Technique

The TEE probe is handled and placed the same way as a gastroscope. The risks are low [19]. The probe is advanced into the esophagus after anesthesia of the pharynx, which can be combined with intravenous administration of a sedative. Usually the patient has been left fasting for at least 6 h and is positioned in the left decubitus position (Fig. 3).

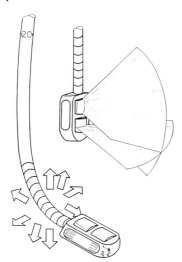

Fig. 1. Bi-plane TEE transducer

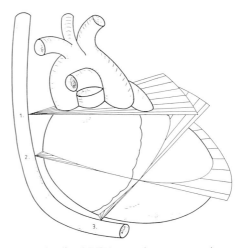

Fig. 2. Standardized TEE scanning center points.
1, Aortic root;
2, ventricular level;
3, gastric fund

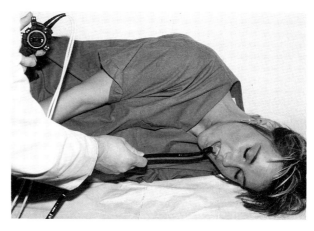

Fig. 3. Esophageal intubation. Other positions or respiration result in small topographical variations of the organs within the standardized scan planes.

"Classical" Indications and Findings

The TEE approach has two major advantages:
1. New scanning planes enable intrathoracic structures to be analyzed (e.g., left atrial appendage, thoracic aorta) which could be studied only incompletely by TTE.
2. The closer vicinity of the structures of interest to the transducer brings about a better lateral resolution. Furthermore, high frequency transducers which have better axial resolution can be used, refining representation of morphology.

Disadvantages of TEE are its increased logistic expense and the distinct discomfort for the patient. The mentioned advantages and limitations implicate the TEE indications. TEE should not be used for screening, but is an especially valuable tool for those questions in echocardiography that cannot be answered by TTE. A short description of the "classical" indications for TEE follows.

Source of Embolism. TTE only permits the positive evaluation of an atrial thrombus, whereas its exclusion can only be proved using TEE [9] by examining the left atrial appendage (Fig. 4). Further sources of embolism can be detected by TEE: A patent foramen ovale [9] becomes evident after intravenous administration of a contrast agent (Fig. 5). Spontaneous echocardiographic contrast [6], as a sign for arising thrombosis, can be made visible. Embolism of arteriosclerotic and thrombotic plaques of the ascending aorta are a possible cause for cerebral ischemias (transient ischemic attacks, prolonged reversible ischemic neurological deficit, stroke Fig. 6).

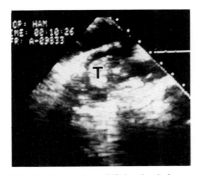

Fig. 4. Thrombus (*T*) in the left atrial appendage

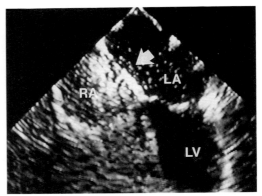

Fig. 5. Contrast bubbles shunting (*arrow*) through a patent foramen ovale. *RA*, right atrium, *LA*, left atrium; *LV*, left ventricle

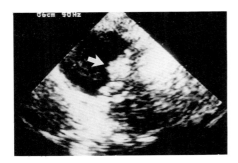

Fig. 6. Arteriosclerotic plaques (*arrow*) in the descending aorta

Valvular Endocarditis. On TTE not all endocarditic vegetations [7] can be observed. Due to the improved structure resolution of TEE diagnostic reliability for endocarditis is very high. This includes examination of valvular prosthesis.

Pathology of the Thoracic Aorta. The ascending and descending aorta and the aortic arch can be explored precisely due to their topographical proximity. Dissecting aneurysms [1] can be demonstrated in transversal (Fig. 7) and sagittal sections (Fig. 8). Additional CFM exhibits the flow in the various lumina [13]. Concerning the sensitivity in the diagnosis of dissecting aortic aneurysms, TEE is superior to computed tomography [18].

Pathology of the Atrial Septum. Defects of the atrial septum can be classified as septum-primum, septum-secundum and sinus-venosus defects. Postoperative remnants or recurrences can be evaluated. The size of a defect can be measured in two dimensions by BI-TEE; its shunting can be demonstrated qualitatively using CFM (Fig. 9).

Bi-planar Transesophageal Echocardiography

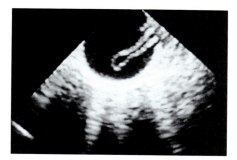

Fig. 7. Transversal section of a dissecting aortic aneurysmn (descending aorta)

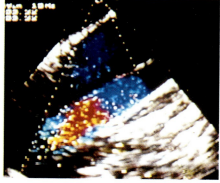

Fig. 8. Sagittal sections with additional CFM marking the flow in both lumina of the dissecting aneurysm

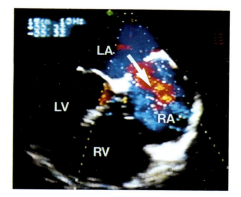

Fig. 9. Atrial septum secundum defect with left-to-right shunting (*arrow*). RA, right atrium; *LA*, left atrium; *RV*, right ventricle; *LV*, left ventricle

Malfunction of Valvular Prosthesis. The reflection artifacts of a mechanical valvular prosthesis are projected into the ventricle, so that regurgitation into the atrium is visualized without artifacts. Valvular insufficiency or malfunction [17] is detected (Fig. 10) easily.

Cardiac and Mediastinal Masses. With TEE mediastinal ultrasound examination is possible. Metastases, mediastinal tumor masses [14], and other structures can be visualized.

Anesthesiological and Critical Care Monitoring. TEE enables echocardiographic examination to be performed during an operative intervention [2] or ventilation to be controlled in an intensive care unit [15]. Left ventricular function can be measured continuously.

Cardiac Surgery and Interventional Cardiology. Surgial interventions to reconstruct heart valves can be optimized by simultaneous TEE [4]. In a similar manner valvuloplasty can be monitored [3].

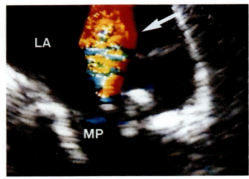 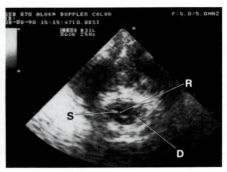

Fig. 10. Regurgitation (*arrow*) through a bioprosthesis (*MP*) in mitral position. LA, left atrium

Fig. 11. Transversal TEE scan of the spinal region. *R* spinal cord; *S*, spinal roots; *D*, dura mater spinalis

Special Indications. The TEE approach makes pathological changes such as subvalvular aortic stenosis, atrioventricular defects and diverticula of the ventricle visible in the same way as the intervertebral disk and the spinal cord [8] (Fig. 11).

Impaired Acoustical Conditions. In all cases where TTE is limited due to impaired acoustical conditions (for example, bandages, emphysema, or pycnic habitus), TEE is an excellent method for cardiac examination. Only gastric hernias, esophageal diverticula or an extreme rotation of the heart may restrict the TEE method.

Perspectives for the Future

Apart from further improvement of transducer design and technology, we expect additional information from digital image analysis. Doppler tomography [12] reconstructs real flow profiles by combining two CFM images under an angle, thereby making all the information about directional flow available. Three-dimensional reconstructions from serial B-scan sections using the program ANAT3D [5] provide special information about the topographic relations between different anatomical and pathological structures (Figs. 12–14) [11]. Finally, hemodynamic measurements deduced from the surface area and volume of the reconstructions also make quantitative information available.

References

1. Boerner N, Erbel R, Braun B, Henkel B, Meyer J, Rumpelt J (1984) Diagnosis of aortic dissection by transesophageal echocardiography. Am J Cardiol 54:1157–1158

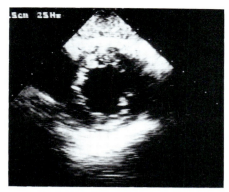

Fig. 12. Transgastric short axis section of the left ventricle

Fig. 13. Three-dimensional reconstruction of the spinal region from five serial sections through an intervertebral disk. (Violet, intervertebral disk; yellow, nucleus pulposus; brown, spinal cord; green, spinal roots; red, central canal; blue, dura mater spinalis)

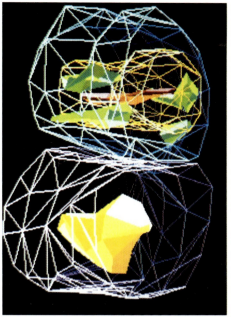

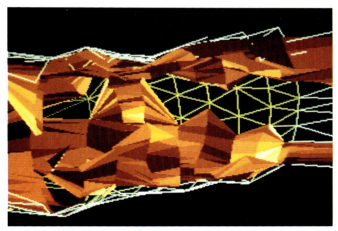

Fig. 14. Three-dimensional reconstruction of an arteriosclerotic descending aorta. (Green, aortic endothelium; red-yellow-shaded, plaques)

2. Bumb KL, Laviolette RJ, Trippi JA, Siderys H, Halbrook HG (1989) Transesophageal echocardiography – a technique for intraoperative monitoring. Indiana Med 82: 452–454
3. Casale PN, Whitlow P, Currie PJ, Stewart WJ (1989) Transesophageal echocardiography in percutaneous balloon valvuloplasty for mitral stenosis. Cleve Clin J Med 56:597–600

4. Drexler M, Erbel R, Dahm M, Mohr-Kahaly S, Oelert H, Meyer J (1986) Assessment of successful valve reconstruction by intraoperative transesophageal echocardiography (TEE). Int J Card Imaging 2:21–30
5. El-Gammal S, Altmeyer P, Hinrichsen K, (1989) ANAT 3D: shaded three-dimensional surface reconstructions from serial sections. Acta Stereol 8:543–550
6. Erbel R, Stern H, Ehrenthal W, Schreiner G, Treese N, Krämer G, Thelen M, Schweizer P, Meyer J (1986) Detection of spontaneous echocardiographic contrast within the left atrium by transesophageal echocardiography: spontaneous echocardiographic contrast. Clin Cardiol 9:245–251
7. Erbel R, Rohmann S, Drexler M, Mohr-Kahaly S, Gerharz CD, Iversen S, Oelert H, Meyer J (1988) Improved diagnostic value of echocardiography in patients with infective endocarditis by transesophageal approach. A prospective study. Eur Heart J 9:43–53
8. Funck M, Schneider B, Igloffstein J, Vogel P, Hanrath P (1989) Transösophageale Echoskopie des Spinalkanals. Dtsch Med Wochenschr 114:529–533
9. Hammentgen R, Winkel B, Fehske W, Nitsch J, Lüderitz B (1989) Patent foramen ovale: precise diagnosis by transesophageal contrast echocardiography. Circulation [Suppl II] 80, no. 4:II-403, 1603
10. Hammentgen R, Bergbauer M, Ricken D (1990) The advantages of bi-plane transesophageal echocardiography. Zbl Haut 157:332
11. Hammentgen R, el-Gammal S, Hausmann M, Bergbauer M, Ricken D (1990) Three-dimensional surface reconstructions of cardiac and paracardiac structures. International Symposium on Echocardiography, Mainz 1990 (Abstr B 33)
12. Hammentgen R (1991) Transösophageale Echokardiographie: monoplan-biplan, Atlas und Lehrbuch. Springer Berlin Heidelberg New York
13. Hashimoto S, Kumada T, Osakada G, Kubo S, Tokunaga S, Tamaki S, Yamazato A, Nishimura K, an T, Kawai C (1989) Assessment of transesophageal Doppler echocardiography in dissecting aortic aneurysm. J Am Coll Cardiol 14:1253–1262
14. Lestuzzi C, Nicolosi GL, Dall'Aglio V, Mimo R, Zanuttini (1990) Mediastinal pathology studied by transesophageal echocardiography. J Am Soc Echo 3:223 (Abstr 3G)
15. Oh JK, Seward JB, Khandheria BK, Freeman WK, Tajik AJ (1988) Transesophageal echocardiography in the intensive care unit. Circulation [Suppl II] 78, no. 4:II-298, 1190

Skin Tumors in 20 MHz Ultrasound

Sonographic Structure of Benign Skin Tumors

E. W. BREITBART and P. MOHR

Biophysical methods of measurement are of growing importance in dermatological diagnosis.

Proper dermatologic diagnosis depends on a precise visual and palpatory description of macromorphologic processes in human skin. However, confirmation of a diagnosis is often only possible by way of histologic examination of a biopsy taken from the dermatologic process in question.

Dermatologic diagnostic methods in use to date include inspection of the skin (macromorphologic) and histology (micromorphologic). In addition, a third investigative method is now available which is new and completely independent of the others: sonography. As an in vivo diagnostic method, sonography makes it possible to determine the elastic behavior of the skin's inner structure. Ultrasound diagnostics thus fill the gap that previously existed between inspection and histology. The following are currently seen as indications for a routine ultrasound examination:

- Measurement of skin thickness [1, 6, 7, 13].
- Measurement of tumor thickness [3, 4].
- Measurement of invasion depth of a malignant melanoma in planning operative therapy [2, 3, 5].
- Preoperative thickness measurement of all tumors to be treated using cryosurgery, laser surgery, or radiation. This can be used to set parameters for determining both cryosurgical depth and intensity and length of radiation and laser therapy [2, 5].
- Determination of the size of cutaneous metastases of a malignant melanoma to evaluate the therapeutic effects of cytostatic drugs [3].
- Checkups and determination of therapeutic effects on chronic inflammatory dermatoses, e.g., psoriasis and mycosis fungoides [3].
- Checkups and determination of therapeutic effects on collagenoses (measurement of elasticity, maximum stretch) [3, 6].
- Studies on the effects of steroids on the skin [12]

The most important dermatological tumor is malignant melanoma (Figs. 1, 2). Sonographically, it is a homogeneous, echo-poor tumor with isolated, weak, internal echoes. A melanoma normally possesses a degree of reflectivity comparable to that of fat (Fig. 3).

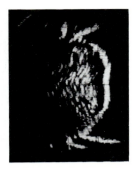

Fig. 1. B-mode ultrasound scan of a malignant melanoma. Note the typical echo-lucent structure of the tumor. Ultrasound imaging system: Ophthalmoscan 200, Sonometrics, NY

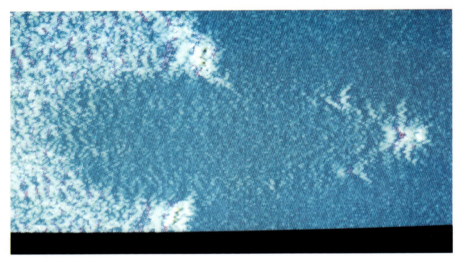

Fig. 2. High frequency-picture of a malignant melanoma. This tumor also has a very low echo density. Ultrasound imaging system: DUB 20, Taberna Pro Medicum, Lüneburg

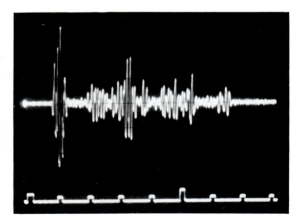

Fig. 3. The same tumor as in Fig. 1 scanned using A-mode. The echo pattern of the tumor is similar to that of fat

In our study of benign tumors, only those that macromorphologically resembled a malignant growth were of interest. We examined a total of 187 benign dermatological tumors, the differential diagnostic evaluation of which led to suspicion of a malignant melanoma. Among these tumors were cases of seborrheic keratosis, angioma, blue nevus, histiocytoma, acanthoma, granuloma pyogenicum as well as actinic and solar keratoses. Patients with seborrheic keratoses were the largest group in our series. Of 90 histologically diagnosed tumors of this type, macroscopic evaluation pointed to seborrheic keratosis in 61 patients; the correct diagnosis was made sonographically 72 times. These results reveal improved in vivo diagnostics of about 12% due to sonography (Fig. 4).

In the group of patients with angiogenic tumors, the combination of visual inspection, palpation, and sonographic examination led to a correct diagnosis in 83%, a diagnostic improvement of 15% (Fig. 5).

Sonography is an important tool in the differential diagnosis of a blue nevus. In such patients, our macroscopic diagnosis was correct in only 31%, whereas sonographic examination resulted in 77% correct diagnoses (Fig. 6).

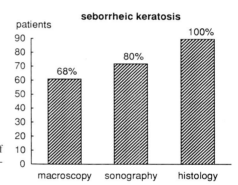

Fig. 4. Number of correct diagnoses of seborrheic keratosis; macroscopy and ultrasound compared to histology

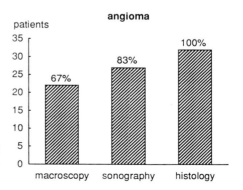

Fig. 5. The number of correct diagnoses of angioma; macroscopy and ultrasound compared to histology

The most difficult lesion to evaluate is the pigmented histiocytoma. Only 20% of the diagnoses obtained using ultrasound and a macroscopic examination were identical with histologic diagnoses (Fig. 7).

These results show that the specificity and sensitivity of sonographic examination can vary from tumor to tumor. Since reflectivity depends on the acoustic impedance at the border between two different tissues, it is possible for completely different tumors to yield similiar ultrasound images, if the tissues happen to show the same relationship between acoustic impedance levels (Fig. 8).

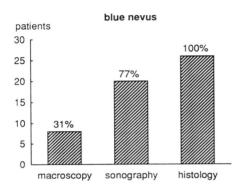

Fig. 6. The number of correct diagnoses of blue nevus; macroscopy and ultrasound compared to histology

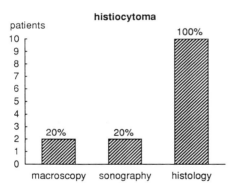

Fig. 7. The number of correct diagnoses of histiocytoma; macroscopy and ultrasound compared to histology

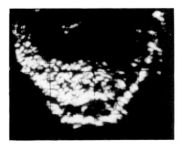

Fig. 8. B-mode scan of a seborrheic keratosis with little hyperkeratosis

The ultrasound signals from several different dermatological lesions will now be considered more closely. In seborrheic keratoses examined in B-mode, strong acoustic impedance at the surface is paired with strong to weak tumorous internal echo images (Fig. 9).

The one-dimensional A-mode also reveals stronger echo signals from the interior of the tumor than from the underlying fat. The tumor appears to be lodged on the otherwise unchanged and noninfiltrated corium. The histologic correlate to this ultrasound pattern is seen in hyperkeratosis and in pseudocysts in the cutaneous horny material such as are found in most seborrheic keratoses (Fig. 10).

Angiogenic tumors up to a certain size can be distinguished quite well from malignant melanomas. Their ultrasonic image is characterized by stronger internal echoes with oval to round low-echo areas that vary in size according to the type of tumor under consideration. In the case of angiokeratomas, stronger surface reflections with dorsal acoustic shadows are also frequently seen (Figs. 11, 12).

Granuloma pyogenicum may be confused with an ulcerated melanotic melanoma. However, it can be distinguished from a low-echo malignant melanoma on the basis of diffuse, strong, intratumorous echo signals (Fig. 13).

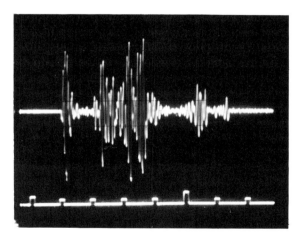

Fig. 9. The same tumor as in Fig. 8 scanned with an A-mode device

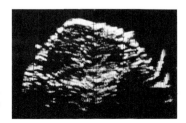

Fig. 10. B-mode scan of an angioma. Typical are round and oval echo-lucid areas combined with the echo-rich tumor

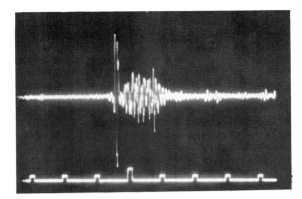

Fig. 11. The same angioma as in Fig. 10 but scanned with the A-mode device. The tumor also appears echo-rich

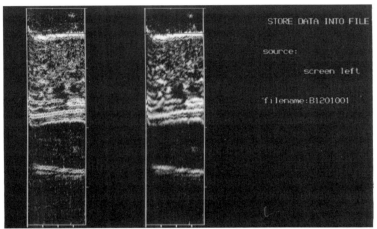

Fig. 12. B-mode scans of an angioma. Ultrasound imaging system: Technological University of Delft

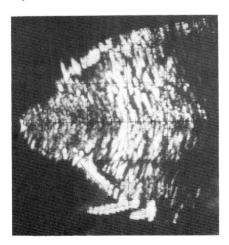

Fig. 13. B-mode scan of a pyogenic granuloma with strong intratumoral reflections

Sonographic Structure of Benign Skin Tumors

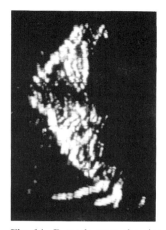

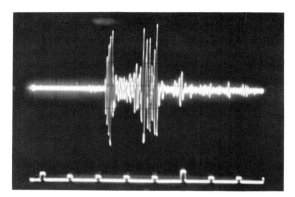

Fig. 14. B-mode scan showing a blue nevus, which ultrasonically appears echo-rich

Fig. 15. The same blue nevus as in Fig. 14 scanned in A-mode. both scanning modes always contribute to the sonographic diagnosis

It is also relatively easy to distinguish a blue nevus from a malignant melanoma using sonography. The histological basis of the rather echo-rich internal structure is provided by the multiple collagen bundles that permeate this tumor (Fig. 14, 15).

In addition to the accoustic patterns that are typical for the tumors mentioned, one also sees several ultrasound images that are not necessarily indicative of a certain tumor. Especially when more than two macromorphologic diagnoses are under discussion, an echo-rich or echo-poor finding often provides the only clinical criterion for exclusion.

We shall now present several atypical findings. The low-echo amplitudes in the A-image shown in Fig. 16 indicate a malignant melanoma; however, not

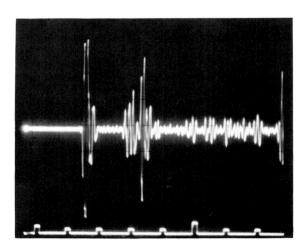

Fig. 16. A-mode scan of a blue nevus that looks like a malignant melanoma

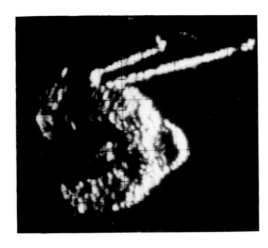

Fig. 17. B-mode scan of the same tumor as in Fig. 16. Often, intratumoral echoes can be detected at the lower part of a blue nevus

until we see the B-scan image do we begin to doubt this tentative diagnosis (Fig. 17). These images in fact show a blue nevus. This example makes clear that, in particular, one-dimensional images can be misleading if the entire tumor is not examined.

The faveolate structure of the ultrasound image shown in Fig. 18 has a surface echo which is reminiscent of a hyperkeratosis; it was diagnosed as an angioma. Histologically, however, it is a mucous cyst.

These examples of sonographically ambiguous lesions make it clear that ultrasound images cannot be properly evaluated unless they can be compared with macroscopic findings (Fig. 19).

The combination of macroscopic and sonographic examination of benign skin tumors was superior to macroscopic diagnosis alone by 17%. We expect that further experience and improved techniques will help us to achieve even better results (Fig. 19).

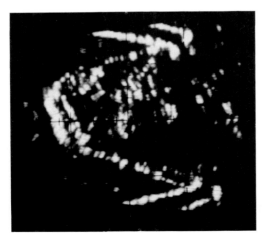

Fig. 18. B-mode scan of a cyst containing mucus. This tumor looks very similar to an angioma

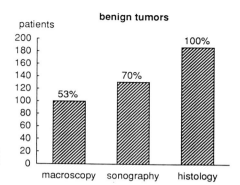

Fig. 19. The number of correct diagnoses of benign tumors: macromorphology and ultrasound compared to histology

At present, sonography is not yet capable of dermatologic tissue differentiation. Tissue structures such as the border between collagen fibre bundles and fatty tissue can be identified. Structural information of this type, however, does not often reveal characteristics specific to the individual dermatologic processes. The morphology of individual cells, mitoses, nuclear plasma relations, etc., cannot be revealed by sonography. It is therefore presently not possible to carry out direct comparisons with histologic diagnostic characteristics. In the future, definite criteria should be developed according to which skin tumors can be classified sonographically. For this purpose, methods must be developed that go beyond subjective visual evaluation of ultrasound images. Irion et al. [9, 10], Decker et al. [8], and Lizzi et al. [11] have made positive steps towards realizing these goals.

To conclude, we would like to emphasize that the future of dermatologic sonography essentially depends on whether this method can be used for in vivo tumor differentiation.

References

1. Alexander H, Miller DI (1979) Determining skin thickness with pulsed ultrasound. J Invest Dermatol 72: 17–19
2. Breitbart EW (1982) Experimentelle Grundlagen zur klinischen Anwendung der Dermatokryochirurgie. Habilitationsschrift, University of Hamburg
3. Breitbart EW, Hicks R (1991) Ultraschall in der Dermatologie. Mediaderm, (in press)
4. Breitbart EW, Rehpenning W (1983) Möglichkeiten und Grenzen der Ultraschalldiagnostik zur in vivo Bestimmung der Invasionstiefe des malignen Melanoms. Z Hautkr 61 (8): 957–987
5. Breitbart EW, Schaeg G, Jänner M, Rehpenning W, Carstensen A (1985) Kryochirurgie – Kontrollmöglichkeiten der Kryochirurgie. Anwendungen in der Dermatologie. Zbl. Haut Geschlechtskr 151 (1): 59–70
6. Breitbart EW, Müller CE, Hicks R, Vieluf D (1989) Neue Entwicklungen der Ultraschalldiagnostik in der Dermatologie. Aktuel Dermatol 15: 57–61
7. Cole GW, Handler SJ, Burnett K (1981) The ultrasonic evaluation of skin thickness in scleroderma. J Clin Ultrasound 9: 501–503

8. Decker D, Trier HG, Irion KM, Lepper RD, Reiner R (1980) Rechnergestützte Gewebsdifferentierung am Auge. Ultraschall 1 (4): 264–296
9. Irion KM (1987) Bestimmung der axialen Auflösung und der frequenzabhängigen Dämpfung von Ultraschallechogrammen unter Berücksichtigung der analytischen Signaldarstellung. Dissertation, University of Stuttgart
10. Irion KM, Faust U, Trier HG, Leppert RD (1984) Digitale Analyse von Ultraschall-B-Bildern zur Ermittlung des dynamischen Verhaltens der Augenrückwand. Ultraschall 5: 126–130
11. Lizzi F, Katz L, Louis LS, Coleman DJ (1979) Application of spectral analysis in medical ultrasonography
12. Maas-Irslinger R, Breitbart EW (1990) Vergleichende Untersuchung der systemischen und lokalen Nebenwirkungen von Prednicarbat und herkömmlichen, halogenierten Kortikosteroiden. Jahrbuch der Dermatologie 1989/90. Biermann Verlag
13. Tam CY, Stathäm B, Marks R, Payne P (1982) Skin thickness measurement by pulsed ultrasound: its reproducibility, validation and variability. Br J Dermatol 106: 657–667

Skin Tumours in High-Frequency Ultrasound

K. Hoffmann, S. el-Gammal, K. Winkler, J. Jung, K. Pistorius, and P. Altmeyer

Introduction

The differential diagnostic classification of skin tumours has always been a special challenge. When making a diagnosis, the dermatologist uses a number of fixed rules. His primary diagnosis is then based on a subjective assessment of the tumour. However, the literature contains little information about the degree of certainty with which dermatologists are able to classify tumours correctly on the basis of clinical examination alone. Grin [11] reports on 13 878 skin tumours examined by dermatologists. In 214 patients a clinical diagnosis of "malignant melanoma" was made and confirmed histologically. In 51 patients a malignant melanoma was not considered clinically but was clearly evident in the histological section. In 79 patients, on the other hand, the diagnosis of malignant melanoma made clinically was not confirmed histologically. These figures are equivalent to a diagnostic accuracy of about 64% and a sensitivity of 85.5%. Similar data have also been reported by other authors [16, 18]. In spite of this unsatisfactory situation no procedure has yet been developed which can assist the dermatologist in tumour diagnosis with a degree of reliability similar, for example, to electrocardiography used in internal medicine to study cardiac diseases [2].

We know today that the skin cancers as a group have the highest incidence of all malignancies in the western world. A procedure which supports the diagnosis of these diseases would thus be highly desirable. Such a procedure must fulfil two important criteria. Firstly, it must provide information quickly and simply. Secondly, on account of the large patient population, the method must be economical to use [2, 3].

In other fields of medicine the search for noninvasive diagnostic methods fulfilling the above postulates led to ultrasound several decades ago. In dermatology ultrasound initially meant a step forward in the search for metastases, particularly of malignant melanomas. The descriptions of ultrasound images of melanoma secondaries vary considerably: they can appear echo-rich or echo-poor, with or without a border zone. Furthermore, sometimes the dorsal echoes are intensified [21]. Figures 1 and 2 show a typical example of a subcutaneous, amelanotic metastasis of a malignant melanoma. The ultrasound scan (Fig. 2) was recorded with a modern 7.5-MHz scanner which has an axial resolution of 0.5 mm and a lateral

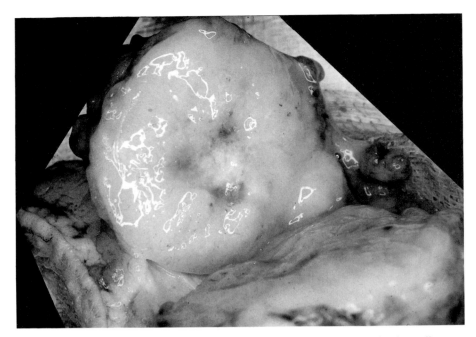

Fig. 1. Surgical specimen from a gluteally located subcutaneous metastasis of a malignant melanoma

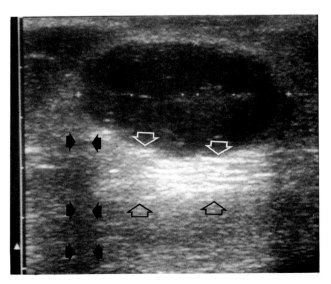

Fig. 2. Ultrasound scan of the metastasis shown in Fig. 1. The *black arrows* indicate a marginal shadow, the *open arrows* subtumoral intensification of echoes

resolution of 1 mm at a depth of 3 cm. In our experience with such scanners metastases measuring 5–6 mm upwards can be visualized. Their resolution is however too low to be suitable for skin tumour examination. A fundamental change was brought about by the "high-resolution" (high frequency) scanners which have recently become available, as these scanners are able for the first time to produce a differentiated two-dimensional image even of individual layers of the skin.

Ultrasound examination of skin tumours was made possible by the fundamental work of Alexander and Miller [1]. In those days the skin was examined mainly with A-mode scanners [1, 4, 5, 8, 9, 17, 25–27]. However, examination of skin tumours using A-scans is not unproblematic, as the investigator obtains only a one-dimensional amplitude image of the skin structure. As far as differentiation of histological structures is concerned it is very difficult to determine from where the individual reflections have arisen. In particular the echopoor hair follicles and finger-like projections of islets of adipose tissue into the corium such as are frequently found on the dorsal aspect of the thighs and the buttocks cannot be differentiated with certainty on the A-scan [15]. As almost all skin tumours always appear more or less echolucent on the ultrasound scan and the method was thus not of genuine differential diagnostic assistance some working groups began to experiment with scanners which we would today describe as low to middle frequency but which permitted B-scan imaging. The dilemma was that for many years although high-frequency A-scanners were available there were no scanners of equally high frequency which provided a sufficiently high-resolution B-scan [33]. On account of the inadequate resolution the malignancies examined could thus usually only be characterized as echo-lucent structures [20, 30–32]. Exact correlation of the sonograms with histological sections or typification of specific reflex patterns was not possible. It is interesting that up to this stage few histopathologists were concerned about the development of Sonography. However, when it was realized that ultrasound procedures could be also be a powerful tool for answering dermatological questions the first studies on the ultrasound characteristics of skin tumours were soon published [6, 12–14, 22, 23]. The discovery that ultrasound measurements of the thickness of skin tumours correlated well with the histometric measurements made high-frequency ultrasound interesting for routine diagnosis. Today there are already two high-frequency ultrasound scanners on the market with frequencies above 20 MHz with A- and B-scan imaging. To date our working group has examined about 7000 skin tumours with these systems. However, on account of the multitude of benign and malignant neoplasms, only a few tumours can be discussed here.

Method

For examination of skin tumours we use two high-frequency ultrasound scanners which operate at frequencies of at least 20 MHz and permit examination in A- and B-mode (DUB 20, Taberna pro medicum, Lüneburg, FRG and Dermascan C, Cortex Technology, Hadsund, Denmark). As comparable sonograms can only be obtained at constant scanner settings all examinations for tumour diagnosis are made with the same settings (amplification of echo amplitudes, colour scales). Only in this manner can we generate comparable ultrasound scans suitable not only for measurement of tumour thickness but also for differential diagnosis. We used a false colour coding where the light colours (white, blue) represent echo-rich regions and the dark colours (black, dark green) echo-poor areas.

Histological Correlation of the Ultrasound Finding

In order to be able to relate the reflex patterns to histological structures of the skin we developed a procedure which on the whole permits correlation between ultrasound scan and histological section [14]. Before the examination, the planes to be examined first by ultrasound and later by light microscopy are marked on that area of skin. When the planes of examination have been marked the region is photographed. One to two ultrasound scans are then made in each plane of examination and stored on hard disk or

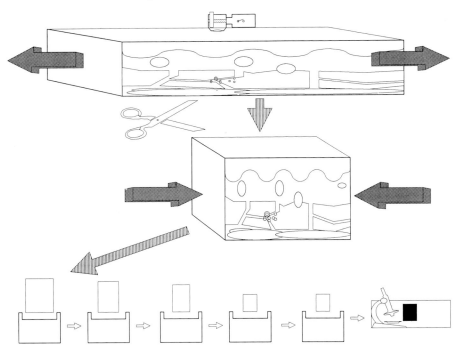

Fig. 3. Schematic representation of the artefacts occurring in thickness measurements. The ultrasound examination is performed with the tissue under physiological tension; this is followed by excision and preparation for histological examination

diskette. Postoperatively the biopsies are then cut to correspond to the planes of examination. Then, in order to determine the histological plane of section, the biopsies are placed on pieces of cardboard to which they adhere firmly and are then fixed in formalin together with the cardboard. Later serial sections are prepared for histological examination. To compare the ultrasound scan and histology, the histological section was examined at a 25-fold magnification and stained with haematoxylin and eosin.

It should be noted that the skin thickness measured in the histological sections are often greater than those measured in vivo [8, 34]. This is attributed to the fact that the biopsy is under less tension after excision (Fig. 3). Due to the work-up of the histological material with dehydration, deparaffinization and the associated shrinkage processes we would, however, expect a reduction in skin thickness. The increased thickness of the biopsy due to the diminished tension evidently more than compensates for the shrinkage artefacts resulting from the histological work-up. It should also be borne in mind that the histological section is 7 μm thick. On the other hand the scanner, in its lateral resolution, subsumes structures along a width of 200 μm to form a sectional image (Figs. 4, 5). We thus cannot expect an

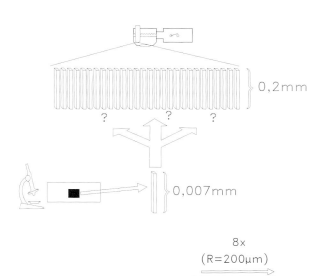

Fig. 4. A histological section is approx. 7 μm thick. The lateral resolution of the scanner is approx. 200 μm. Serial sections must therefore be examined if correlation is required

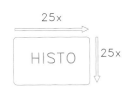

Fig. 5. The ultrasound scan on the monitor (DUB 20) has a lateral magnification × 8 (resolution 200 μm) and an axial magnification × 24 (resolution 80 μm). The image reproduction is therefore compressed. The light microscope magnification is × 25

absolute correlation between ultrasound scan and histological section with respect either to measurement of thickness or to the visualized structures [15].

Examination Procedure

In order to permit later follow-up studies a well-ordered archiving system for collection of images should be set up early. Our working group uses a data base developed for this purpose with the software "dBASE IV".

We recommend the following examination procedure:
- The patient should be well informed about the nature and procedure of the examination as his cooperation will be required.
- Standardized examination conditions must always be observed at all times. As far as possible no changes should be made in the settings for signal intensity, reflex amplitude amplification, etc.. If such changes are necessary a sonogram in the "normal setting" should always be made for reference.
- The examiner should become accustomed as soon as possible to a standardized posture for examining his patients. It is advisable for the patient to lie down during the examination. The skin to be examined should be under moderate tension. For better visualization of structures it may be necessary to examine the skin under various degrees of tension.
- To correlate between the sonogram and the histological section it is imperative to mark the planes to be examined.
- The examiner must on all account avoid exerting pressure on the skin with the transducer during the examinations.
- As far as possible a scan of the contralateral healthy skin should also be made.

Description of Routine Diagnostic Findings

Apart from the customary patient data and the date of examination the report of the ultrasound findings should cover the following fundamental points:

General section

- Clinical diagnosis of the structure to be examined by ultrasound
- Exact anatomical description of the area to be examined
- Account of how many planes of section were examined in which axes

Description of findings

- The reflex characteristics and the thicknesses of entry echo (epidermis), corium, subcutis and muscle fascia must be described in detail.

Table 1. "Bochum nomenclature"
General ultrasound phenomena in B-mode evaluation of skin tumours

Tumour area
echo-rich / same as surrounding tissue (scarcely distinguishable) / echo-poor
Margins
Sharp / indistinct
Border zones
echo-rich / echo-poor
Subtumoral echoes
Attenuation / intensification of dorsal echoes / dorsal acoustic shadow

Internal echoes in tumour area
Intensity (density)
echo-rich (strong) / like surroundings / echo-poor (weak)
Structure
Regular / irregular / ill-defined
Distribution
Homogeneous / inhomogeneous

- Any *structures of interest* (STOI) or *regions of interest* (ROI) should be described (whether pathological or physiological!).
- The location and size of ROI and STOI should be described.
- Evaluation of a tumour area (ROI) should include a description of the density, structure and distribution of the internal echoes. A description should also be given of the demarcation (sharp/indistinct), border zone (present/not present), any echo-lucent or echo-rich processes of the ROI and attenuation or intensification of echoes below the ROI (Table 1).

Evaluation

- The final evaluation of the findings should also take into consideration the clinical and gross morphological information. We must warn strictly against overrating the sonogram: physicians inexperienced in the method are often too quick to use it as differential diagnostic tool.

Malignant Skin Tumours

Malignant Melanoma

Case Study

Superficial spreading melanoma on the upper arm was examined in a 42-year-old woman (Fig. 6). The marked and numbered planes correspond to the areas examined.

The ultrasound scan (Fig. 7) shows an echo-rich entry echo with a homogeneous reflex pattern. Above the echo-poor area corresponding to

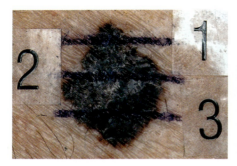

Fig. 6. Superficial spreading melanoma on the upper arm of a 45-year-old woman. The *lines* drawn correspond to the planes of examination for ultrasound and histology

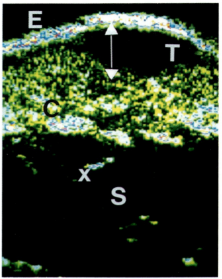

Fig. 7. Ultrasound scan of the tumour, corresponding to plane 2 in Fig. 6. E, entry echo; T, tumour; C, corium; S, subcutis; X, bands of connective tissue in the subcutis; *arrows*, sonometrically measured tumour thickness

the tumour it appears slightly more intense. The oval tumour region is echo-poor and contains no internal echoes. The basal demarcation is well defined, and the lateral demarcation cannot be identified with certainty as there is a narrow echo-poor band below the entry echo which was also found in the healthy skin surrounding the tumour. The corium is moderately echogenic and unremarkable. At the border with the subcutis, echo-rich islets can be distinguished which are separated from the remaining corium by slightly less echo-intense areas. In the completely echolucent subcutis there are only isolated echoes which correspond to bands of connective tissue. Histologically we found a superficial spreading melanoma, Clark level IV, with a tumour thickness of 1.2 mm. Below the tumour was a dense round-cell infiltrate.

When the sonogram is compared with the histological section (Fig. 8) it strikes us first that in the ultrasound scan the tumour region appears more spherical and compact than in the histological section. The reason for this is that the scanner (DUB 20) depicts the image on the monitor with a 24-fold axial magnification and an 8-fold lateral magnification, i.e. the image is compressed (Fig. 3). The histological section on the other hand was photographed at a 25-fold magnification. The depth of the echo-poor area was measured sonographically as 1.8 mm. Comparison of the sonogram and the histological section shows that this is explained by the presence of a subtumoral infiltrate which also appears echo-poor. The scanner is thus

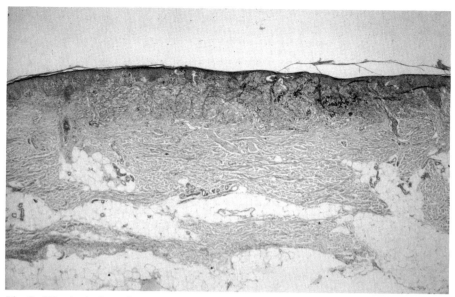

Fig. 8. Histological section corresponding to plane 2 in Fig. 6. On account of the proportionately correct reproduction the tumour appears more elongated than in the ultrasound scan (H & E, × 25)

unable to distinguish between tumour parenchyma and peritumoral infiltrate and depicts both as a single echo-poor area. This phenomenon has already been described and is also found in other tumours which are accompanied by peritumoral infiltration [12–14]. Comparison between histometry and computer-aided determination of tumour thickness in the sonogram, which we call „*sonometry*", shows the fundamental problem of distinguishing between the tumour itself and similarly echo-poor structures situated very close to the tumour, which also explains the differences in the measured results. In our experience this problem arises mainly in respect of hair follicles and bands of adipose tissue projecting finger-like into the corium. In the A-scan a distinction is only possible in exceptional cases. High-frequency B-mode scanners of the first generation were likewise not always capable of producing a topographically correct image of these structures. With the Dermascan C or the DUB 20, however, the experienced examiner can obtain good differentiation of follicles and bands of fatty tissue. In a comparison of the thickness measurements made in 83 malignant melanomas we found a high correlation between the histometrically and sonometrically determined thicknesses ($r = 0.89$). On average the sonometric thicknesses were 0.4 mm greater than the histometric measurements when the entire echo-poor area, including indistinct borders and classifiable projections (hair follicles) was measured. When the boundaries of the echo-poor areas were determined subjectively (exclusion of hair follicles and islands of fatty tissue) it was possible, without knowledge of the light microscopic findings, to improve the correlation to $r = 0.93$ and the average difference between the measurements to 0.15 mm. This demonstrates very clearly the importance of experience for the satisfactory use of ultrasound. An argument which can be held against this procedure, which we have termed "*weighted (sonometric) measurement*" of the ultrasound scan, is that precisely in the case of malignant melanomas agglomerates of tumour cells are sometimes found in the hair follicles. However, on account of its better correlation and the resulting greater clinical relevance, weighted measurement is currently the sonometric method of choice.

The information contained in the ultrasound scan is available in the form of digital information. It has been shown that, using three-dimensional reconstructions, it is possible to calculate the surface area and volume of the tumour [24]. These two parameters can then be used to calculate the "invasive tumour mass" as a new prognostic criterion. It is not yet clear what significance this criterion will have in future. But even today there is no doubt that ultrasound decisively improves the planning of surgery in the management of the malignant melanoma [10, 13, 23, 28].

Kaposi's sarcoma

Case Study

Initial Kaposi's sarcoma on the upper arm was investigated in a 28-year-old man with AIDS (Fig. 9). The ultrasound scan (Fig. 10) corresponds to the plane of section marked in black in Fig. 9. The area corresponding to the Kaposi's sarcoma is echo-poor with good basal demarcation and only poor lateral demarcation. The echo-poor area is filled with homogeneously distributed, strong internal echoes. The border between the corium and the subcutis is only indistinct. In the subcutis there are some bands of connective tissue. On account of the patient's cachectic general state the subcutis is rather thin so that the muscle fascia can be distinguished at the bottom of the picture. Because of the spread of the AIDS pandemy Kaposi's sarcoma has gained particular significance in dermatology. It is a multicentric tumour which is sometimes difficult to distinguish from other skin diseases on the basis of its macroscopic features alone. We have been able to examine about 75 Kaposi's sarcomas to date. We have not found a distinct or characteristic reflex pattern. Although the sarcomas were mostly less echogenic than the surrounding connective tissue the tumour margins were often not clearly identifiable; there were no border zones. Interestingly, the basal demarcation of the tumour areas was often sharper than the lateral demarcation, an unusual feature in tumours located in skin without actinic damage. The reflex characteristics of the tumours ranged from completely echolucent to strong internal reflexes such as in Fig. 7. The reflex pattern is not related to the tumour thickness, as in the case of the malignant melanoma or the naevus cell

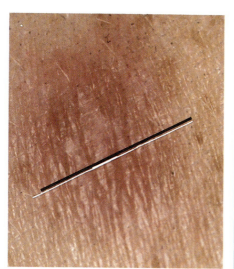 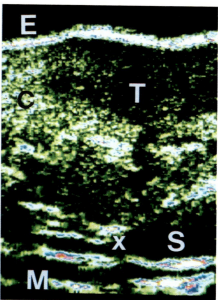

Fig. 9. Initial Kaposi's sarcoma on the upper arm of a 28-year-old patient. The *line* marks the selected plane of examination

Fig. 10. Ultrasound scan corresponding to the plane of examination marked in Fig. 6. *E*, entry echo; *T*, tumour; *C*, corium; *S*, subcutis; *X*, band of connective tissue; *M*, muscle fascia

naevus for example. We did, however, observe that longer-standing sarcoma nodules were more often echolucent than those which had developed more recently.

The early stages of Kaposi's sarcoma are often treated by laser. The condition for success of this treatment is that the sarcoma has not invaded further than the upper corium as the laser is not able to reach deeper portions of the sarcoma with certainty. Thus, high-frequency ultrasound is at present the only noninvasive diagnostic procedure which can provide us with relevant information to help decide whether to apply this tumour thickness-dependent method of treatment. But ultrasound can also be of use in monitoring the progress of treatment. When examining individual nodules under interferon treatment the response of the tumour to the interferon can be verified by monitoring the size of the echo-poor area.

Such treatment monitoring can of course also be employed for cutaneous metastases of other malignomas. An important field of application is, for example, the response of cutaneous metastases of malignant melanomas to chemotherapy or radiation treatment.

192   K. Hoffmann et al.

Benign Skin Tumours

In dermatological patients we often find benign skin tumours which frighten the patients and lead them to consult a doctor. As a rule these tumours can be diagnosed unequivocally by clinical examination so that ultrasound does not appear necessary. However, as already mentioned in the introduction, the dermatologist's supposed certainty is not always justified so that ultrasound examination can help to provide additional information.

Naevus Cell Naevi

Case Study

Papillomatous naevus cell naevus was seen on the abdomen of a 35-year-old man (Fig. 11). In the sonogram (Fig. 12) we see a slightly widened entry echo beneath which there is a roundish, echo-poor area with weak, inhomogenously distributed internal reflexes. The echo-poor area is sharply demarcated on all sides but has an indistant border. Below is the corium with echoes which are not typical of this region. This is followed by the echo-poor subcutis and then by the muscle fascia. The corresponding histological section (Figs. 13, 14) shows a papillomatous naevus cell naevus with embedded horny cyst. The rete ridges are elongated and ramified. Between the rete ridges we find normal corium, naevus cell nests and tumour stroma.

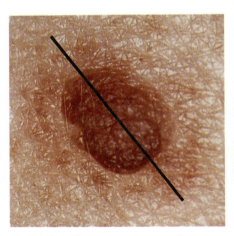

Fig. 11. Papillomatous naevus cell naevus on the back of a 45-year-old woman. The *line* shows the plane of scan

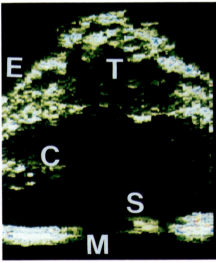

Fig. 12. Ultrasound scan corresponding to the plane of examination shown in Fig. 11. *E*, entry echo; *T*, tumour; *C*, corium; *S*, subcutis; *M*, muscle fascia

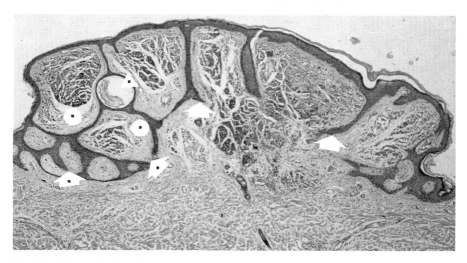

Fig. 13. Histological section corresponding to the plane of examination shown in Fig. 11. The rete ridges are elongated and ramified (bridging phenomena; *arrows*. In between are naevus cell nests, stroma and corial connective tissue, *circle*. On *top left* a horny cyst (*arrow head*) is seen (H&E × 25)

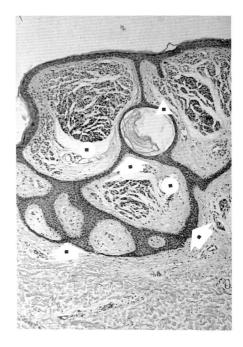

Fig. 14. Detail from Fig. 13 (H&E × 50)

The broadened entry echo results from a large impedance jump from water to epidermis and the subsequent impedance jump when the signal leaves the epidermis and strikes the underlying naevus cell nests and tumour stroma. The signal thus passes through several interfaces one after the other, each of which scatters part of the signal. The most likely explanation for the internal echoes often found in the naevi is that they are produced by the highly echogenic normal connective tissue lying between the rete ridges and the naevus cell nests. Ramified rete ridges lying at 90° to the signal could also produce echoes. The closely packed corium on the back leads to increased absorption of sound. The result is a relatively echo-poor corium in the sonogram.

In some naevi the histological examination showed horny cysts which gave rise to internal reflexes. A surprising finding was that, in contrast to the corial connective tissue, the naevus stroma was echo-poor. The scanner is not able to distinguish between naevus cells (nestss) and stroma – the sonogram shows both as a single echo-poor area. This phenomenon is found not only in naevus cell naevi but also in basal cell carcinomas. Papillomatous naevus cell naevi in particular often lead to an attenuation of dorsal echoes which can be explained by the scattering and absorption of the signal within the tumour. This phenomenon can, however, only be seen in a highly echogenic, thin corium such as that of the forearm. It is not usually identifiable in the echo-poor corium of the back. Other working groups also found similar reflex behaviour in naevus cell naevi [6, 23]. In our opinion differentiation between histologically remarkable "dysplastic" naevi and "harmless" naevi, which has been considered possible elsewhere [6], is not possible with the currently available scanners. After evaluation of the ultrasound scans of 700 naevus cell naevi, we can specify the following characteristics: all naevi with the exception of naevoid lentigo appear as an echo-poor area and the large majority of naevi contain weak, inhomogeneously distributed internal reflexes within the echo-poor, usually sharply demarcated areas. No other particular sonographic features were found.

Seborrhoeic Keratosis

Practically pathognomonic acoustic characteristics of seborrhoeic keratosis on high-frequency ultrasound were described very early [4, 5, 23]. They do not apply to all forms of seborrhoeic keratosis. We were only able to confirm a typical pattern for the hyperkeratotic type. As a rule this type shows massive attenuation of dorsal echoes, sometimes even a complete acoustic shadow. Such a pathognomonic acoustic pattern is not always found in purely acanthotic or adenoid types. The reflex characteristics are not influenced by the pigmentation of the seborrhoeic keratosis but are by the frequently found horny cysts.

Figure 15 exhibits a pigmented seborrhoeic keratosis on the back of a 55-year-old man. The ultrasound scan (Fig. 16) shows the typical picture of

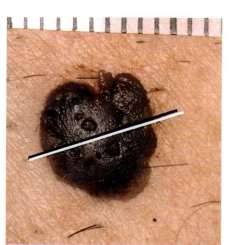 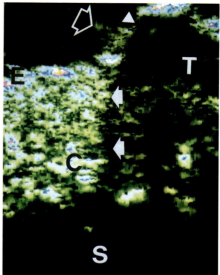

Fig. 15. Pigmented seborrhoeic keratosis on the back of a 55-year-old man. The *line* marks the chosen plane of examination

Fig. 16. Ultrasound scan corresponding to the plane of examination shown in Fig. 12. *E*, entry echo; *T*, tumour; *C*, corium; *S*, subcutis; *arrowhead*, lateral scattering of signal; *open arrow*, pagoda echoes; *white arrows*, lateral boundaries of the dorsal acoustic shadow

a seborrhoeic keratosis. The entry echo is widened and partly interrupted. These interruptions arise when the signal is scattered laterally at the obliquely rising edges of the tumour. The tumour edges show a reflex pattern which resembles the shape of a Chinese pagoda (*"pagoda echo"*). The echo-poor tumour area contains only few marginally situated, weak internal echoes. The corium is under slight tension on account of the patient's posture during the examination and is thus slightly more echogenic than we would otherwise expect in this region. On account of the increased reflectivity there is a clear demarcation between the corium and the subcutis, which appears black. Below the echo-poor tumour area the dorsal echoes are attenuated. As in all cases of dorsal attenuation or acoustic shadows the lateral demarcation is sharp. The histological section (Fig. 17) can be correlated well with the ultrasound image. The acanthosis is echolucent. The marginally located internal echoes in the tumour area correspond to the readily distinguishable horny cysts in the histological section. Together with the hyperkeratosis and acanthosis, they are also responsible for the scattering and absorption of the acoustic signal which then appears as acoustic shadow. The attenuation of echoes beneath a papillomatous naevus cell naevus is generally weaker. In borderline cases evaluation of the internal echoes and the entry echoes can help distinguish between the reflex patterns.

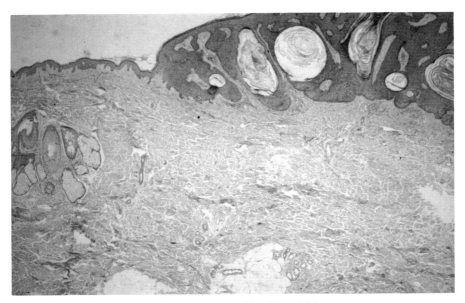

Fig. 17. Histological section corresponding to Fig. 13 and 14

Sometimes patients present with seborrhoeic keratosis which is irritated, rubbed smooth, or even bleeding to have skin cancer ruled out. These lesions usually display the reflex characteristics described in the above case and can thus be distinguished clearly from other skin tumours. In such cases high-frequency ultrasound can provide a reliable further information for diagnosis.

Histiocytomas

As a rule the experienced dermatologist has no trouble distinguishing histiocytomas from other skin tumours. The differential diagnosis becomes more difficult, however, when a new histiocytoma develops in a patient with a malignant melanoma as it must then be distinguished from an amelanotic metastasis. Histiocytomas do not display a uniform reflex pattern either. In these tumours, however, the differences lie in the nature and distribution of the internal echoes rather than the alternatives echo-rich/echo-poor. Histiocytomas particularly often contain marginally located internal echoes within an otherwise echo-poor tumour area. In the majority of cases the boundary between the tumour area and the surrounding tissue can be identified. Some histiocytomas, however, display homogeneously distributed strong internal reflexes similar to the surrounding corium so that exact determination of the lateral boundaries is difficult.

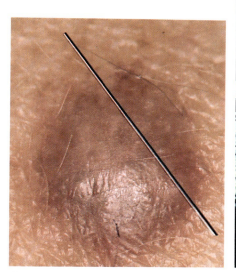 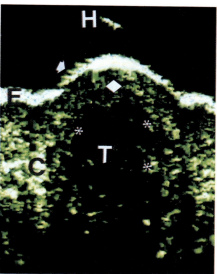

Fig. 18. Histiocytoma on the forearm of a 74-year-old woman. The *line* marks the chosen plane of examination

Fig. 19. Ultrasound scan corresponding to the plane of examination shown in Fig. 18. *E*, entry echo; *C*, corium; *T*, tumour; *H*, hair; *diamond*, band with reflectivity similar to that of corium (*asterisk*, inhomogenously distributed, marginally located internal echoes)

A retikulohistiocytoma measuring 1.5 × 1.8 cm on the forearm was examined in a 74-year-old woman (Fig. 18). The patient had had a malignant melanoma removed 2 years previously (tumour thickness according to Breslow 4.9 mm). In the ultrasound scan (Fig. 19) we see above the entry echo an oblique reflex which corresponds to a hair above the tumour. The entry echo is only slightly widened. At the left ascending edge there are signs of a pagoda echo. The reflex pattern of the corium is rather weak, corresponding to the low skin tension. Below the entry echo is a narrow band of strong, homogeneously distributed reflexes. Below this band, indistinctly demarcated from it, we see an echo-poor area extending as far as the subcutis. The lateral demarcation is indistinct, and the basal demarcation cannot be identified. The echo-poor area contains marginally situated strong internal reflexes. In contrast to this, the amelanotic secondaries of a malignant melanoma which are to be considered in the differential diagnosis are usually sharply demarcated and contain no internal reflexes.

The histological section (Fig. 20) confirms the clinical and ultrasound diagnosis of a "histiocytoma". The retikulohistiocytoma is separated from the epidermis by a narrow band of unchanged connective tissue which corresponds to the echo-rich band below the entry echo in the ultrasound image.

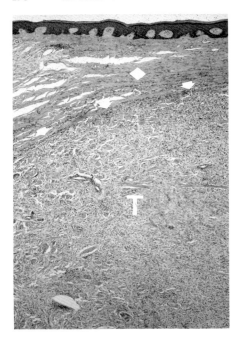

Fig. 20. Histological section corresponding to Figs. 15 and 16. *Diamond*, round-cell infiltration of corium; *arrows*, tumour boundaries; *T*, tumour

Other Tumours

Angiomas do not show a uniform reflex pattern. In most cases the angioma appears echo-poor to echolucent. Below thrombosed angiomas we sometimes find streaky acoustic attenuation (with a beginning in the tumour area) extending far into the subtumoral corium. We have not yet seen this acoustic pattern in any other tumour. Unfortunately this phenomenon cannot be considered pathognomonic as it is only found in 10%–20% of the tumours examined.

Visualization of calcification in skin tumours is easy. The calcifications frequently appearing as hyperreflective spots on the ultrasound scan are a useful aid to topographic orientation when comparing ultrasound and histological sections. However, if the entire tumour is complete calcified, there is a complete acoustic shadow and internal echoes are no longer visible, so that a diagnostic is only possible in conjunction with the findings made on palpation. Fluid-filled cysts also have a pathognomonic acoustic appearance. The fluid causes considerably less deceleration of the signal than does the surrounding corium so that the corium beneath the cyst appears more echogenic than the surroundings. In these cases we speak of intensification of dorsal echoes. As a result of the greater velocity of sound in the fluid the echoes produced by the corium beneath the cyst return to the transducer earlier. This leads to a "shortening phenomenon" on the B-scan image, the corium below the cyst appearing closer to the skin surface than is in fact the case in vivo. With sebum-filled cysts we have a completely different situation. Here the spectrum of reflex patterns ranges from echolucent to hyperreflective. The sharply defined edges permit us sometimes to distinguish these cysts from other tumours.

Lipomas are often completely echolucent. Apart from differential diagnostic purposes, ultrasound examination is helpful to determine whether a lipoma is encapsulated, as encapsulated lipomas can be managed simply by enucleation via a simple skin incision.

Summary

High-frequency ultrasound is still a very new method which will no doubt undergo very rapid further development. Its principal advantage is that it is a noninvasive procedure which can provide the examiner with valuable information on a tumour. As we still have too little experience with the currently available scanners, which in addition require modification in some points, some important problems such as reliable differential diagnosis have not yet been solved. Scanners with higher frequencies (50–150 MHz) or acoustic microscopes (1–2 GHz) operating in vitro can be expected to provide additional information [7, 19, 35]. Magnetic resonance tomographs designed specially for the skin also appear promising [29]. It can be expected that self-learning, "intelligent" computer programs will soon be available for image evaluation. There is, however, no doubt that high-frequency ultrasound is a useful procedure for measurement of tumour thickness/width and for monitoring the progress of treatment. In these questions the method is at present unmatched so that, at least in hospitals working in the field of oncology its use must be strongly recommended.

References

1. Alexander H, Miller DL (1979) Determining skin thickness with pulsed ultrasound. J Invest Dermatol 72: 17–19
2. Altmeyer P (1989) Dermatologische Ultraschalldiagnostik – gegenwärtiger Stand und Perspektiven. Z Hautkr 64: 727–728 (editorial)
3. Altmeyer P, Hoffmann K, el-Gammal S (1990) Sonographie der Haut. Münch Med Wochenschr 132 (18): 14–22
4. Breitbart EW, Hicks R, Rehpennig W (1985) Möglichkeiten der Ultraschalldiagnostik in der Dermatologie. Z Hautkr 61: 522–526
5. Breitbart EW, Rehpennig W (1983) Möglichkeiten und Grenzen der Ultraschalldiagnostik zur in vivo Bestimmung der Invasionstiefe des malignen Melanoms. Z Hautkr 58: 975–987
6. Breitbart EW, Müller CH, Hicks R, Vieluf D (1989) Neue Entwicklungen der Ultraschalldiagnostik in der Dermatologie. Aktuel Dermatol 15: 57–61
7. Buhles N, Altmeyer P (1988) Ultraschallmikroskopie an Hautschnitten. Z Hautkr 64: 926–934

8. Dines KA, Sheets PW, Brink JA, Hanke CW, Condra KA, Clendenon JL, Goss SA, Smith JS, Franklin TD (1984) High frequency ultrasonic imaging of skin: experimental results. Ultrason Imaging 6: 408–434
9. Fornage DW, Deshaynes JL (1986) Ultrasound of normal skin. J Clin Ultrasound 14: 619–622
10. Gassenmeier G, Kiesewetter F, Schell H, Zinner M (1990) Wertigkeit der hochauflösenden Sonographie für die Bestimmung des vertikalen Tumordurchmessers beim malignen Melanom der Haut. Hautarzt 41: 360–364
11. Grin CM, Kopf AW, Welkovich B, Bart RS, Levenstein MJ (1990) Accuracy in the clinical diagnosis of malignant melanoma. Arch Dermatol 126: 763–766
12. Hoffmann K, el-Gammal S, Altmeyer P (1989) 20 MHz B-scan Sonographie an Händen und Füßen. In: Altmeyer P et al. (eds) Handsymposium: Dermatologische Erkrankungen der Hände und Füße. Edition Roche, Basel, pp 285–300
13. Hoffmann K, el-Gammal S, Matthes U, Altmeyer P (1989) 20 MHz Sonographie der Haut in der präoperativen Diagnostik. Z Hautkr 64: 851–858
14. Hoffmann K, Stücker M, el-Gammal S, Altmeyer P (1990) Digitale 20-MHz-Sonographie des Basalioms im b-scan. Hautarzt 41: 333–339
15. Hoffmann K, el-Gammal S, Altmeyer P (1990) Ultraschall in der Dermatologie. Hautarzt 41: W7–W15
16. Hoffmann K, Matthes U, Stücker M, Segerling M, Altmeyer P (1990) "Prevention week." in Bochum 1989 for malignant melanoma information. Öff Gesundheitswes 52: 9–13
17. Kirsch JM, Hanson ME, Gibson JR (1984) The determination of skin-thickness using conventional ultrasound equipment. Clin Exp Dermatol 9: 280–285
18. Koh HK, Lew RA, Prout MN (1989) Sreening for melanoma/skin cancer: theoretical and practical considerations. J Am Acad Dermatol 20: 159–172
19. Kolosov OV, Levin VM, Myev RG, Senjushkina TA (1987) The use of acoustic microscopy for biological tissue charakterization Ultrasound Med Biol 13: 477–483
20. Kraus W, Nake-Elias A, Schramm P (1985) Diagnostische Fortschritte bei malignen Melanomen durch die hochauflösende Real-time-Sonographie. Hautarzt 36: 386–392
21. Miyauchi S, Murikami S, Miki Y (1988) Echographic studies of superficial lymphadenopathies. J Dermatol 15: 263–267
22. Miyauchi S, Tada M, Miki Y (1983) Echographic evaluation of nodular lesions of the skin. J Dermatol 10: 221–227
23. Murikami S, Miki Y (1989) Human skin histology using high-resolution echography. J Clin Ultrasound 17: 77–82
24. Pawlak F, Hoffmann K, el-Gammal S, Altmeyer P (1990) Three-dimensional reconstruction of ultrasonic images of the skin. Zentralbl Hautkr 157: 330
25. Payne PA (1983) Non-invasive skin measurement by ultrasound. RNM Images 13: 24–26
26. Payne PA (1985) Medical and industrial applications of high resolution ultrasound. J Phys E Sci Instrum 18: 465–473
27. Price R, Jones TB, Goddard J Jr, James AE (1980) Basic concepts of ultrasonic tissue characterization. Radiol Clin North Am 18: 21–30
28. Querleux B, Léveque JL, de Rigal J (1988) In vivo cross-sectional ultrasonic imaging of human skin. Dermatologica 177: 332–337
29. Querleux B, Yassine MM, Darasse L, Saint Jalmes, Sauzade M, Leveque JL (1988) Magnetic resonance imaging of the skin: a comparison with the ultrasonic technique. Bioeng Skin 4: 1–14
30. Rukavina B, Mohar N (1979) An approach of ultrasound diagnostic techniques of the skin and subcutaneous tissue. Dermatologica 158: 81–92
31. Schwaighofer B, Pohl-Markl H, Frühwald F, Stiglbauer R, Kokoschka EM (1987) Der diagnostische Stellenwert des Ultraschalls beim malignen Melanom. Fortschr Röntgenstr 146: 409–411

32. Strasser W, Vanscheidt W, Hagedorn M, Wokalek H (1986) B-scan Ultraschall in der Dermatologie. Fortschr Med 25: 495–498
33. Tan CY, Marks R, Payne P (1981) Comparison of xeroradiographic and ultrasound detection of corticosteroid induced dermal thinning. J Invest Dermatol 76: 126–128
34. Tan CY, Statham B, Marks R, Payne PA (1982) Skin thickness measurement by pulsed ultrasound: its reproducibility, validation and variability. Br J Dermatol 106: 657–667
35. Tanaka M (1985) The development and medical application of a ultrasonic microscope. Nippon Rinsh 43: 2713

Assets and Limitations of High-Frequency Ultrasound in the Analysis of Basal Cell and Squamous Cell Carcinomas

D. VIELUF and H. C. KORTING

Noninvasive assessment of skin tumors has mainly been based on history, clinical analysis, and, rarely, surface microscopy, which assess only two dimensions of the lesion. To get an idea of the third dimension surgical removal of the lesion and histologic examination are needed. However, particularly in older patients, this is often not considered to be the treatment of choice. Thus, there clearly is a need for other noninvasive procedures of analysis. Ultrasound imaging might fill the gap [3, 5, 6, 10, 12], as it has already proven helpful in the analysis of tumors of inner organs. Detailed ultrasound analysis of skin lesions nowadays seems feasable due to the advent of devices with a frequency of up to 20 MHz [4, 13], a frequency markedly higher than the one considered ideal for the analysis of internal organs, for physical reasons. With the analysis of skin tumors it seems especially rewarding if a device is able to provide both A-mode and B-mode images. One of these new devices is the DUB 20 system manufactured by Taberna Pro Medicum, Lüneburg. This system has been described in more technical detail elsewhere [4].

In dermatological oncology it is important to determine the actual thickness and spread of the tumor. Pertinent information would not only help to optimize surgical treatment with respect to safety margins, but also radiotherapy, cryotherapy and laser therapy. In this context one could imagine that B-mode images would be useful in finding the best site to assess the extension of a lesion using A-mode. Additionally, in certain cases, ultrasound analysis of skin tumors might be helpful in differential diagnosis and in the differentiation of the tumor mass and inflammatory border. Practical clinical use, however, has to be based on sufficient knowledge of the limitations of this method which may be, e.g., due to topography or to interference by other structures of the skin close to the lesion, leading to amplitudes which might be misinterpreted [4, 13].

We have been using the DUB 20 system for about 1 year. In order to define the potential role of ultrasound imaging in the dermatologic care of basal cell and squamous cell carcinomas the following assessments had to be made: Potential assets and limitations of ultrasound imaging in the clinical care of basal cell carcinomas and squamous cell carcinomas
1. Thickness and lateral extension of the tumor
2. Type of tumor
3. Limitations due to localization, irregular surface, and hyperkeratosis

During a period of 6 months we clinically evaluated skin tumors suspected of being either basal cell or squamous cell carcinomas. In all cases ultrasound analysis was compared with histologic examination of the biopsies. The following discussion is based on an analysis of a total of about 30 tumors.

In some patients tumor thickness could be unambiguously determined, i.e., a clear-cut region lacking any echo or showing a more or less regular pattern of discrete echos that could be differentiated from surrounding tissue showing the well-known typical aspects of corium and/or subcutis (Fig. 1). In the A-mode the lower border of the lesion was characterized by a high amplitude signal (Fig. 2). Such a clear-cut differentiation between tumorous and nontumorous skin tissue could be made in about 50% of all basal cell carcinomas, but only in a minority of squamous cell carcinomas. If the lower border of the lesion did not differ clearly from the surroundings, it seemed helpful to try to determine a "maximum tumor thickness", i.e., the distance between the skin surface and the uppermost point within the skin where a definitely normal skin structure could be found sonographically. Using this modified value, the tumor thickness could be determined in about an additional 25% of patients with basal cell carcinoma. The corresponding figure for patients with squamous cell carcinomas reached about 30%. Figure 3 shows the typical B-mode image of a basal cell carcinoma lacking a clear-cut lower border, so that maximum tumor thickness can be not determined.

There are several reasons why only a maximum tumor thickness, as defined above, and not the actual tumor thickness can be assessed. Sometimes it is due to the type of basal cell carcinoma, as characterized by histologic features. In particular, multicentric superficial and sclerodermiform basal cell carcinomas are difficult to assess. Moreover, a marked inflammatory reaction may cause problems in differentiation. A major obstacle in connection with the assessment of skin tumor thickness is superficial hyperkeratosis. This is particularly true for squamous cell carcinomas, but the problem is also seen with basal cell carcinomas. As hyperkeratosis more or less completely reflects the ultrasound waves, the area beneath it cannot be judged. This is demonstrated in Fig. 4, which shows a typical squamous cell carcinoma. A major aim in the development of the DUB 20 system was to achieve high resolution of the upper parts of the skin. In general, the lower parts are difficult to analyze; hence, tumors thicker than 18 mm cannot be exactly assessed.

Determination of the lateral borders of the tumor seems to be possible; however, with the DUB 20 system, a lot of time is required to assess the tumor extension, since a series of various scans must be analyzed. Moreover, the same problems addressed in connection with determination of tumor thickness also apply to determination of the lateral extension of the tumor.

Ultrasound analysis, especially using the B-mode in connection with the A-mode, may sometimes be helpful in differentiating skin tumors [1, 4]. For example, a pigmented basal cell carcinoma that clinically resembles a malignant melanoma is highly echogenic in a more or less homogeneous

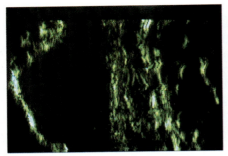

Fig. 1. B-mode image of a basal cell carcinoma with a well-defined lower border

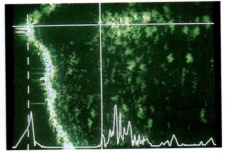

Fig. 2. A-mode image of a basal cell carcinoma. High amplitude signal represents the border between lesioned and underlying normal skin

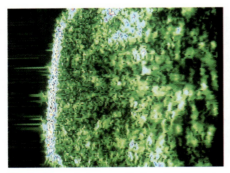

Fig. 3. B-mode image of a basal cell carcinoma lacking a well-defined lower border not allowing the determination of maximum tumor thickness

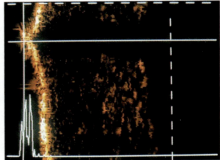

Fig. 4. B-mode image of a squamous cell carcinoma with marked hyperkeratosis leading to complete reflection of the ultrasound beam

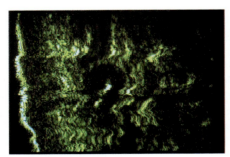

Fig. 5. B-mode image of a basal cell carcinoma on the right cheek characterized by an echo-poor zone

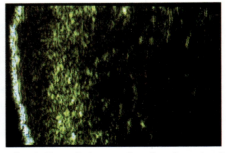

Fig. 6. B-mode image of a solar elastosis of the left cheek resembling the image of the basal cell carcinoma shown in Fig. 5

pattern, while a malignant melanoma rather tends to be more or less echo-free [1, 2, 4, 8, 9, 11, 12]. In most cases, however, a clear-cut differentiation of basal cell carcinoma from squamous cell carcinoma or other types of skin tumors is difficult, if possible at all. In rare cases, it can even be impossible to differentiate between a tumorous and nontumorous skin lesion by ultrasound. Figures 5 and 6 show B-mode images of a basal cell carcinoma and of aged skin in a symmetric location, i.e., on the right and left cheek. In this particular example, the similarity between aged skin and a basal cell carcinoma is due to the echo pattern of elastotic tissue. Furthermore, since edema, as judged by ultrasound, more or less resembles elastosis, it can be difficult to differentiate between the two.

For several reasons, skin tumors localized in certain parts of the body are difficult to analyze with the DUB 20. This obviously applies to regions where the skin to be analyzed is occluded by other structures, in particular, by nail plates. This is partially due to the configuration of the applicator of the DUB 20 system, which makes a plane surface obligatory for accurate analysis. Thus, those parts of the human body which are not planar are difficult to assess. Unfortunately, this is quite often the case when it comes to the analysis of skin tumors, especially tumors localized on the lateral nose, the inner angle of the eye, on the upper and/or lower eye lid, on the jaw close to the ramus mandibulae, on the ear, and also on parts of the capillitium. For similar technical reasons, tumors with an irregular surface, such as mainly found in exophytic tumors or lesions characterized by hyperkeratosis, are also problematic to access. Here too it might be difficult to attach the applicator firmly to the skin.

In spite of the numerous difficulties and limitations of the analysis of tumorous skin lesions of the basal cell or squamous cell type by ultrasound, this noninvasive in vivo method completes the conventional diagnostic approach [1, 3–5, 10]. Ultrasound analysis can be especially helpful when planning therapeutic procedures in topographical terms. So far, exposure area and half-value thickness of X-ray therapy could only be determined based on estimation. Ultrasound analysis that gives clear-cut data concerning the extension of the tumor may help to reduce or extend both the intensity and the area of X-ray application, leading to reduced harm to collateral tissues; thus the therapeutic safety can be increased. The same, in fact, is true for other, increasingly used, nonsurgical, therapeutic procedures, such as cryotherapy and laser therapy [4, 7, 13].

In general, the results of ultrasound analysis of skin tumors depend on the experience of the investigator. Furthermore, future development of ultrasound devices will add to the value of using ultrasound in dermatologic oncology. In this connection, one has to develop smaller applicators and devices, with the possibility of systematic scanning of surfaces and increased depth of analysis. In addition, use of a gel as contact medium instead of water might be helpful in the analysis of uneven surfaces.

References

1. Al-Aboosi M, Edwards C, Marks R (1987) Diagnosis and assessment of small skin tumors using pulsed A-scan ultrasound. J Invest Dermatol 89: 334–335
2. Breitbart EW, Rehpenning W (1983) Möglichkeiten und Grenzen der Ultraschalldiagnostik zur in vivo Bestimmung der Invasionstiefe des malignen Melanoms. Z Hautkr 58: 975–987
3. Breitbart EW, Hicks R, Rehpenning W (1986) Möglichkeiten der Ultraschalldiagnostik in der Dermatologie. Z Hautkr 61: 522–526
4. Breitbart EW, Müller CE, Hicks R, Vieluf D (1989) Neue Entwicklungen der Ultraschalldiagnostik in der Dermatologie. Aktuel Dermatol 15: 57–61
5. Brenner S, Ophir J, Weinraub Z (1984) Thickness of basal cell epithelioma measured preoperatively by ultrasonography. Arch Dermatol 120: 252–253
6. Hughes BR, Black D, Srivastava A, Dalziel K, Marks T (1987) Comparison of techniques for the non-invasive assessment of skin tumours. Clin Exp Dermatol 12: 108–111
7. Kimmig W, Kröger HJ, Hicks R, Breitbart EW (1987) Ultraschall-kontrollierte Nd-YAG-Lasertherapie von Viruspapillomen. Aktuel Dermatol 13: 231–233
8. Kraus W, Schramm P, Hoede N (1983) First experiences with a high-resolution ultrasonic scanner in the diagnosis of malignant melanomas. Arch Dermatol Res 275: 235–238
9. Kraus W, Nake-Elias A, Schramm P (1985) Diagnostische Fortschritte bei malignen Melanomen durch die hochauflösende Real-Time-Sonographie. Hautarzt 36: 386–392
10. Miyauchi S, Tada U, Miki Y (1983) Echography evaluation of nodular lesions of the skin. J Dermatol 10: 221–227
11. Schweigkofer B, Pohl-Marke H, Frühwold F, Stiglbauer R, Kokoschka EM (1987) Der diagnostische Stellenwert des Ultraschalls beim malignen Melanom. Fortschr Rontgenther 146: 409–411
12. Shafir R, Itzehak Y, Heyman Z, Azizi B, Tsur H, Hiss J (1984) Preoperative ultrasonic measurement of the thickness of cutaneous malignant melanoma. J Ultrasound Med 3: 205–208
13. Vieluf D, Breitbart EW, Hicks R (1988) Ultraschalldiagnostik maligner Tumoren der Haut. Zentralbl Hautkr 154: 659

The Acoustic Characteristics of the Basal Cell Carcinoma in 20-MHz Ultrasonography

M. STÜCKER, K. HOFFMANN, S. EL-GAMMAL, and P. ALTMEYER

Introduction

The basal cell carcinoma is the most common skin tumour in the central European population [12]. In Japan its incidence has increased 1.8-fold within the past 30 years [11]. The standardised incidence rate for the basal cell carcinoma in Australia is 657/100000 (6). On account of this considerable worldwide significance it is important that treatment of this tumour be optimised. It would be desirable if preoperative information on the spread, depth and malignancy status of the tumour were as detailed as possible. Ultrasound, as a non-invasive, indefinitely repeatable procedure already established in many fields of medicine, appears suitable to provide such information. However, ultrasound scanners with resolutions sufficiently high for imaging of the skin have only recently become available [2, 15]. The possibilities of ultrasound measurement of skin thickness have already been well studied [17] and there have been individual case reports on the morphology of the basal cell carcinoma in ultrasound scans [3, 5, 8, 13]. In this study the ultrasound properties of the basal cell carcinoma were examined systematically in a larger population.

Patients and Methods

Patients

We studied the acoustic behaviour of 75 basal cell carcinomas of various clinical and histological types (Figs. 1, 2). Of these 36 were in female patients and 39 in male patients. The patients were between 37 and 88 years of age, with a mean age of 70 years.

Equipment and Methods

We performed the examinations with the digital 20-MHz B-mode ultrasound scanner DUB 20 (Taberna pro Medicum, Lüneburg, FRG). Each basal cell carcinoma was examined in 4 to 12 planes. In the interpretation of the

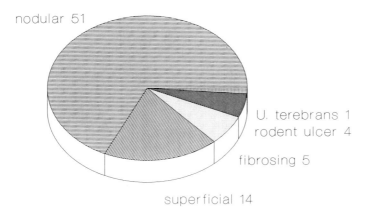

Fig. 1. Material studied: clinical types of basal cell carcinoma ($n = 75$)

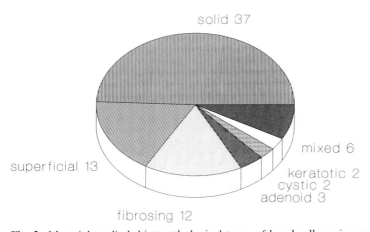

Fig. 2. Material studied: histopathological types of basal cell carcinoma ($n = 75$)

ultrasound images one ultrasound section per tumour corresponded exactly to the histological plane of section (method see [9]). The sonograms were first described individually. Then the ultrasound phenomena were coded and evaluated in a second computer system. In each case the ultrasound image corresponding to the histological preparation and the respective perpendicular image were used. The following sonographic properties were evaluated: echogenicity of the tumour in the false colour representation and in densitometry; structure and distribution of the internal echoes; shape, borders and demarcation of the tumour; dorsal (subtumoral) acoustic behaviour.

Results

Two perpendicular ultrasound scans from each of 59 basal cell carcinomas were included in the overall analysis. Seventeen basal cell carcinomas were so unfavourably situated (e.g. on the bridge of the nose) that it was not possible to examine them in two planes perpendicular to each other. In these cases only the scan corresponding to the histological plane of section was evaluated. The total number of scans evaluated was thus 133. The examples in the illustrations are a basal cell carcinoma with sclerodermiform areas (Figs. 3–6), a superficial basal cell carcinoma (Figs. 7–9) and a solid basal cell carcinoma (Figs. 10–12), in each case showing the clinical, ultrasound and histological features. In 131 scans the basal cell carcinoma could be distinguished from the surrounding corium as a echo-poor structure. These structures contained weak, inhomogeneously distributed internal echoes. In five scans, apart from interference echoes also found in the water path, no internal echoes were found. Only one tumour reflected the ultrasound waves almost as strongly as the surrounding healthy corium in both planes examined. Altogether the acoustic reflection by tumour parenchyma, tumour stroma and inflammatory infiltrate was equally weak, giving an echo-poor area. Although, having a thickness of 294 µm, the size of the parenchymal buds in Fig. 9 was well above the axial resolution of about 80 µm, these structures could not be demonstrated by ultrasound (Fig. 8). The decisive, contour-forming structure was thus the inflammatory infiltrate.

The shapes of the structures in the ultrasound scans varied considerably but due to the regular outline provided by the inflammatory infiltrate, well-defined geometric shapes occurred in 59% of the cases (Fig. 13). The shapes longitudinal ellipse, transverse ellipse, semicircle and circle occurred only in nodular basal cell carcinomas. The band-shaped structures included a disproportionate number of clinically and histologically superficial basal cell carcinomas (Fig. 14). In contrast, 23 to 25 ultrasound scans showed the superficial basal cell carcinomas as band-shaped structures. The two remaining cases were also band-shaped but there were also circumscript arciform indentations in the direction of acoustic entry which represented hair follicles. Otherwise no correlation was found between the histological findings and the outline of the tumour in the ultrasound scan. 66.7% (36) of the shapes under the heading "other" were complex-structured figures which did not fit into any geometric category. In a smaller number of cases there were definable figures such as cotyloid (2), helical (1), triangular with entry echo as the base of the triangle (3), ovoid (1), bean-shaped (3), band-shaped with arcs pointing upwards (2), thick band-shaped to botuliform (1), resembling a target (1), resembling a beehive (4).

Corresponding to the high incidence of defined shapes, the basal cell carcinomas in 79% of the ultrasound scans had smooth margins. In three of these scans the structures were relatively echo-rich but an echo-poor border rendered them readily distinguishable from their surroundings. Hyporeflec-

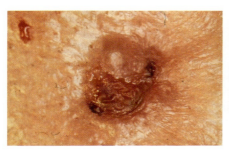

Fig. 3. Nodular basal cell carcinoma in a 75-year-old patient, preauricular

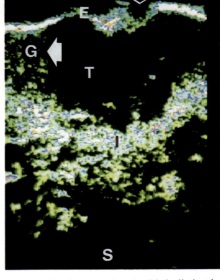

Fig. 4. Ultrasound image of the basal cell carcinoma shown in Fig. 3. *E*, entry echo with well-defined depressions (*open arrow*); *T*, tumour: irregular border with hypoechoic projections, well-defined basal boundary, indistinct lateral boundary; *I*, intensification of dorsal echoes; *S*, subcutis; *G*, loosely structured echo-poor band with indistinctly demarcated, echo-poor regions (dark green-black; *closed arrow*)

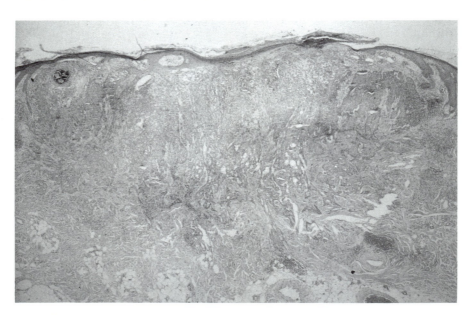

Fig. 5. Basal cell carcinoma with sclerodermiform growth in the deeper regions. Same plane of section as Fig. 4. Eroded regions of epidermis are filled with fibrin (depressions in the entry echo of the ultrasound scan). Sclerodermiform bands of basaloid cells extend well into the corium. The degree of inflammatory infiltration varies and is less marked in the deeper regions. H&E, × 25

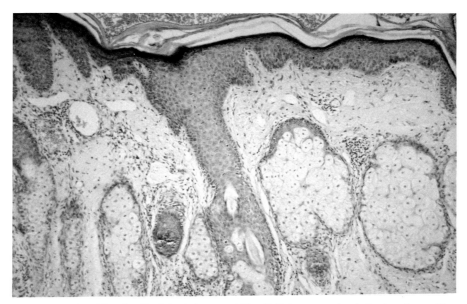

Fig. 6. Healthy skin, detail of the left part of Fig. 5. Sebaceous glands in the plaque-like material of actinic elastosis. H&E, × 100

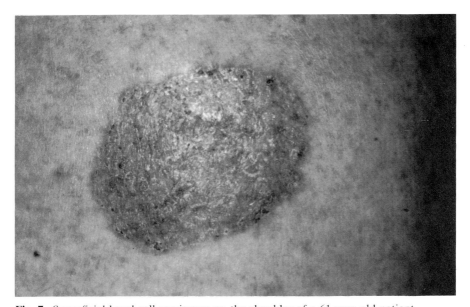

Fig. 7. Superficial basal cell carcinoma on the shoulder of a 61-year-old patient

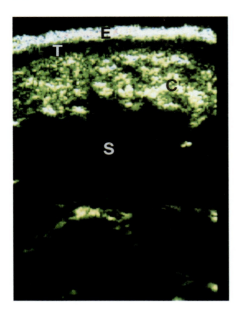

Fig. 8. Ultrasound scan of the superficial basal cell carcinoma shown in Fig. 7. *E*, strong entry echo; *T*, tumour: band-shaped echo-poor area containing few weak, inhomogeneously distributed internal echoes, regular borders and sharp basal demarcation. *C*, corium; *S*, subcutis with projections into the corium. Distance from skin surface to border between lesion and corium: not more than 616 μm

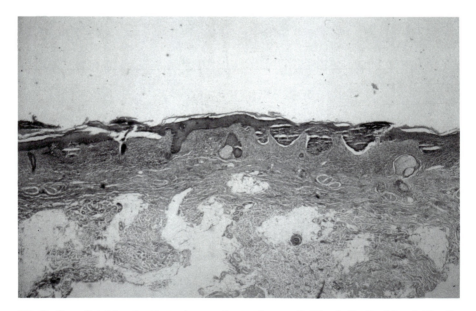

Fig. 9. Superficial basal cell carcinoma. Same plane as in Fig. 8. Buds of basaloid cells, surrounded by tumour stroma and pronounced round-cell infiltrate. Thickness of tumour buds max. 294 μm; thickness of complex consisting of buds, stroma and inflammatory infiltrate max. 600 μm. Numerous fatty tissue projections into the corium. H&E, × 25

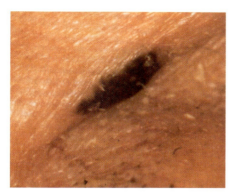

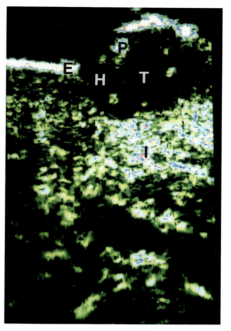

Fig. 10. Pigmented, nodular basal cell carcinoma in the nasolabial fold in a 79-year-old patient

Fig. 11. Ultrasound scan of the pigmented basal cell carcinoma shown in Fig. 10. *E*, entry echo; *T*, tumour, sharp demarcation, irregular border; *I*, intensification of dorsal signals; *H*, hair follicle; *P*, horn pearl; *arrow*, subepidermal echolucent band in healthy skin

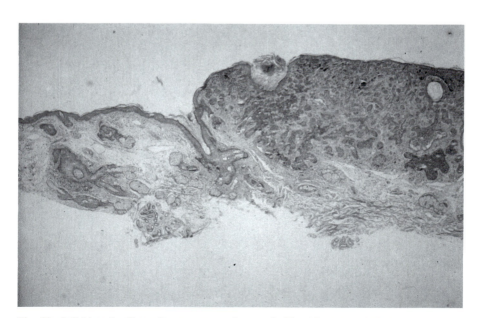

Fig. 12. Solid basal cell carcinoma, same plane as in Fig. 10. A hair follicle can be seen between tumour and healthy skin. The healthy corium next to the tumour is oedematous and loosely structured. Regard horn pearl. H&E, × 25

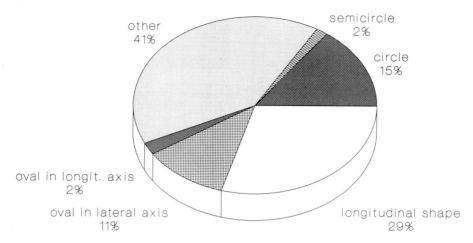

Fig. 13. Shape of basal cell carcinoma on ultrasound ($n = 133$)

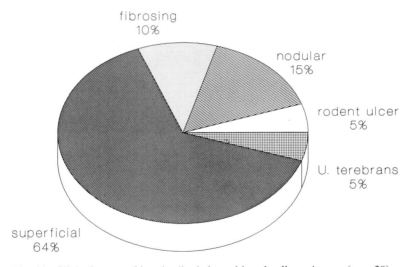

Fig. 14. Clinical types of longitudinal-shaped basal cell carcinoma ($n = 39$)

tive projections were only seen in 21% (Figs. 4, 11). 72% of the basal cell carcinomas were sharply demarcated basally, 56% laterally.

Altogether 18 sonograms depicted basal cell carcinomas of the sclerodermiform type. Here, as in the total population, the basal demarcation was in most cases sharp (78%). Well-defined lateral demarcation, on the other hand, was only found in 28%. However, *all* the sclerodermiform basal cell carcinomas were situated in actinically exposed facial skin while this was only the case in 56% of the total sample. In all the lesions with indistinct demarcation there was an adjacent subepidermal, echo-poor band in the surrounding tissue which was shown by the histological preparations to be either actinic elastosis (Fig. 6) or loosely structured oedematous corium (Fig. 12), e.g. in rosacea.

In 74% the echoes in the corium beneath the lesions were at least partially altered compared with the surroundings. Attenuated echoes or acoustic shadows were projected onto thickened regions of the entry echo. The histological preparations showed hyperkeratosis in these cases. Frequently the echoes were enhanced (Figs. 4, 11, 15). At least partial enhancement of

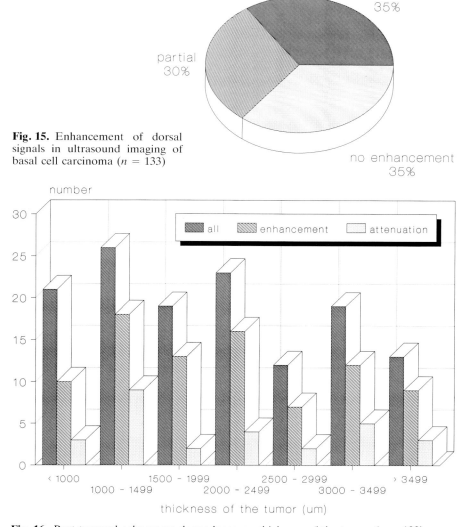

Fig. 15. Enhancement of dorsal signals in ultrasound imaging of basal cell carcinoma ($n = 133$)

Fig. 16. Post-tumoral echoes: no dependence on thickness of the tumor ($n = 133$)

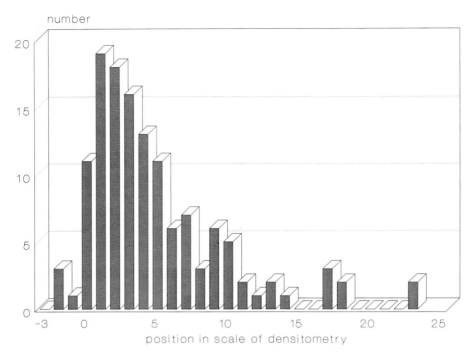

Fig. 17. Densitometry of basal cell carcinoma ($n = 133$)

dorsal echoes was found about three times more often than at least partial attenuation. Neither phenomenon increased with increasing or decreasing tumour thickness (Fig. 16). The dorsal acoustic behaviour was thus not dependent on the thickness of the tumour.

The echogenicity of the lesions as determined by densitometry was between -1.50 and 23.81. This is equivalent to a range of 25.31 (Fig. 17). The mean value was 5.08. The standard deviation of 4.66 gave a coefficient of variation of 91.7%. The particularly echo-poor basal cell carcinomas included mainly adenoid and cystic forms with mean densitometry values of 2.65 and 0.77. The superficial and sclerodermiform varieties, on the other hand, were rather echo-rich, with mean densitometer values of 7.41 and 7.17 (Fig. 18). The wide dispersion of the densitometer values, reflected in high standard deviations, should be noted. Corresponding to the low densitometry values, the black colour standing for echolucence predominated in 96%.

Basal cell carcinomas with hyperpigmentation were seen on 17 ultrasound scans. They displayed the same properties as the total sample described above (Fig. 11). The pigment had no effect on the acoustic behaviour.

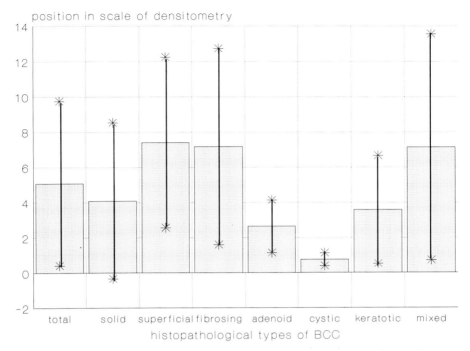

Fig. 18. Histopathological types of basal cell carcinoma in densitometry ($n = 133$)

Discussion

The 20-MHz ultrasound scan shows the basal cell carcinoma as an echo-poor structure containing weak, inhomogeneously distributed internal echoes and does not permit any differentiation between tumour parenchyma, tumour stroma and inflammatory infiltrate [8, 9]. Only in exceptional cases the internal echoes can be correlated with particular structures in the histological sections, a finding which is confirmed by other authors [5]. Grey-scale images in higher frequency ranges of 25 and 40 MHz also depict basal cell carcinomas as echo-poor structures beneath a surface echo [13]. Ultrasonic differentiation between tumour parenchyma and inflammatory infiltrate appears to be a fundamental problem in the 20-MHz range as typical inflammatory skin diseases such as lichen planus and lichenification in eczema also appear as echolucent subepithelial bands on the ultrasound scan [7].

In our own material, hyporeflective projections were rare (21% of the scans) as the margin-forming infiltrate usually had a smooth border. On the other hand, in ultrasonography of other infiltrating tumours such as mammary carcinomas irregular borders with echo-poor and echo-rich projections are an important criterion of malignancy [4].

The regular border of the infiltrate is also the reason for the frequent circumscript geometric shapes.

An important question is whether ultrasound permits non-invasive delimitation of basal cell carcinomas. Precise basal delimitation was possible in 72% of the scans. Especially in actinically exposed skin, lateral demarcation is confounded by the presence of subepidermal, echo-poor bands adjacent to the tumour area (Figs. 4, 11). In these cases the histological preparations show either the plaque-like corium of actinic elastosis or loosely structured oedematous corium. Two factors facilitate differentiation from tumour tissue: firstly we find relatively evenly distributed internal echoes; secondly the subepidermal, echo-poor bands are also found contralaterally in definitely healthy skin. Indistinct lateral demarcation is found strikingly often in sclerodermiform basal cell carcinomas (72%). It is not yet entirely clear whether this is due to the histopathological structure of the tumour itself or to the tissue surrounding the tumour as all basal cell carcinomas of the sclerodermiform type were located in particularly actinically exposed facial skin containing the subepidermal, echo-poor bands described above. Here, too, differential diagnosis was possible on the basis of the criteria described.

We were able to relate attenuation of dorsal echoes to the presence of parakeratosis or hyperkeratosis. This was also the case in verrucae seborrhoeicae and in squamous cell carcinomas with superficial keratosis [8]. The enhanced entry echo indicates enhanced reflection, which is considered to be the origin of acoustic shadowing [16]. Enhancement of dorsal echoes is considered a typical characteristic of cysts which cause less attenuation of the sound waves than their surroundings. The sound thus strikes the tissue lying posterior to the cyst with higher energy and depicts this as more highly echogenic than the environment [14]. It has not yet been established conclusively whether the enhancement of dorsal echoes frequently found in basal cell carcinomas is due to a comparable artefact or to some different mechanism. As there have been no reports to date on enhancement of dorsal echoes in other skin tumours, this phenomenon might attain differential diagnostic significance.

Measurement of the echogenicity of the basal cell carcinoma by means of densitometry provides quantitative confirmation of the markedly echo-poor picture already imaged. The densitometer values show a wide range of 25.31, i.e. 9.89% of the entire length of the scale. Differentiation from other skin tumours which also usually appear echo-poor [3, 8] thus appears to be problematic using densitometry alone. There are two conceivable reasons for the wide dispersion of the values. On the one hand, it is possible that the measuring procedure lacks sufficient precision. On the other hand, we must bear in mind the varied structure of the basal cell carcinoma as fibroepithelial mixed tumour containing individually varying proportions of more echogenic connective tissue and more echolucent structures such as tumour parenchyma and inflammatory infiltrate. In conformity with this latter hypothesis the mean densitometer values of adenoid and cystic forms of basal cell carcinoma are particularly low (Fig. 18). Here we find secretion-filled cavities which contain only few echogenic structures. Particularly high densitometer values, on the other hand, are found in superficial and sclerodermiform basal cell carcinomas. Both contain more highly echogenic connective tissue within the echo-poor areas. However, even after classification by tumour type the densitometer values are still widely dispersed and the standard deviations show overlapping intervals (Fig. 18). Differential diagnosis of the various histological types is thus not possible by means of densitometry alone.

The high precision and validity of ultrasound measurement of skin thickness or tumour thickness has already been demonstrated in several other studies [1, 10, 18]. Together with the sharp basal demarcation of the basal cell carcinoma demonstrated here we can conclude that ultrasound can improve the application of radiation therapy and cryosurgery. On account of the good lateral delimitation, safety margins can be minimised. Further studies should examine whether consistent preoperative use of high-frequency ultrasound is in fact able to significantly reduce the relapse rate of treated basal cell carcinomas.

References

1. Alexander H, Miller DL (1979) Determining skin thickness with pulsed ultrasound. J Invest Dermatol 72: 17–19
2. Altmeyer P (1989) Dermatologische Ultraschalldiagnostik – gegenwärtiger Stand und Perspektiven. Z Hautkr 64: 727–728
3. Breitbart EW, Müller CE, Hicks R, Vieluf D (1989) Neue Entwicklungen der Ultraschalldiagnostik in der Dermatologie. Aktuel Dermatol 15: 57–61
4. Bücheler E, Friedmann G, Thelen M (1983) Real-time-Sonographie des Körpers. Thieme, Stuttgart, pp 99–110
5. Dines KA, Sheets PW, Brink JA, Hanke CW, Condra KA, Clendenon JL, Goss SA, Smith DJ, Franklin TD (1984) High frequency ultrasonic imaging of skin: experimental results. Ultrason Imaging 6: 408–434
6. Giles GG, Marks R, Foley P (1988) Incidence of non-melanocytic skin cancer treated in Australia. Br Med J [Clin. Res] 296: 13–17
7. Hoffmann K, el-Gammal S, Altmeyer P (1989) 20 MHz B-scan Sonographie an Händen und Füßen. In: Altmeyer P, Schultz-Ehrenburg U, Luther H (eds) Handsymposium: Dermatologische Erkrankungen der Hände und Füße. Roche, Basel, pp 285–300
8. Hoffmann K, el-Gammal S, Matthes U, Altmeyer P (1989) Digitale 20 MHz Sonographie der Haut in der präoperativen Diagnostik. Z Hautkr 64: 851–858
9. Hoffmann K, Stücker M, el-Gammal S, Altmeyer P (1990) Digitale 20 MHz Sonographie des Basalioms im b-scan. Hautarzt 41: 333–339
10. Hughes BR, Black D, Srivastava A, Dalziel K, Marks R (1987) Comparison of techniques for the non-invasive assessment of skin tumours. Clin Exp Dermatol 12: 108–111
11. Ikeda S, Kiyohara Y, Mizutani H (1989) Comparative aspects of melanoma and non-melanoma skin cancers in Japan. J Invest Dermatol [Suppl 5] 92: 204–209
12. Levi F, La Vecchia C, Te VC, Mezzanotte G (1988) Descriptive epidemiology of skin cancer in the Swiss canton of Vaud. Int J Cancer 42: 811–816
13. Murakami S, Miki Y (1989) Human skin histology using high-resolution echography. JCU 17: 77–82
14. Pernice H, Braun B (1989) Sonographische Untersuchungstechnik. In: Braun B, Günther R, Schwerk W (eds) Ultraschalldiagnostik, 6th edn. ecomed, Landsberg

15. Querleux B, Léveque JL, De Rigal J (1988) In vivo cross-sectional ultrasonic imaging of human skin. Dermatologica 177: 332–337
16. Rosenfield AT, Taylor KJW, Jaffe CC (1980) Clinical applications of ultrasound tissue characterization. Radiol Clin North Am 18: 31–58
17. Serup J (1984) Localized skleroderma (morphoea): thickness of sclerotic plaques as measured by 15 MHz pulsed ultrasound. Acta Derm Venereol (Stockh) 64: 214–219
18. Tan CY, Statam B, Marks R, Payne PA (1982) Skin thickness measurement by pulsed ultrasound: its reproducibility, validation and variability. Br J Dermatol 106: 657–667

Value of High-Frequency Sonography in Determination of Maximal Vertical Tumor Thickness in Primary Malignant Melanoma of the Skin

G. GASSENMAIER, F. KIESEWETTER, and H. SCHELL

Introduction

Diagnosis of malignant melanomas of the skin is performed primarily by clinical examination and confirmed by histology. With regard to surgical treatment of the tumor, the minimum lateral excision margins have to be determined by measuring the maximum vertical tumor thickness [2, 3, 4].

A desirable improvement in planning surgical therapy would be a noninvasive preoperative determination of the maximum tumor thickness in patients with malignant melanoma. Sonography offers an ideally suited method: Traditional ultrasound systems do not provide the resolution required for use on the skin; however, the development of high-resolution systems (frequencies of about 20 MHz) has provided the technical conditions for sonographic evaluation of the skin, e.g., benign and malignant tumors [1, 7].

The aim of our investigation was to answer the following questions:
1. Does an acceptable correlation exist between preoperative sonometry and postoperative histometry of malignant melanoma? In particular, can sonography determine tumor thickness for planning subsequent surgical treatment?
2. Which histological conditions lead to a disagreement between preoperative sonographic and postoperative histometric measurements of tumor thickness?

Material and Methods

Equipment. An experimental ultrasound system (Siemens) with a 20 MHz B-mode sector scanner was used. This system had a maximum scan rate of three images per second and a resolution of 0.1 mm vertically and 0.5 mm laterally. A dual image display, black and white monitor system was used for imaging. Distance measurements between two selectable points had an accuracy of 0.1 mm.

Methods. We examined 493 patients with a total of 532 benign and malignant skin tumors. Histologically, in 144 patients a malignant melanoma was diagnosed.

All patients were preoperatively examined using sonography in at least two planes, including sonometric evaluation of the maximum vertical tumor diameter. All tumors were surgically removed and histologically examined, including histometric evaluation of the maximum vertical tumor thickness. In cases of differences between sonometric and histometric measurements of tumor thickness serial slices of the tumor were prepared.

Results

Sonography of Normal Skin

Image reconstruction is carried out from left to right (Fig. 1). The left border of the image shows a slight echo from the applicator membrane. Following an almost echo-free area caused by the ultrasound gel, more intensive entry echo on the skin surface is found. Adjacent dermis leads to a homogeneous, echo-rich, band-like region. Next to it, the subcutaneous fat shows an echo-poor pattern with reflection lines from connective tissue septa.

Sonographic Pattern of Malignant Melanoma

Malignant melanoma can be well-contrasted sonographically (Fig. 2). These tumors are homogeneously echo-free in comparison to surrounding echo-rich dermis, from which they can be well defined. As a rule, a sharp border

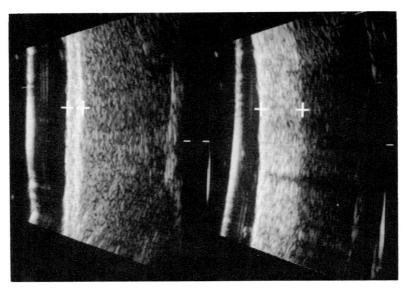

Fig. 1. Ultrasound image of normal skin. *Left*, inner side of upper arm; *right*, back. The thickness of dermis is marked with *crosses*

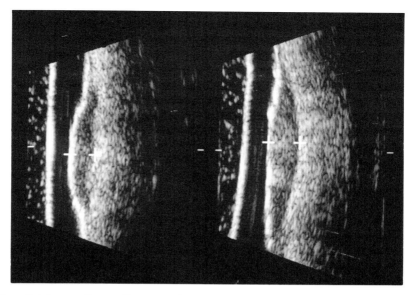

Fig. 2. Superficial spreading malignant melanoma. Sonographically low echo intensity compared to the dermis. Well-defined tumor with a maximum vertical diameter of 2.0 mm marked with *crosses*

between the echo-poor tumor structures and the echo-rich corium is seen at the region of the tumor base. This border is significant for determining the maximum vertical tumor diameter (TD_{max}).

Correlation Between Sonometry and Histometry in Malignant Melanoma of the Skin

To determine the reliability of the sonometric tumor diameter we have plotted the sonographic and histologic results on a scatter diagram (Fig. 3). A strong correlation between sonometric and histologic measurements of tumor thickness (r = 0.95) was obtained for all tumors.

Currently, tumor resection is performed with modified excision margins [5, 6]. Therefore, we classified our sonometric data into four groups, according to the histometric tumor thickness values of Breslow [2]. The correlation between sonometric and histometric tumor thickness measurements was then calculated. These evaluations showed, especially in thin melanoms (TD_{max} <0.76 mm), that the correlation coefficient decreases with decreasing histometric tumor thickness. In general ultrasound frequently overestimates the maximum tumor thickness (Tables 1 and 2).

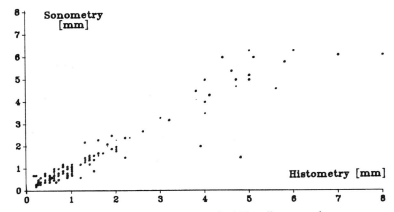

Fig. 3. Correlation between histometry and sonometry in 144 malignant melanomas; $n = 144$, $r = 0.95$

Table 1. Reliability of preoperative sonographic determination of maximum vertical tumor diameter in malignant melanoma compared to histometry. Overview through a 3×3 field table

Histometry Sonometry	<0.76 mm	0.76–1.5 mm	>1.5 mm	Sum
<0.76 mm	46	4	–	50 (34.7%)
0.76 mm–1.5 mm	8	37	2	47 (32.6%)
>1.5 mm	–	4	43	47 (32.6%)
Sum	54 (37.5%)	45 (31.3%)	45 (31.3%)	144 (100%)

Table 2. Correlation coefficient between histologic and preoperative sonographic determination of the maximum vertical tumor diameter in all malignant melanomas and subgroups

Tumor thickness[a] (TD_{max})	Count (n)	r
>1.5 mm	144	0.95
≤1.5 mm	45	0.87
≤1.5 mm	99	0.85
≥0.75 mm	45	0.70
<0.76 mm	54	0.63

r, correlation coefficient; TD_{max}, maximum vertical tumor diameter
[a] All malignant melanomas

Histomorphologic Analysis

In 126 (87%) of the 144 patients with a single malignant melanoma, the correct preoperative classification of the maximum histometric tumor thickness could be obtained by sonography.

In six patients, histological examination revealed a higher tumor thickness than the sonographically determined value. In such cases, histology showed small tumor islands or subtumoral aggregates of tumor cell remnants below the tumor mass. Subsequent histometric measurement of their diameter yielded values below the resolution of the ultrasound transducer.

The preoperative tumor thickness was sonographically overestimated in 12 patients. This can be explained by:

Association of subtumoral, band-like, lymphohistiocytic infiltrates, which were included in sonographic tumor diameter evaluation. These inflammatory infiltrates with a low-echo intensity could not sufficiently be distinguished by sonography from the tumor mass (five tumors).

Dermal nevus components side by side with malignant melanoma. Nevus cell aggregations with a low-echo intensity similar to malignant melanoma cells or associated inflammatory infiltrates also could not be differentiated from the tumor mass. This leads to an overestimation of the tumor thickness (three tumors).

Formalin fixation and paraffin embedding caused tumor shrinkage. Despite strong correlation in tumor diameters in the range of 0.75 mm and 1.5 mm, four tumors were misclassified. These had histometric tumor thickness values just below these thresholds, whereas sonometric values were just above.

Conclusion

The evaluation of tumor thickness in malignant melanoma is required for preoperative planning of therapy and, furthermore, is a direct indicator of prognosis. Our investigations demonstrated that ultrasound examination of tumor thickness in malignant melanoma can be done quickly and reliably without discomfort for the patient. The sonometrically determined tumor thickness values show a strong correlation with the histometric values (Figs. 4 and 5).

In general, there is a tendency of the sonographic method to overestimate the tumor thickness. The reasons for this are:
a) shrinkage of the tissue after excision;
b) association of lymphocytic infiltrates at the tumor base; and
c) dermal nevus components at the tumor base. A subtumoral association of lymphocytic infiltrate or components of a dermal nevus cannot always be differentiated from malignant melanoma.

Thin tumor islands invading the deeper dermis as well as separated subtumoral melanoma cells may escape the sonographic detection, leading to an underestimation of the tumor thickness (Fig. 6).

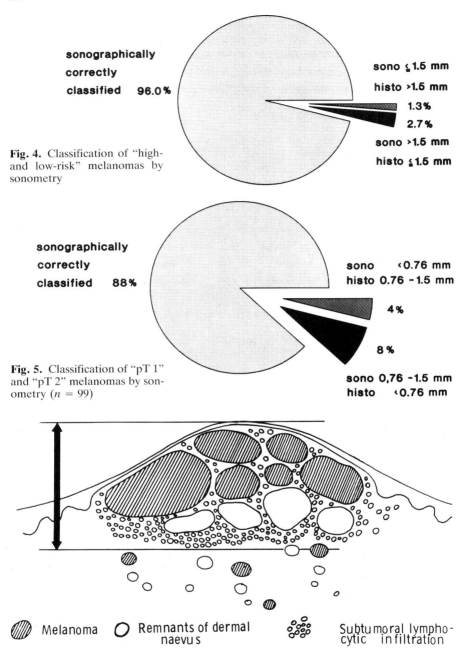

Fig. 4. Classification of "high- and low-risk" melanomas by sonometry

Fig. 5. Classification of "pT 1" and "pT 2" melanomas by sonometry ($n = 99$)

Fig. 6. Limits of sonography in evaluation of maximum vertical diameter of malignant melanoma. Overestimation of tumor thickness by subtumoral corial nevus components or by inflammatory infiltrates. Underestimation of tumor thickness because of adjacent subtumoral melanoma cell islands

Even in spite of the above-noted limitations, high-resolution sonography provides a noninvasive preoperative estimation of tumor thickness in malignant melanoma of the skin, valuable in preoperative therapy planning. Clearly, the benefits of ultrasound cannot be directly compared with those of histology, in which additional staining or immunohistochemical tests provide the definitive diagnosis. It is therefore difficult to imagine that cellular differentiation in the microscopic level can be made solely on ultrasound reflection behaviour.

References

1. Breitbart EW, Müller CE, Hicks R, Vieluf D (1989) Neue Entwicklungen in der Ultraschalldiagnostik. Aktuel Dermatol 15: 57–61
2. Breslow A, Mach SD (1977) Optimal size of resection margin for thin cutaneous melanoma. Surg Gynecol Obstet 145: 691–692
3. Day CL, Lew RA, Mihm MC (1981) The natural break points for primary tumor thickness in clinical stage I melanoma. N Engl J Med 305: 1155
4. Garbe C, Stadler R, Orfanos CE (1986) Prognose-orientierte Therapie beim malignen Melanom. Hautarzt 37: 365–372
5. Hundeiker M, Drepper H (1987) Therapie der malignen Melanome. Dtsch Med Wochenschr 112: 553
6. Schmoeckel C (1985) Der Sicherheitsabstand bei der Melanomexcision. In: Wolff HH, Schmeller W (eds) Fehlbildungen, Nävi, Melanoma. Springer, Berlin Heidelberg New York, p 207
7. Hoffmann K, el-Gammal S, Matthes U. Altmeyer P (1989) Digitale 20 MHz Sonographie der Haut in der präoperativen Diagnostik. Z Hautkr 64: 851–858

Inflammatory Diseases in 20 MHz Ultrasound

Examination of Circumscribed Scleroderma Using 20-MHz B-Scan Ultrasound

K. HOFFMANN, S. EL-GAMMAL, U. GERBAULET, H. SCHATZ, and P. ALTMEYER

Instrumental technology has not gained great importance in the diagnosis of skin diseases. Especially in chronic dermatoses such as circumscribed scleroderma only limited possibilities are offered to quantify its manifestations using objective criteria [3]. Therefore, evaluations of the dynamic progression of these diseases are still mainly based on clinical and subjective investigations [4]. Over the past few years, we used ultrasound extensively on our patients with morphea [19–22]. We already knew that with the aid of B-scan ultrasound we could visualize infiltrations and quantify skin thickness [1, 2, 6–8, 12–14, 16, 32]. So far, those capabilities did not influence our decisions regarding the therapy of this disease [15, 17, 18, 22, 23, 26, 28, 29]. The following investigations were designed to evaluate the importance of high-frequency (> 20 MHz) ultrasound for clinical routine use.

Equipment

In our experiencce 20-MHz scanners with an axial resolution ob about 80 μm are especially suited to investigate patients with circumscribed scleroderma. As a rule, the skin and the subcutaneous fat can be visualized up to a depth of 0.7–1.0 cm. Higher-frequency scanners do offer a better resolution, but as the depth of invasion is antiproportional to the frequency, the subcutaneous tissue cannot be examined with frequencies above 20 MHz [5, 9, 10].

We used a DUB 20 (Taberna pro medicum, Lüneburg, FRG) and a Dermascan C (Cortex Technology, Hadsund, DK) for our investigations. Both units were suitable for our investigations, but they are configured differently and have various advantages and drawbacks. The DUB 20 fully digitally processes the signals, but it takes about 5 s for this procedure. The Dermascan C, however, is able to perform almost in real-time. The random access memory (RAM) of the DUB can store ten sonograms, the Dermascan C stores two pictures in its RAM, after a second external computer unit has been attached even more. The coupling water bath of the Dermascan C is encapsulated by foil. This actually makes the routine work easier as the troublesome sealing of the coupling water bath container can be omitted. However, the foil causes a dispersion of signals, reflections and absorptions which sometimes cannot be differentiated from the entry echo. Comparing the images, the DUB 20 seems to produce a slightly higher axial resolution than the Dermascan C. In contrast, the Dermascan C software offers several interesting options. Our team uses both instruments in routine diagnosis with satisfactory results.

Circumscribed Scleroderma

In 1753, more than 200 years ago, "scleroderma" was first mentioned by the Italian Curzio. As a matter of fact, our knowledge about pathogenesis, chemical findings, and clinical morphology have increasingly grown. Basically we distinguish between two types: progressive systemic scleroderma and circumscribed scleroderma. The term "morphea" or "morphoea" which was established by Erasmus Wilson is often synonymously used for circumscribed scleroderma. Due to the involvement of inner organs one must attach major importance to progressive systemic scleroderma *quoad vitam*. In contrast to the progressive systemic scleroderma circumscribed scleroderma is generally a prognostically harmless skin disease, which proceeds episodically without involvement of inner organs and with a tendency to spontaneous healing. It presents clinically as a regional and temporally delimited condensation of the subcutaneous fat tissue and possibly the muscles. Up to this point we did not have reliable and easily accessible parameters for a safe quantification of involvement and progression of this disease. For that reason, several research groups attempted to make those therapeutically important data available for the medical practitioner by means of modern medical technology [1, 32–36, 38].

Patients and Method

Within 1 year some of the patients in our hospital (n=63) who attended our special consultation hours for scleroderma were examined by ultrasound. Nineteen patients regularly made use of a sonographic control every 3 months. The clinical typing of scleroderma was according to the ADF (Arbeitsgemeinschaft Dermatologische Forschung, Germany) classification [4] (Table 1). Some 93% were of the plaque type of circumscribed scleroderma (morphea). The following results refer to this type.

All sclerotic plaques of examined patients were sonographically compared with the contralateral healthy skin. If possible, the central and a peripheral area of the plaque were examined. In several cases sonography and histology taken from the same level could be compared. With the help of an exact anatomical description and picture documentation the examined plaques and examination levels were topographically recorded to ensure that the following measurements took place in the same area. The patient was examined in standardized body positions for each measurement as the tension of the skin possibly influences the echogenity. The skin thickness was measured as the distance extending from the entry echo to the deepest corium region in the subcutaneous fat.

Table 1. Clinical division of circumscribed (localized) scleroderma as suggested in the ADF classification

Type	Name
1	Plaque-type a <5 focuses b <5 focuses
2	Guttate circumscribed scleroderma
3	Erythematous circumscribed scleroderma (Atrophodermia idiopathica et progressiva – Pasini Perini)
4	Linear circumscribed scleroderma
5	1 Scleroderma "en coup de sabre" 2 Facial hemiatrophy (Parry-Romberg-Syndrome)
6	Nodular circumscribed scleroderma
7	Subcutaneous circumscribed scleroderma
8	Eosinophilic fasciitis of Shulman

Table 2. Clinical division of patients examined in this study corresponding to the ADF classification

Type	Number of patients	%
1	58	93
a	28	45
b	30	48
3	2	3
4	2	3
8	1	3

Cases

Case 1: Localized Scleroderma in a 19-Year-Old Woman. The first examination showed a slightly indurated, clearly circumscribed and moderately red plaque in the right inguen which existed for 4 months as the patient stated. Four months later we found an ivory-colored center and as surrounding violaceous halo in the same area which on palpation gave the impression of being more solid than in the primary investigation. Both sonograms were taken from exactly the same level in the center of the plaque.

Figure 1 shows the findings at first evaluation. The sonogram shows an almost not demarcated entry echo and an only moderately echogenous corium. At the corium-subcutis borderline only a few echo-rich amplifications are visible as they are not atypical for this region. The following subcutaneous fat is presented with a limited number of reflections. Fibers of

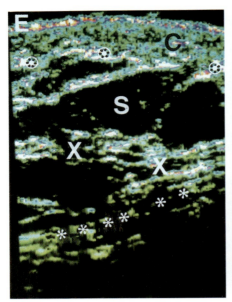

Fig. 1. Circumscribed scleroderma in a 19-year-old woman (initial findings in case 1).
E, entry echo; *C*, corium; *circles*, reflex amplifications; *S*, subcutaneous fat; *X*, subcutaneous trabeculae; *asterisks*, inguinal ligament

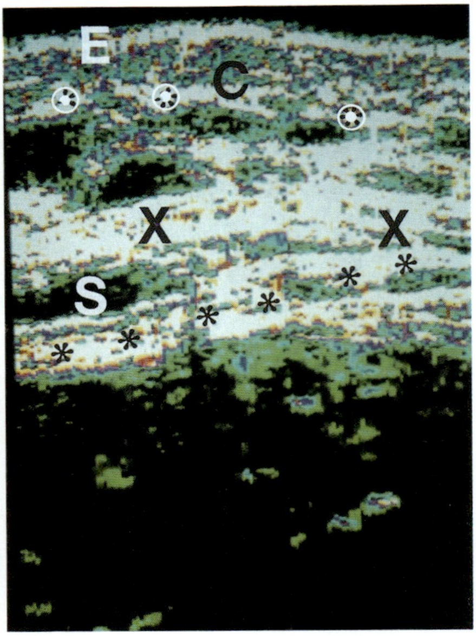

Fig. 2. Findings in case 1, 3 months later.
E, entry echo; *C*, corium; *circles*, reflex amplifications; *S*, subcutaneous fat; *X*, subcutaneous trabeculae; *asterisks*, inguinal ligament

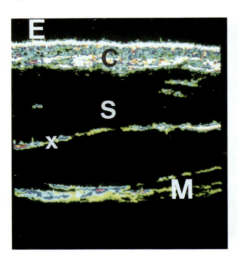
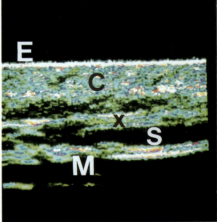

Fig. 3. Circumscribed scleroderma in a 9-year-old child (initial findings in case 2).
E, entry echo; *C*, corium; *S*, subcutaneous fat; *X*, subcutaneous trabeculae; *M*, musculous fascia

Fig. 4. Findings in case 2, 4 months later.
E, entry echo; *C*, corium; *S*, subcutaneous fat; *M*, musculous fascia; *X*, subcutaneous trabeculae

connective tissue can be found from the lower corium to the inguinal ligament.

Figure 2 shows the same area 3 months later. The entry echo is clearly thickened and turned out to be an echo-rich white band. The corium, however, seems to be a little thinner than in the initial picture. An increase of echogenity is demonstrated by a preponderance of blue and white signals. The reflex amplification at the corium-subcutis borderline grew thicker and condensated. The ultrasound findings of the corium are possibly a result of its increased tension. The subcutaneous fat can hardly be defined. Fibers of connective tissue are distinctly condensated and thickened. They are hardly separated from the inguinal ligament.

The ultrasound examination also showed clinically clear progression of the circumscribed scleroderma.

Case 2: The sonograms show an area of the lower abdominal region which corresponds exactly to that of Case 1. Localized Scleroderma in a 9-Year-Old Child. The finding shows only a slight macroscopic change. An ivory-colored, bright and sharply circumscribed plaque was found which on palpation was more solid at second evaluation (Fig. 4).

Figure 3 shows the initial ultrasound finding. The horizontally running entry echo is reflexogeneous and homogeneous. The corium is thin; at the corium-subcutis borderline we see moderate reflex amplifications. The subcutaneous fat is presented echo-poor with trabeculae running through the middle part. The muscle fascia is well defined. The corium appears typical for a child of this age. As a rule, the skin is thinner and more reflexogeneous than that of an adult. Figure 4 shows the same area 4 months later. The reflex pattern of the entry echo is almost unchanged. In contrast, the corium is distinctly thickened. Reflex- amplifications in the depth of the corium have almost disappeared. The subcutaneous fat is extremely thinned. The clearly thickened subcutaneous trabeculae are now connected with the muscle fascia on one side and with the lower corium on the other.

The clinical findings of rapid progression of the disease could sonographically be confirmed.

Case 3: Localized Scleroderma in a 49-Year-Old Woman. Both sonograms are taken from the central part of a plaque in the upper abdominal region. On account of an adipositas per magna the clinical quantification of the induration was particularly difficult. The patient was treated with Adsulfidine during the investigation time.

Figure 5 shows the initial finding. The entry echo is homogeneously echo-rich. The underlying corium shows a clear echosignal amplification. Especially the lower corium shows a massive increase of echogenity. Within the echo-poor subcutaneous fat of the adipose patient only few reflexes can be detected. They correspond to fibers of connective tissue.

Figure 6 shows the same finding 6 months later. The entry echo remains almost unchanged. In contrast to healthy skin, the corium is still echogen-

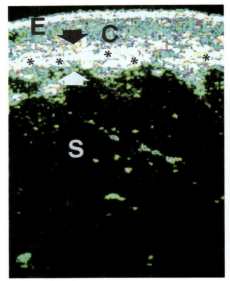 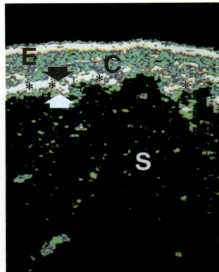

Fig. 5. Circumscribed scleroderma in a 49-year-old woman (initial findings in case 3).
E, entry echo; *C*, corium; *asterisks/arrows*, massive increase of reflexogenity in the lower corium; *S*, subcutaneous fat

Fig. 6. Findings in case 3, 6 months later. *E*, entry echo; *C*, corium; *asterisks/arrows* reflex amplifications in the lower corium-, *S*, subcutaneous fat

ous, but it shows distinctly less reflexes than at initial examination. This can be interpreted as a reduction of condensation. The echo signals from the corium-subcutis borderline have also decreased and became thinner.

General Findings

The sclerotic plaques of the 63 patients examined showed a thickened corium in contrast to contralaterally located healthy areas of the skin ($p \leq 0,001$). The extension of the increase of the corium depended upon the localization in question and on the thickness of the originally healthy skin (Fig. 7). In the inguen where the skin is comparatively thin to other areas, the relative increase of the skin thickness is indicative. The average thickness of the corium of healthy skin amounted to 0.91 mm; the average increase of the thickness of the corium was 61 % in a sclerotic plaque ($p \leq 0.001$). In the lower regions of the back (average skin thickness = 2 mm), the mean increase of the thickness of the corium in a sclerotic plaque was 21 % ($p \leq =0.001$).

Compared to normal skin, ultrasound showed an additional echo-signals in the lower corium (Fig. 8). Their frequency was dependent on

Examination of Circumscribed Scleroderma Using 20-MHz B-Scan   237

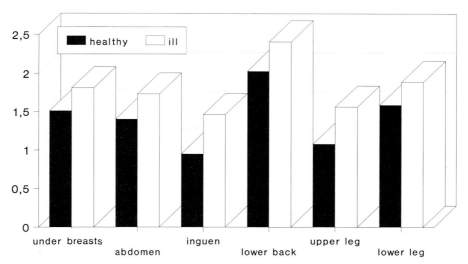

Fig. 7. Thickness of the skin (in mm) at various body localizations

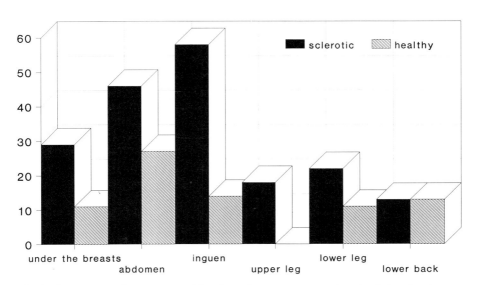

Fig. 8. Percentage of sonograms with echo enhancement at various body localizations

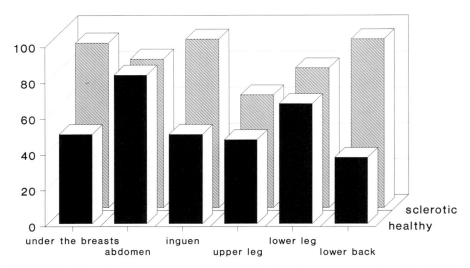

Fig. 9. Number of sonograms on which thick trabeculae were seen at various body localizations

the investigated regions. Echo-rich spots in the lower corium were found in 96 % of the cases in the inguen. In contrast only 44 % of the corresponding healthy regions of the skin showed similar echo-rich spots. A further characteristic of localized scleroderma is the increase in number and/or width of subcutaneous trabeculae, which originate in the corum-subcutis borderline region and pass through the subcutaneous fat. Such echo-rich trabeculae were found particularly often in sclerotic lesions in the inguen. Some 57 % of the examined plaques of this region showed those trabeculae, but only 11 % of healthy skin presented those structures (Fig. 9).

Sclerotic plaques of nine of our patients showed a decrease in the thickness of the corium in the course of examination, projecting a regression. In contrast, the sclerotic plaques of nine other patients showed an increase of the thickness of the corium, in the sense of a progression. One female patient did not show progression by increase of skin thickness but rather a strong increase of trabeculae of connective tissue in the subcutaneous fat. Evaluating the sonogramms over the course of time, patients with progressions often show an increase of echogenity at the corium-subcutis borderline (Fig. 8).

The corium of those nine patients with regressive sclerotic plaques became 0.49 mm thinner on the average. This corresponds to a reduction of the corial thickness of 24 % ($p \leq 0.001$). In the abdominal and thoracal regions the average reduction of the corial thickness was 0.60 mm. This is equivalent to a regression of 27 % ($p \leq 0.001$). Plaques on the inguen and lower extremities presented a mean increase of the corium of 0.42 mm. This is equivalent to a relative progression of 31 % ($p \leq 0.001$).

In this study the results of ten ultrasound examinations corresponded to those of the clinical assessment, in two cases clinical, and ultrasound results were contradictory, and in seven cases the clinical observation did not allow an assessment of the process of the disease and its tendency while ultrasound could visualise clear changes of the sclerotic plaques.

Discussion

In histology the different types of localized scleroderma are as difficult to distinguish from one another as they can be separated from the progressive systemic sclerosis [30]. However, it is possible to detect progression of the disease, characterized by an inflammatory early phase with continuous change into sclerosis as the final result as a consequence of formation of new collagen fibers. The differentiation into different types of scleroderma is clinically possible. In clinical routine diagnosis objective parameters for the follow-up and quantification of the disease are required. For this purpose, different procedures have been suggested in the past years.

Serup and Northeved described a method to quantify the elasticity of the skin in patients with localized scleroderma [36]. Measurements of the elasticity of the skin could detect functional changes (elasticity) of sclerotic plaques, but they did not give further detailed information about histological changes. Other disadvantages were that a minimal remaining elasticity of the skin was necessary for reproducible readings and that not every location of the body is suited for this kind of examination.

Histological examinations are invasive and strain the patients. Furthermore, tissue once excised cannot be examined over time. Excision and further preparation of the sections also lead to shape changes and do not allow exact evaluation of in vivo conditions [21, 22]. Examinations over the course of time are nearly impossible.

Besides, methods to measure the thickness of the skin and skinfolds exists. The measurement of skinfolds by means of the "Harpenden Skinfold Caliper" has been frequently described [13, 14, 24, 41, 42]. The main disadvantage of this method is the inclusion of subcutaneous fat into the measured skinfold. Moreover, the caliper cannot be applied in every region of the body. Because of these insufficiencies the method did not fully assert itself in daily routine. A very precise method to measure the thickness of the skin is the radiographic technique by Black [7]. With the use of xeroradiography [14] this procedure was optimized; nevertheless, the problem of exposure to radiation remained. A noninvasive method to measure the skin thickness and density is ultrasound. The sonographic estimation of skin thickness was initially performed in the A mode [2, 14, 28, 39]. Finally, innovations in microelectronics (hardware and software), transducer technology and scanners made two-dimensional B-scan investigations with a high resolution possible. In addition to the ability to measure the skin thickness it also gives information about the micromorphology of the skin. A special advantage lies in the clear presentation of the corium-subcutis borderline and the subcutaneous fat, which is frequently not shown in the histologic sections.

A Danish group quantified the extent of a sclerotic plaque in A mode with a 15-MHz scanner [33–35]. Another group used a 10-MHz B-mode unit to measure the thickness of sclerotic skin on patients who were afflicted by acrosclerosis [1]. Subsequently, even a 25-MHz B-mode unit was used for this purpose [27].

By use of the above-mentioned recently developed high-resolution 20-MHz B-scan ultrasound a better evaluation of physiological and pathological structures of the skin and the subcutaneous fat was possible [19].

In localized scleroderma and progressive systemic sclerosis ultrasound examinations were performed to evaluate the thickness of sclerotic plaques. It could be proved that the skin in sclerotic plaques is distinctly thickened [11, 18, 23, 36, 38].

The sclerotic plaques of our patients suffering from localized scleroderma showed an increase of the corial thickness ranging from 1% to 294% compared to contralateral skin sites. These results correspond to the findings of the Danish group who found increases of the skin thickness of 13% to 310% [1]. Our high standard variations (ranging from 0.1 mm to 0.5 mm) were due to great individual deviations [18]. To interpret the extent of changes in skin thickness in localized scleroderma we had to compare the involved skin (plaques) to healthy contralaterally located corresponding areas on the same patient. It is inadmissible to use skin thickness measurements of healthy subjects as a standard.

The extent of the differences in the corial thickness between healthy and sclerotic skin were dependent on the location of the affliction. Thinner skin as it can be found in the inguen region and the lower extremities was relatively more greatly affected by the sclerosis than the comparatively thicker skin of the abdominal region, the thoracal region and the back. In the inguen (average thickness 0.91 mm), the mean increase of the corial thickness showed a maximum of 61%. Our results are well in line with the findings of other research groups in this respect [38].

Beside an increase of the corial thickness the sclerotic plaques showed an increase in echo signal amplifications in the lower corium and in subcutaneous trabeculae. Both phenomena are not exactly pathognomonic as they could also be found in healthy skin to lesser extent. These echo-rich spots in the lower corium could be explained as follows:
1. The collagen fibers in the lower corium are tightly packed, depending on the location and
2. an inflammatory progression zone, which is clinically observed at the borders of scleroderma plaques [30].

This inflammatory process can lead to homogenized collagen connective tissue and increase the echogenity of the lower corium.

The increase of collagen fibers and their compact arrangement in the lower corium is responsible for the higher echogenity of sclerotic plaques in comparison to healthy skin. Especially the sclerotic plaques of the inguen showed these scattered echo reflexes, probably based on increased sclerosis in this region. The high tendency of progression of localized scleroderma in the inguen also explains the distinct and frequent appearance of echo-rich subcutaneous trabeculae in this region. Other research groups described the appearance of these echo-rich trabeculae on the B-scan images of morphea as well [38].

In many cases the entry echo and the subcutaneous fat is thinner than in contralateral, healthy skin. The entry echo mainly is irregular and not comparable with histometry regarding the thickness of the epidermis. We found only a minimum correlation of the entry echo and the histometric measurement of the epidermal thickness. The subcutaneous fat often is not distinguishable in the depth of the tissue as the muscle fascia is not always detected as a whole. This is basically due to the limited penetration caused by absorption. Furthermore, subcutaneous trabeculae frequently found in the sclerotic plaques are responsible for limited sound-energy reaching the muscle fascia. The 20-MHz scanners in their present state of technology are not suited for an exact demarcation of the subcutaneous fat.

The average progression of plaques in the thoracal and abdominal regions was 28% and 29% in the inguen and lower extremities. These almost identical results suggest that progression is not dependent on the location of the plaques. This is also true for the regression of sclerotic plaques.

Patients with regression and duration of more than 32 months showed an about 20% greater decrease in the thickness of the corium than those with shorter durations. Those patients with progression of the plaques and a duration of less than 16 months showed a 13% higher increase of the thickness of the corium than those with a longer duration of disease. With increasing duration and therapy, the extent of regression of the sclerotic plaques increased, while the extent of progression was reduced. This result was conform with the clinical experience that long duration of disease and therapy corresponds to regression or stable condition while progressive sclerosis normally occurs in patients with a recently developed or shortly treated morphea.

The advantage of noninvasive ultrasound observation of localized scleroderma is the possibility to objectively evaluate the course of development of sclerotic plaques. Myers [27] and Akesson [1] recommended ultrasound for the evaluation of the process of this disease due to the objectivity and exact reproducibility of this technique. Fornage and Deshaynes [17] also recognized ultrasound as an important method to study skin diseases associated with an increase of skin thickness.

The 20-MHz B-scan ultrasound is presently the best suited method to investigate localized scleroderma. The course of development of the disease can be clearly recorded and in addition to the sonographic measurement of the skin thickness further important criteria can be provided.

Information about changes of the corium, subcutis and muscle fascia deal important information concerning quality and quantity of the sclerotic process which was not available until now. Especially in deciding on the appropriate therapeutic treatement this precise diagnostic method must not be withold from the patient.

References

1. Åekesson A, Forsberg L, Hedeström N, Wollheim F (1986) Ultrasound examination of skin thickness in patients with progressive systemic sclerosis (scleroderma). Acta Radiol Diagn 27: 91–94
2. Alexander H, Miller DL (1979) Determining skin thickness with pulsed ultrasound. J Invest Derm 72: 17–19
3. Altmeyer P (1989) Dermatologische Ultraschalldiagnostik – gegenwärtiger Stand und Perspektiven (Editorial). Z Hautkr 64: 727–728
4. Altmeyer P. Goerz G, Goertz J, Holzmann H, Staudt R, Mensing H, Krieg T (1990) Zur Klassifikation der circumskripten Sclerodermie. Hautarzt 41: 16–21
5. Altmeyer P, Hoffmann K, el-Gammal S (1990) Sonographie der Haut. MMW 132 (18): 14–22
6. Beck S, Spence VA, Lowe JG, Gibbs JH (1986) Measurement of skin swelling in the tuberculin test by ultrasonography. J Immunol Methods 86: 125–130
7. Black MM (1969) A modified radiographic method for measuring skin thickness. Br J Dermatol 81: 661–666
8. Brazier S, Shaw S (1986) High-frequency ultrasound measurement of patch test reactions. Contact Dermatitis 15: 199–201
9. Breitbart EW, Hicks R, Rehpennig W (1985) Möglichkeiten der Ultraschalldiagnostik in der Dermatologie. Z Hautkr 61: 522–526
10. Breitbart EW, Müller CH, Hicks R, Vieluf D (1989) Neue Entwicklungen der Ultraschalldiagnostik in der Dermatologie. Akt Dermatol 15: 57–61
11. Cole GW, Handler SJ, Burnett K (1981) The ultrasonic evaluation of skin thickness in scleroderma. J Clin Ultrasound 9: 501–503
12. Dines KA, Sheets PW, Brink JA, Hanke CW, Condra KA, Clendenon JL, Goss SA, Smith JS, Franklin TD (1984) High frequency ultrasonic of skin: experimental results. Ultrason Imaging 6: 408–434
13. Dykes PJ, Marks R (1976) Measurement of dermal thickness with the Harpenden skinfold caliper. Arch Dermatol Res 256: 261–263
14. Dykes PJ, Mark R (1976) Measurement of skin thickness: a comparison of two in vivo techniques with a conventional histometric method. J Invest Dermatol 21: 418–429
15. El-Gammal S (1990) Experimental approaches and new developments with high frequency ultrasound in dermatology. Zentralbl Haut 157: 327
16. Feldmann S, Hoffmann K, el-Gammal S, Altmeyer P (1990) Sonographic quantification of the tuberculin-type reaction. Zentralbl Haut 157: 320–321
17. Fornage DW, Deshaynes JL (1986) Ultrasound of normal skin J Clin Ultrasound 14: 619–622
18. Görtz S, Hoffmann K, el-Gammal S, Altmeyer P (1990) High frequency b-scan sonography and skin-thickness measurement of normal skin. Zentralbl Haut 157: 319–320
19. Hoffmann K, el-Gammal S, Altmeyer P (1989) 20 MHz B-scan Sonographie an Händen und Füßen. In: Altmeyer P et al. (eds) Handsymposium: Dermatologische Erkrankungen der Hände und Füße. Edition Roche, pp 285–300

20. Hoffmann K, el-Gammal S, Matthes U, Altmeyer P (1989) 20 MHz Sonographie der Haut in der präoperativen Diagnostik. Z Hautkr 64: 851–858
21. Hoffmann K, Stücker M, el-Gammal S, Altmeyer P (1990) Digitale 20-MHz-Sonographie des Basalioms im b-scan Hautarzt 41: 333–339
22. Hoffmann K, Stücker M, el-Gammal S, Altmeyer P (1990) b-scan Sonographie in der Dermatologie. Hautarzt 41: W7–W16
23. Kirsch JM, Hanson ME, Gibson JR (1984) The determination of skin-thickness using conventional ultrasound equipment. Clin Exp Dermatol 9: 280–285
24. Lawrence CM, Shuster S (1985) Comparison of ultrasound and caliper measurements of normal and inflamed skin thickness. J Dermatol 112: 195–200
25. Miyauchi S, Tada M, Miki Y (1983) Echographic evaluation of nodular lesions of the skin. J Dermatol 10: 221–227
26. Murikami S, Miki Y (1989) Human skin histology using high-resolution echography. J Clin Ultrasound 17: 77–82
27. Myers SL, Cohen JS, Sheets PW (1986) B-mode ultrasound evaluation of skin thickness in progressive systemic sclerosis. J Reumatol 13: 577–550
28. Payne PA (1985) Medical and industrial applications of high resolution ultrasound. J Phys E Sci Instrum 18: 465–473
29. Querleux B, Léveque JL, de Rigal J (1988) In vivo cross-sectional ultrasonic imaging of human skin. Dermatologica 177: 332–337
30. Rieger H, Wolter M, Marsch WCh (1987) Histologie der Sklerodermien in Dermatologie und Rheuma, Holzmann et al. [editor], Springer (pp 235–240)
31. Rigal J, Escoffier C, Querleux B, Faivre B, Agach P, Leveque JL (1989) Assessment of aging of the human skin by in vivo ultrasonic imaging. J Invest Dermatol 93: 621–625
32. Schuster S, Black MM, McVitie E (1975) The influence of age and sex on skin thickness, skin collagen and density. Br J Dermatol 93: 639–643
33. Serup J (1984) Quantification of acrosclerosis: measurement of skin thickness and skin-phalanx distance in females with 15 MHz Pulsed Ultrasound. Acta Dermatol Venereol 64: 35–40
34. Serup J (1984) Localized scleroderma: thickness of sclerotic plaques measured by 15 MHz pulsed ultrasound. Acta Dermatol Venerol 64: 35–40
35. Serup J (1985) The sclerotic centre of morphea plaques, In: Serup J – Localized Scleroderma, 16–26, Almquist & Wiksell periodical Company, Stockholm
36. Serup J, Northheved A (1985) Skin elasticity in localized scleroderma (morphea). J Dermatol 12: 52–62
37. Serup J, Staberg B, Klemp P (1984) Quantification of cutaneous oedema in patch test reactions by measurement of skin thickness with high frequency pulsed ultrasound. Contact Dermatitis 10: 88–93
38. Sondergaard J, Serup J, Tikjob G (1985) Ultrasonic a- and b- scanning in clinical and experimental dermatology. Acta Dermatol Venereol (Stockh) 65 [Suppl 120]: 76–82
39. Tan CY, Statham B, Marks R, Payne PA (1982) Skin thickness measurement by pulsed ultrasound: its reproducibility, validation and variability. Br J Dermatol 106: 657–667
40. Tanner JM, Whitehouse RH (1955) The harpenden skinfold caliper. Am J Physiol Anthropol 13: 743–746
41. Wahlberg JE (1983) Assessment of skin irritancy: measurement of skin fold thickness. Contact Dermatitis 9: 21–26
42. Wahlberg JE, Nilsson G (1984) Skin irritancy from propylene glycol. Acta Dermatol Venereol (Stockh) 64: 286–290

Examination of Psoriasis Vulgaris Using 20-MHz B-Scan Ultrasound

K. Hoffmann, S. el-Gammal, H. Schwarze, T. Dirschka, and P. Altmeyer

With a prevalence of 1%–2% psoriasis vulgaris is one of the most frequent skin diseases. As a rule, the clinical diagnosis of this disease is not particularly difficult, apart from several rare types. It was the idea from the very beginning to use ultrasound in the study of psoriasis to search for characteristic sonographic phenomena.

Psoriasis vulgaris exhibits several morphological changes which separates it from other dermatoses by histological evaluation. Hyperparakeratosis and acanthosis associated with elongation and clumping of the epidermal rete belong to those changes. In the dermal papillae, located between the epidermal rete, an edema sometimes develops. The capillaries within the papillae are dilated, resulting in a hyperemia. Inflammatory infiltrations can regularly be found within epidermis and corium. On account of these considerable changes in the histological morphology it should be possible to establish sonographic characteristics for this disease. Following this concept ultrasound could be a new promising approach for future investigations of dermatological diseases.

Case Studies

Figure 1 shows the results of clinical investigation of a patient with psoriasis vulgaris of the chronic stationary type. The black line shows the ultrasound investigation level on the right side of the chest. The sonogram (Fig. 2) corresponding to Fig. 1 shows a typical view of a psoriasis plaque.

The entry echo is clearly thickened. At several places there is dorsal echo attenuation. Directly underneath the entry echo an echolucent band is recognized which shows irregularly distributed internal echoes. The underlying corium can be well distinguished from the subcutaneous fat and shows a homogeneous corium whose echoreflexes are weaker and fainter with increasing depth. The histological section corresponding to Fig. 1 and 2 (Fig. 3) indicates severe acanthosis with subepidermal inflammatory infiltration. Islands of connective tissue embedded in the epidermis are possibly responsible for internal reflexes within the echolucent band.

Figure 4 shows the sonogram of another patient's plaque who has already been treated (salicylic vaseline) to reduce the parahyperkeratosis. As a

Examination of Psoriasis Vulgaris Using 20-MHz B-Scan Ultrasound 245

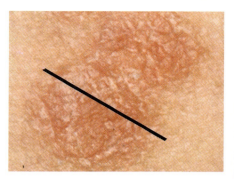

Fig. 1. Psoriasis vulgaris of the chronic stationary type, *black line* shows the sonographical investigation level

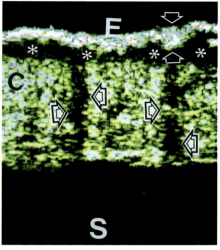

Fig. 2. Corresponding sonogram to Fig. 1. E, entry-echo; C, corium; S, subcutaneous fat; *closed arrows/open arrows*, area with dorsal echo attenuation; *asterisks*, echolucent band

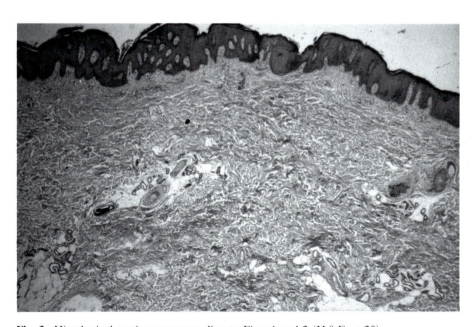

Fig. 3. Histological section corresponding to Figs. 1 and 2 (H&E, ×25)

Table 1. ELB – echo-lucent bands can be found in various dermatoses

- actinic elastosis
- psoriasis vulgaris
- severe type IV-reaction
- atopic dermatitis
- lichen planus
- skin cancer

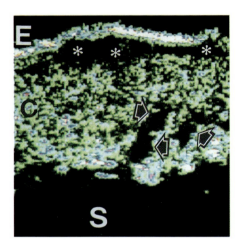

Fig. 4. Sonogram of a patient who has been treated with salicylic vaseline. *E*, entry echo; *C*, corium; *arrows*, hair follicles

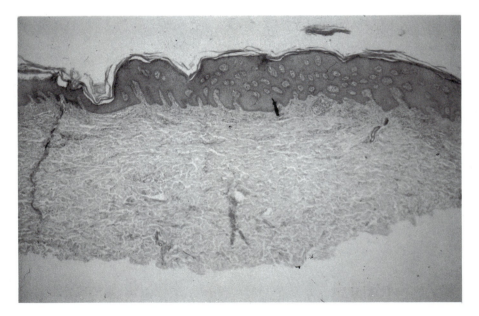

Fig. 5. Histological section corresponding to Fig. 4 (H & E, ×25)

result, the entry echo is distinctly thinner. The underlying echolucent band again shows faint, inhomogeneously distributed internal echoes. The corium gives the impression of being slightly dispersed. In the lower right part of the picture one finds two oblique echolucent structures (arrows) which correspond to hair follicles the histological section. Fig. 5 corresponds to the sonogram of Fig. 4, but does not show these hair follicles. However, severe acanthosis with underlying inflammatory infiltration is apparent. Both are most likely responsible for the echolucent band.

Discussion

To understand and interpret these findings it is important to discuss the basic sonographic phenomena and artifacts that can occur on the path of the signal on its way through the psoriasis plaque:

1. Coupling water bath

Especially when evaluating a psoriasis plaque unexperienced investigators are inclined to use a high-energy signal or a strong amplification of the received echoes. This frequently causes echoes in the coupling water bath.

2. Parahyperkeratosis / stratum corneum

The parahyperkeratosis in psoriasis (or the healthy stratum corneum) represents the first important borderline to the ultrasound signal entering the skin and causes reflections. We call this reflection "entry echo". The micromorphological aspect of the parahyperkeratotic stratum corneum of a psoriatic plaque appears to be inhomogeneous in contrast to normal stratum corneum (as far as it can be evaluated in the histological section). Both show air inclusions to a different extent. Since the axial resolution of a 20-MHz scanner is close to 80 μm, the normal horny layer and epidermis appear as one echo zone. The thickened, parahyperkeratotic stratum corneum in psoriasis plaques, however, can be differentiated from the acanthotic epidermis. Following the entry echo, the parahyperkeratotic structures provide further borderlines causing echoes and dispersion of ultrasound signals.

3. Acanthosis / epidermis

The epidermis has a mainly homogeneous structure. The distances between keratinocytes are clearly above 80 μm so that only few echoes can be expected from this layer. This applies to the acanthosis as well, but it can be differentiated from the entry echo on account of its thickness, of distinctly above 80 μm in most cases. Both epidermis and acanthosis are presented as an echo-poor band as a rule.

4. Edema / infiltration

From oncology as well as from investigations of allergic reactions it is known that both edema or inflammatory infiltration are presented echo poor.

In our experience it is possible to describe a psoriatic plaque by B-scan ultrasound [21]. The method is limited by the pattern of reflections of the first borderline which consists of the psoriatic parahyperkeratosis or the stratum corneum. The reflexogeneous echo band of this layer (entry echo) is indeed dependent upon the thickness of the borderline. Comparative sonometrical and histometrical thickness measurements of the epidermis of healthy skin (secondary excisions of malignant melanoma) lead to differences of up to 35% and a correlation of only $r=0.32$. Even the sonometrical thickness measurements of parahyperkeratotic stratum corneum do not correspond well to histometry or in vivo conditions. Nevertheless, we can observe changes in the reflex patterns of the entry echo during therapy. It is conceivable that better sonographic evaluation of the epidermis will be achieved in the future by means of high-frequency scannerss (> 50 MHz) equipped with time-gain compensation amplifiers.

The echo-poor band following the entry echo can possibly be explained in the presence of acanthosis. Sonographically we cannot differentiate acanthosis from echo-poor infiltration or edema. It is known that the local application of steroids reduces inflammatory infiltration. In pilot studies we applied topical steroids on psoriatic lesions. The following sonographic evaluation revealed no difference in the thickness of the echo-poor band. We assume that the acanthosis represents the main morphological correlation of the echo-poor band underneath the entry echo. However, the echo-poor band is not pathognomonic for psoriasis as it is also found in other dermatoses (Fig. 2).

Investigating healing plaques on treated patients we detected an echo-poor band, although clearly thinner, even after complete clinical clearing of the lesion.

We made these observations on three of seven patients who were evaluated by sonography for various times within several weeks.

This observation will be a major aspect of our investigations in the future ultrasound as 20 MHz proved to be an effective tool to study progression and the effects of treatment in this disease. Whether sonographically achieved parameters are also superior to clinical parameters as is the case with circumscribed scleroderma must be analyzed in further studies.

References

1. Alexander H, Miller DL (1979) Determining skin thickness with pulsed ultrasound. J Invest Derm 72: 17–19
2. Altmeyer P (1989) Dermatologische Ultraschalldiagnostik – gegenwärtiger Stand und Perspektiven (Editorial). Z Hautkr 64: 727–728
3. Altmeyer P, Hoffmann K, el-Gammal S (1990) Sonographie der Haut. MMW 132 (18): 14–22

4. Brazier S, Shaw S (1986) High-frequency ultrasound measurement of patch test reactions. Contact Dermatitis 15: 199–201
5. Breitbart EW, Hicks R, Rehpennig W (1985) Möglichkeiten der Ultraschalldiagnostik in der Dermatologie. Z Hautkr 61: 522–526
6. Breitbart EW, Müller CH, Hicks R, Vieluf D (1989) Neue Entwicklungen der Ultraschalldiagnostik in der Dermatologie. Acta Dermatol 15: 57–61
7. Dines KA, Sheets PW, Brink JA, Hanke CW, Condra KA, Clendenon JL, Goss SA, Smith JS, Franklin TD (1984) High frequency ultrasonic of skin: experimental results. Ultrason Imaging 6: 408–434
8. El-Gammal S (1990) Experimental approaches and new developments with high frequency ultrasound in dermatology. Zentralbl Haut 157: 327
9. Feldmann S, Hoffmann K, el-Gammal S, Altmeyer P (1990) Sonographic quantification of the tuberculin-type reaction Zentralbl Haut 157: 320–321
10. Fornage DW, Deshaynes JL (1986) Ultrasound of normal skin. J Clin Ultras 14: 619–622
11. Görtz S, Hoffmann K, el-Gammal S, Altmeyer P (1990) High frequency b-scan sonography and skin-thickness measurement of normal skin. Zentralbl Haut 157: 319–320
12. Hoffmann K, el-Gammal S, Altmeyer P (1989) 20 MHz B-scan Sonographie an Händen und Füßen. In: Altmeyer P et al. Handsymposium: Dermatologische Erkrankungen der Hände und Füße, Edition Roche: 285–300
13. Hoffmann K, el-Gammal S, Matthes U, Altmeyer P (1989) 20 MHz Sonographie der Haut in der präoperativen Diagnostik. Z Hautkr 64: 851–858
14. Hoffmann K, Stücker M, el-Gammal S, Altmeyer P (1990) Digitale 20- MHz-Sonographie des Basalioms im b-scan. Hautarzt 41: 333–339
15. Hoffmann K, el-Gammal S, Altmeyer P (1990) b-scan Sonographie in der Dermatologie. Hautarzt 41: W7–W16
16. Kirsch JM, Hanson ME, Gibson JR (1984) The determination of skin-thickness using conventional ultrasound equipment. Clin Exp Dermatol 9: 280–285
17. Lawrence CM, Shuster S (1985) Comparison of ultrasound and caliper measurements of normal and inflamed skin thickness. J Dermatol 112: 195–200
18. Murikami S, Miki Y (1989) Human skin histology using high-resolution echography. J Clin Ultras 17: 77–82
19. Querleux B, Léveque JL, de Rigal J (1988) In vivo cross-sectional ultrasonic imaging of human skin. Dermatologica 177: 332–337
20. Rigal J, Escoffier C, Querleux B, Faivre B, Agach P, Léveque JL (1989) Assessment of aging of the human skin by in vivo ultrasonic imaging. J Invest Dermatil 93: 621–625
21. Schuster S, Black MM, McVitie E (1975) The influence of age and sex on skin thickness, skin collagen and density. Br J Dermatol 93: 639–643
22. Sondergaard J, Serup J, Tikjob G (1985) Ultrasonic a- and b-scanning in clinical and experimental dermatology. Acta Dermatol Venereol 65 [Suppl 120]: 76–82
23. Tan CY, Statham B, Marks R, Payne PA (1982) Skin thickness measurement by pulsed ultrasound: its reproducibility, validation and variability. Br J Dermatol 106: 657–667

Ultrasound Assessment of the Comparative Atrophogenicity of Potent Fluorinated and Nonfluorinated Topical Glucocorticoids

H.C. Korting, D. Vieluf, and M. Kerscher

Upon prolonged application of prednicarbate to normal human skin no signs of skin atrophy were seen either on clinical or histopathological inspection [5]. This finding deserved further investigation, as prednicarbate has been found to be about as potent in controlled clinical trials as the well-known conventional glucocorticoid betamethasone-17-valerate [8]. In fact, these two findings hint at an increased benefit/risk ratio for prednicarbate as the first clinically applied congener of the new class of glucocorticoids of the nonfluorinated double ester type [6].

As early as 1981, Tan and co-workers proposed using ultrasound analysis of the skin to assess the reduction of skin thickness brought about by the application of topical glucocorticoids [7]. More recently, Dykes et al. [2] demonstrated a clear-cut reduction of skin thickness upon repeated application of both betamethasone-17-valerate and fluocinolone acetonide, but not prednicarbate. In fact, the slight reduction of skin thickness due to the prednicarbate preparation used was about the same as with the corresponding vehicle. These findings, however, are in conflict with the more recent ones by Lubach and Grüter [4], who reported marked skin atrophy due to the application of prednicarbate. Atrophy was similar to that found using the conventional potent glucocorticoid amcinonide. Both these trials were based on ultrasound analysis of the skin using only the A-mode, as initially proposed by Tan and co-workers [7]. Therefore, we found it rewarding to initiate one further trial using both the A- and B-mode to get additional insight into the problem.

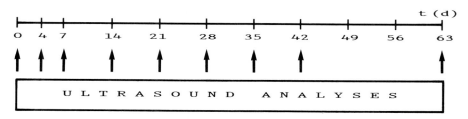

Fig. 1. Schedule of the application of the various topical treatment modalities and of ultrasound analyses (treatment time: 6 weeks)

As described earlier [3], 24 healthy volunteers were enrolled in a randomized double-blind trial. Four different treatment modalities were used: 1. prednicarbate cream 0.25 % (A); 2. the corresponding vehicle (B); 3. betamethasone-17-valerate cream 0.1 % (C); and 4. clobetasol-17-propionate cream 0.05 % (D).

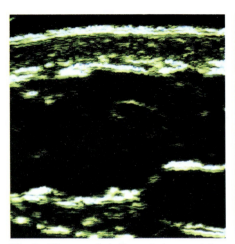

Fig. 2. Characteristic B-mode image at the start of the study

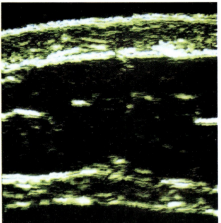

Fig. 3. Characteristic B-mode image after application of prednicarbate cream for a period of 6 weeks

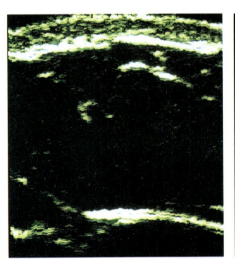

Fig. 4. Characteristic B-mode image after application of betamethasone-17-valerate cream for a period of 6 weeks

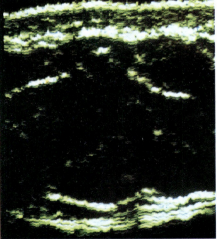

Fig. 5. Characteristic B-mode image after application of clobetasol 17-propionate cream for a period of 6 weeks

The proximal flexor part of the forearm is particularly prone to skin atrophy, according to clinical experience, and is also a site of predilection of atopic eczema, a prime indication for topical glucocorticoids. Thus, an area of 4 × 4 cm square on the most proximal part of the volar side of the forearm was chosen as the test area. The preparations analyzed were applied twice daily using 0.1–0.2 ml per site. All volunteers either received preparation A or B on one of their forearms and preparation C or D on the other. Skin thickness, defined as the thickness of epidermis and dermis, was assessed along a straight line between the input echo and the output echo. To identify representative parts of the skin, the sites for the assessment of skin thickness using A-mode were selected by using B-mode images. At each time point, six straight lines were analyzed at each test site, two of them lying at the very center at right angles, the other two parallel to the four borders. The thickness value was obtained as an arithmetic mean. Both for B- and A-mode analysis the DUB 20 system (Taberna Pro Medicum, Lüneburg, FRG) was used, as described recently [1]. The schedule of application of the various drugs and analyses is given in Fig. 1. In some volunteers, i.e. 8 in 12 applying clobetasol-propionate cream, eczema craquelé made discontinuation of application necessary before the end of the pre-fixed application period.

Figures 2–5 show B-mode images of the skin at the start and after 6 weeks' application of prednicarbate, betamethasone-17-valerate, and clobetasol-propionate cream. Figure 6 shows the corresponding image following long-term application of the prednicarbate cream vehicle; the corresponding A-mode image is superimposed on the B-mode image. Mean values of skin thickness before, during, and after application of the various treatment modalities are given in Fig. 7–10. According to multivariate analysis, there was no statistically significant difference with respect to the values for prednicarbate cream and the corresponding vehicle. Such a difference, however, could be demonstrated with the two conventional glucocorticoids from day 7 onward. If marked skin atrophy was seen after prolonged application of a conventional glucocorticoid, it took more than 2 weeks for nearly complete regeneration.

Although 0.25% prednicarbate cream and 0.1% betamethasone-17-valerate cream are about equipotent [8] in treating inflammatory skin disease, in particular eczema, clear-cut differences are found with respect to

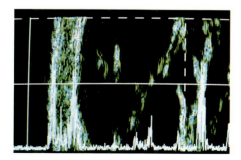

Fig. 6. Characteristic B-mode image after application of the prednicarbate cream vehicle for a period of 6 weeks. The corresponding A-mode image is superimposed

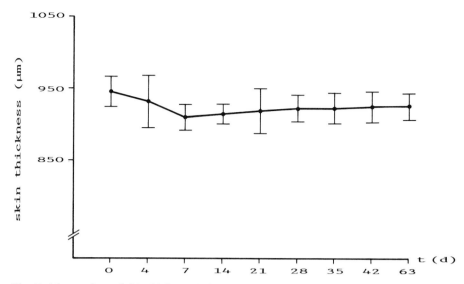

Fig. 7. Mean values of skin thickness before, during, and after application of prednicarbate cream

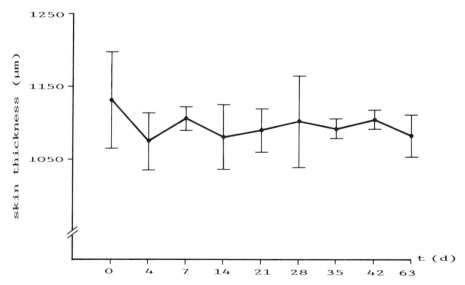

Fig. 8. Mean values of skin thickness before, during, and after application of the prednicarbate cream vehicle

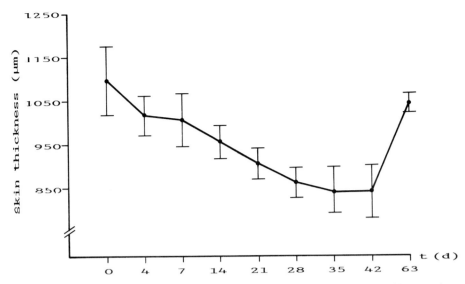

Fig. 9. Mean values of skin thickness before, during, and after application of betamethasone-17-valerate cream

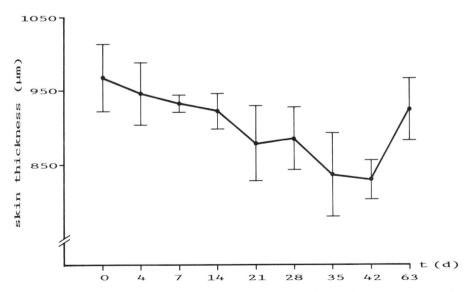

Fig. 10. Mean values of skin thickness before, during, and after application of clobetasol-17-propionate cream

the atrophogenic potential, at least in normal skin. This is even more relevant from a clinician's point of view, as there was no clear-cut difference between prednicarbate cream and the corresponding vehicle, i.e. a bland cream. This deserves further study, as skin atrophy due to potent fluorinated conventional glucocorticoids such as betamethasone-17-valerate seem to turn up even after short periods of application, i.e., the 7 days frequently required as the minimum amount of time needed to treat atopic eczema. The persistence of skin atrophy for a few weeks is important, since inflammatory skin diseases requiring treatment with glucocorticoids often tend to relapse early. Further investigations addressing other congeners of the nonfluorinated double ester type of topical glucocorticoids will have to determine whether, at the highest dose, the low atrophogenic potential of prednicarbate reflects a common quality of the entire group of substances. The present findings make it clear that ultrasound analysis is a valid tool to discriminate the atrophogenic potential of various glucocorticoids for topical use. Based on our experience, assessment of skin thickness should be done using data based on A-mode analysis of straight lines chosen from previously obtained B-mode images. This helps to avoid consideration of sites which are not representative of the entire test area.

References

1. Breitbart EW, Müller ChE, Hicks R, Vieluf D (1989) Neue Entwicklungen der Ultraschalldiagnostik in der Dermatologie. Aktuel Dermatol 15: 57–61
2. Dykes PJ, Hill S, Marks R (1988) Assessment of the atrophogenicity potential of corticosteroids by ultrasound and by epidermal biopsy under occlusive and nonocclusive conditions. In: Christophers E, Schöpf E, Kligman AM, Stoughton RB (eds) Topical corticosteri od therapy. Raven, New York, pp 111–118
3. Korting HC, Vieluf D, Kerscher M (1990) o.25 % Prednicarbate cream and the corresponding vehicle induce less skin atrophy than 0.1 % betamethasone 17-valerate cream and 0.05 % clobetasol propionate cream. Eur J Clin Pharmacol (in press)
4. Lubach D, Grüter M (1988) Vergleichende Untersuchungen über die hautverdünnende Wirkung von Amcinonid und Prednicarbat an unterschiedlichen Körperregionen des Menschen. Aktuel Dermatol 14: 197–200
5. Schröpl, F, Schubert C (1988) Long-term study on local steroids using thee example of prednicarbate. In: Christophers E, Schöpf E, Kligman AM, Stoughton RB (eds) Topical corticosteroid therapy. Raven, New York, pp 155–168
6. Stache U, Alpermann HG (1986) Zur Chemie und Pharmakologie von Prednicarbat (Hoe 777), einem halogenfreien, topischen antiinflammatorisch wirksamen Kortikosteroid. Haut Geschlechtskr 61 [Suppl 1]: 3–6
7. Tan C, Marks, R, Payne P (1981) Comparison of xeroradiographic and ultrasound detection of corticosteroid induced dermal thinning. J Invest Dermatol 76: 126–128
8. Vogt HJ, Höhler Th (1988) Controlled studies of intraindividual and interindividual design for comparing corticoids clinically. In: Christophers E, Schöpf E, Kligman AM, Stoughton RB (eds) Topical corticosteroid therapy. Raven, New York, pp 169–180

Ultrasound: Applications in the Study of Human Skin Disorders and the Response to Treatment

H. Schatz, T. Stoudemayer, and A.M. Kligman

Scanning Specifications

We emphasize the usefulness of the B-scan mode to obtain comparative information on the area, thickness, and echo characteristics of skin. B-scans show the skin as a two dimensional structure, allowing an overview, and facilitating the judgement of where to make measurements. Due to their one dimensional nature A-scans are not suitable for these assessments. For precise thickness measurements, we utilize the range of interest (ROI) function on our instrument by tracing the whole dermis with a trackball. The computer calculates the area in square millimeters and displays the mean intensity and standard deviation according to the 256 gray levels in the image. We then divide the area measure by the transducer range of 22.3 mm. If we use the highest B-scan resolution, the resulting distance represents the mean of 224 single measurements, procured by one automated procedure. Comparative echo intensity assessments require the use of a uniform swept gain throughout the study. Since every transducer has different characteristics it is not reliable to compare intensity measurements, obtained using different instruments, not even of the same model. The choice of a horizontal swept gain helps to minimize the error due to inconsistent skin-transducer distance.

Selection of the appropriate color scale is crucial. We prefer a scale that provides high definition in the lower echo domain, where black and white displays do not reveal subtle echo changes.

Characterization of Normal Skin

The interpretation of pathologic changes requires the establishment of values in reference to the normal state. We have detected a wide individual range of skin thickness and echo distribution in normals (Fig. 1). Apart from these individual variations, we found that different body sites show different echo characteristics.

In a study of 40 normal persons, encompassing young men, old men, young women, and old women (n=10 per group), we found significant differences ($p<0.0001$) among the mean skin thickness of the dorsal forearm (1.56 mm),

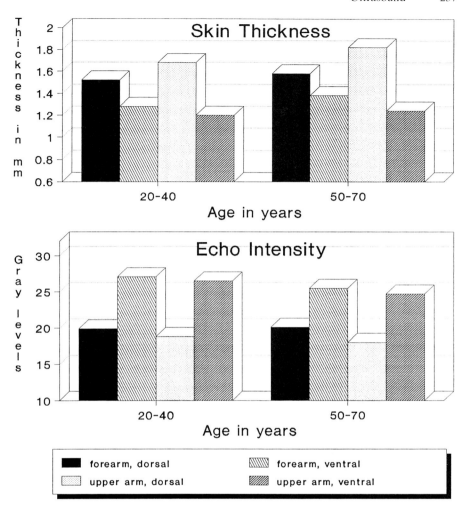

Fig. 1. Mean skin thickness and mean dermal echo intensity on the arms and forearms of normal individuals. Besides the wide variations at different body sites, note the negative correlation between the mean values for skin thickness and echo intensity

ventral forearm (1.39 mm), dorsal upper arm (1.80 mm) and ventral upper arm (1.26 mm). There were also differences among the test sites within each group ($p<0.02$). The standard deviation ranged between 0.05 mm and 0.3 mm. Thus the skin thickness for the dorsal upper arm covers the wide range of 1.70 mm to 2.70 mm. We found wide variations in dermal echo intensity. Various body regions showed significant differences. Generally, thicker skin tends to be less echo intense than thinner skin.

Aging

Aging changes can be monitored by evaluating the distribution of echoes throughout the dermis. In 1989, de Rigal et al [4] observed a characteristic nonechogenic sub-epidermal band as a common finding in progressively aged skin [4]. We could not demonstrate this to be a uniform finding, but there was a reduction of dermal echo amplitude and an increased interecho spacing below the epidermis at some body sites. Measurements of the thickness and

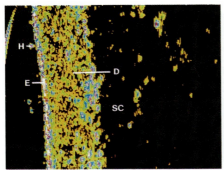

Fig. 2. Scan of the dorsal forearm of a 35-year-old subject with normal skin, E = epidermis, D = Dermis, SC = subcutaneous tissue, H = hair

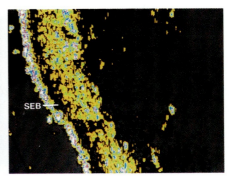

Fig. 3. Scan of the dorsal forearm of a 66-year-old subject. SEB = subepidermal band ("aging band")

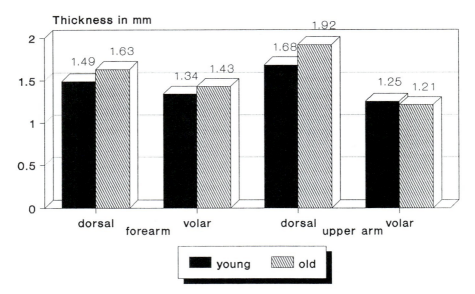

Fig. 4. The influence of sun exposure on skin thickness. Only on the dorsal (sun exposed) aspects of the forearms and upper arms significant thickening of the dermis was found

intensity of this band showed a significant decrease of echo with increasing age, especially on the dorsal aspect of the forearm. In contrast to de Rigal's findings, this band did not expand with increasing age, but decreased in echo intensity. The width of this band seems to depend more on skin thickness and body site. Some body regions, like the inner upper arm, show these echo patterns even in young subjects.

The presence of this subepidermal band (aging band) and the evaluation of its acoustic density can serve as a marker for age related skin changes.

Actinic Changes

Dermal thickness was measured on the arms and forearms of 25 old subjects (56–68 years) and 25 young subjects (17–29 years). We observed a significant increase with age only on the "sun-exposed" dorsal aspects of the arms ($p<0.05$ for the forearm and $p<0.01$ on the upper arm). The "sun-protected" volar aspects did not differ significantly. The low-intensity subepidermal band was characteristic of the dorsal aspect of the aged forearm and was found to be broader ($p<0.01$) and lower in echoes ($p<0.02$).

Osteoporosis

Experience suggested to us that the skin of osteoporosis patients is thinner than that of age matched normals. We compared various skin sites in osteoporosis patients and normal subjects (equal age groups). In a pilot study with 10 patients suffering from osteoporosis, we found a reduction in skin

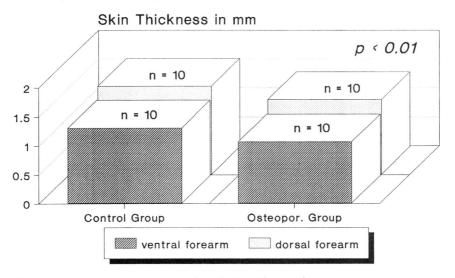

Fig. 5. Skin thickness in osteoporosis patients and normals

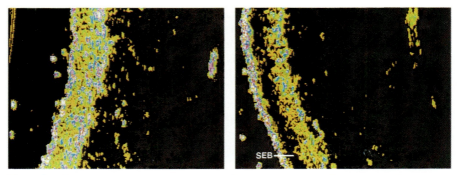

Fig. 6, 7. B-scans of dorsal upper arm of a 45-year-old patient (Fig. 6) and a 72-year-old patient (Fig. 7), both suffering from osteoporosis. The skin thickness is reduced to only 1.1 mm in both cases, compared to an average thickness of 1.8 mm. The older patient exhibits a clear subepidermal band (SEB)

thickness of 35% compared to the control group ($p<0.01$). Thus, in osteoporosis there may be a generalized loss of collagen. Accordingly, ultrasound assessment of the skin may be a useful prognosticator.

Wound Healing

Monitoring reepithelialization, formation of granulation tissue and contraction of wounds by means of ultrasound has many advantages. The effects of location, age, disease, or wound dressings can be determined objectively. Suction blisters and shave biopsies can serve as split-thickness test wounds. Punch biopsies create full-thickness wounds for studying repair by secondary

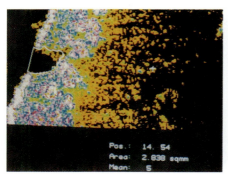

Fig. 8. Scan for the evaluation of wound volume after punch biopsy

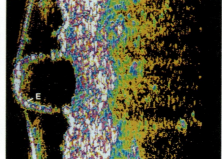

Fig. 9. Scan of a suction blister as a model for wound healing. The epidermis is separated from the dermis. After removal of the blister roof the reepithelialization process can be followed by B-scan imaging. E = epidermis (blister roof)

intention. Area measurements directly on the image allow calculation of the wound volume and the degree of regrowth of the epithelium (Fig. 8). A unique wound is the subepidermal blister (Fig. 9) raised by a suction device. After removal of the blister roof, the deepithelialized area can serve as a model to study reepithelialization or as a test area for topically applied drugs.

Scleroderma

The increased deposition of collagen in systemic scleroderma, morphea, and other sclerosing disorders are readily reflected in the ultrasonic image [5]. However, ultrasound examinations have still not come into use for grading the degree of involvement or for following up the response to therapeutic interventions. A-scans are unsatisfactory for this purpose.

Figure 10 presents a typical image of sclerodermatous skin. The wide high-intensity band in the lower two thirds of the dermis probably reflects the broad, parallel collagen bundles with diminished spacing. These collagen bundles are also reaching into the subcutaneous tissue.

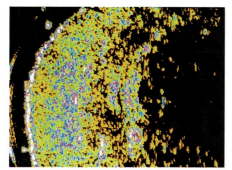

Fig. 10. Scan of the volar forearm of a 40-year-old woman with systemic scleroderma (skin thickness 2.1 mm)

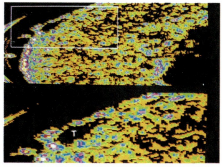

Fig. 11. Scan of a superficial spreading malignant melanoma 5 mm in diameter. T = tumor

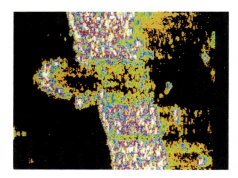

Fig. 12. Scan of a dermatofibroma penetrating the entire dermis

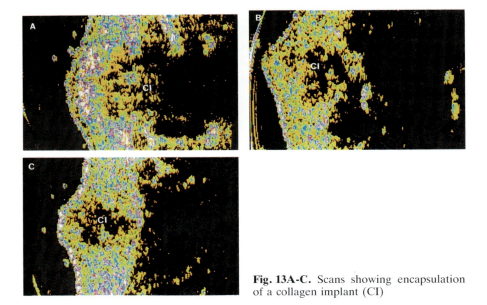

Fig. 13A-C. Scans showing encapsulation of a collagen implant (CI)

Tumors

Due to their cellular homogeneity, most skin tumors are presented as low echo areas and cannot be differentiated [2, 3]. Only the depth, area, and demarcation from the adjacent structures can be defined, possibly affecting prognosis. Ultrasound may help in determining the best surgical approach. Caution is necessary with tumors growing in an infiltrating way, since small satellites cannot be detected.

Fate of Collagen Implants

Bovine collagen is often used to correct scars and age wrinkles, but the long term results are unpredictable owing to variable resorption. We injected 0.1 ml of Zyplast (Collagen Corp) into volar forearm dermis and followed the progress of the implant by B-scan imaging. The freshly injected collagen was not confined to the dermis but actually dispersed into the subcutis (Fig. 13A). After one week the host dermis had partially encapsulated the implant (Fig. 13B). This process was complete by 3 weeks. At this time the implant became more prominent and firmer on palpation (Fig. 13C). The ultimate fate of the implant will be determined over 6 months.

Conclusion

The B-scan technique provides new opportunities for studying human skin in health and disease. The benefits for experimental dermatology are great and as of yet mainly unexplored. We are far from understanding how the different tissue structures contribute to the composition of the final image. However, measurements of thickness and area in B-scan mode have proved reliable for monitoring progressive changes and responses to treatment in a variety of disorders. More information can be extracted by analyzing the intensity patterns in the various skin layers. Closer interaction between researcher and clinician is required to improve applicability of this promising technique.

References

1. Alexander H, Miller DL (1979) Determining skin thickness with pulsed ultrasound. J Invest Derm 72: 17–19
2. Breitbart EW, Rehpennig W (1982) Möglichkeiten und Grenzen der Ultraschalldiagnostik zur in vivo Bestimmung der Invasionstiefe des malignen Melanoms. Z Hautkr 58: 975–987
3. Hughes BR, Black D, Sriastava A, Dalziel K, Marks R (1987) Comparison of techniques for the non-invasive assessment of skin tumors. Clin Exp Derm 12: 108–111
4. de Rigal J, Escoffier C, Querleux B, Faivre B, Agache P, Leveque J-L (1989) Assessment of aging of the human skin by in vivo ultrasonic imaging. J Invest Derm 93:621–625
5. Serup J (1984) Localized scleroderma (morphea): thickness of sclerotic plaques as measured by 15 MHz pulsed ultrasound. Acta Derm Venereol 64: 214–219

Experimental Approaches in 20 MHz Ultrasound

Ultrasound Evaluation of Wound Volume as a Measure of Wound Healing Rate

P.T. Pugliese, F. Moncloa, and R.T. McFadden

Introduction

Wound healing has traditionally been determined by the decrease in surface area of the wound. The tattoo technique of Abercrombie et al. [1] and wound area planimeter techniques are frequently employed [2, 3]. These methods are all subject to numerous errors and require meticulous attention to detail [4].

Wound volume, as a measurable parameter of wound healing, has been difficult to measure because many variables are required in calculating the volume of a changing wound. This article reports on a method to evaluate wound healing by the reduction in wound volume as determined by ultrasound measurements.

Method and Materials

The study population included 15 normal male volunteers, 51–66 years of age. A medical history, physical examination, and laboratory tests were performed on all subjects. Each subject underwent four punch biopsies in the lumbar parasacral region previously infiltrated with lidocaine 1%. The punch had a 4 mm internal diameter and was calibrated to a 4 mm depth with a depth-stop. The wounds were numbered 1–4 from left to right in each subject and were allocated as treated or untreated wounds. Each of the treated wounds received 0.05 mls of porcine omental extract during the 28 days of the study. All wounds were dressed with dry gauze.

Measurements were made on days 1, 2, 3, 7, 10, 14, 17, 21, and 28 by the following methods.
1. External diameter using a micrometer (Mitutoyo-Digimatic)
2. External area using a transparent acetate sheet tracing of the wound and estimation of the area with a planimeter
3. Depth and internal diameter by ultrasound imaging by B-scan using a DUB 20 (TPM, Lüneberg, FRG) (Fig. 1)

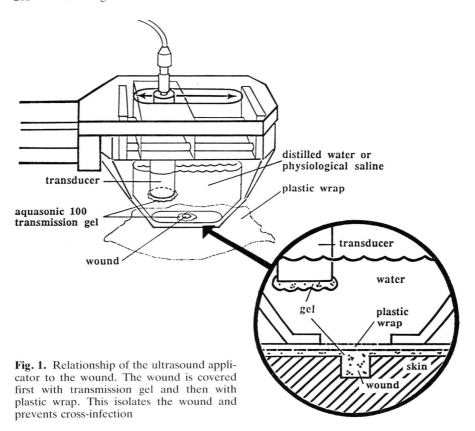

Fig. 1. Relationship of the ultrasound applicator to the wound. The wound is covered first with transmission gel and then with plastic wrap. This isolates the wound and prevents cross-infection

The volume of each wound was calculated using the following formula:

$$V = \pi D_1 + D_1 D_2 + D_2^2$$

where h = wound depth, D_1 = external diameter, and D_2 = internal diameter (Fig. 2).

Measurements were made directly from the video screen using the internal program of the DUB 20.

Results

The results are reported as the rate of wound closure of treated vs untreated wounds, as measured by both the external diameter and the wound volume. These results are plotted on a semilog scale. Figure 3 shows the separation of the two rates after day 10; in Fig. 4, an identical pattern is seen for the plot of

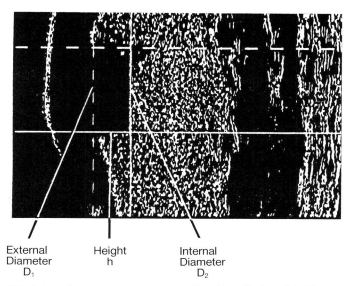

Fig. 2. Relationship of the internal measurement system to the video display of the B-scan of the wound. The location of the measurement parameters D_1, D_2, and h are indicated on the diagram

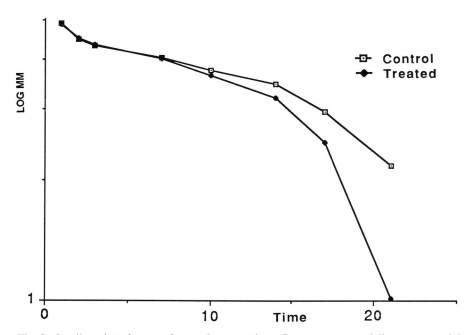

Fig. 3. Semilog plot of external wound area vs time. Curve appears to follow exponential rate

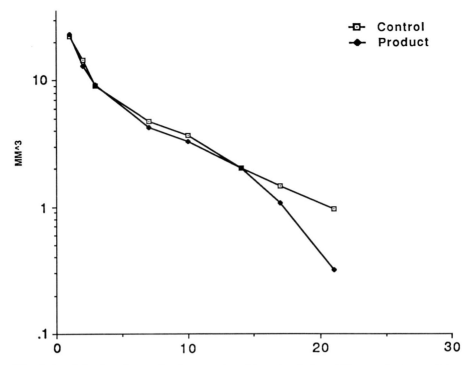

Fig. 4. Semiolg plot of wound volume vs time. Note the distinct difference in shape of the curve as compared to Fig. 3. A polyexponential function appears operative in wound volume reduction

wound volume. It appears from these graphs that the untreated wounds follow an exponential curve while the treated wounds follow a polyexponential curve.

The technique of applying the ultrasound applicator in this study proved to be an important variable. Careful pressure was needed to seal the edges of the applicator to the plastic wrap covering the wound. It was necessary to scan the wound at least three times in order to assure that the maximum wound depth had been scanned and that the scan was reproducible. One scan was selected for this series for wound evaluation.

Discussion

While the physical dimensions of the wound are fundamental in wound healing, the quality of the wound is also important. The amount of collagen and elastin laid down with the wound relates to the amount of fibrosis developed within the wound site. The ultrasound B-scan measurements not

Ultrasound Evaluation of Wound Volume as a Measure   271

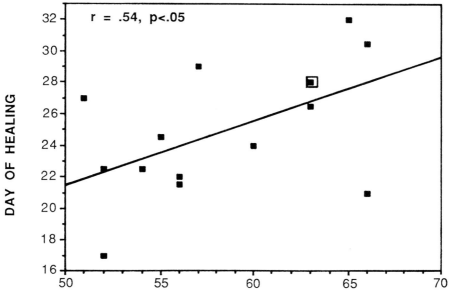

Fig. 5. Correlation plot between days of healing vs subject age with control wounds. Longer healing time is apparent for older subjects

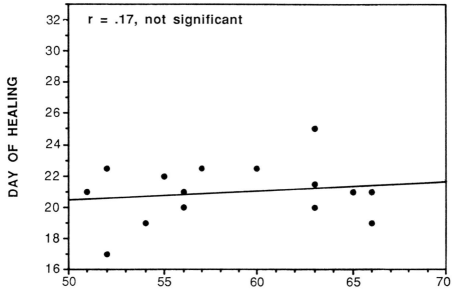

Fig. 6. Correlation plot between days of healing vs subject age with porcine omental extract treated wounds. The age differential is removed, indicating efficacy of the porcine omental extract as a wound healing agent

only allow an accurate determination of the physical dimensions of a healing wound, but also provide an index to structural components of the wound. At present we cannot define with great accuracy the individual dermal components as seen in the B-scan. Greater tissue resolution, perhaps 10–15 μm, would aid in reaching this goal.

These preliminary studies also reveal the well-established delayed healing in aging skin, as seen in Fig. 5. This graph of the wound healing rate vs subject age shows a linear increase in wound healing time with age [5]. This effect is almost obliterated by the use of porcine omental extract (Fig. 6).

Conclusions

The ultrasound B-scan is a valid method to measure wound volume over time. The use of wound volume is as reliable as surface measurement of wound closure, but provides more information. Ultrasound scans for evaluation of wound healing is a new technique and should extend the utility of wound healing models both for the assessment of product efficacy and the understanding of the physiology of wound healing.

References

1. Ambercrombie M, Flerit MH, James DW (1954) Collagen formation and wound contraction during repair of small excised wounds in the skin of rats. J Embryol Exp Morphol 2: 264
2. Lerpziger LS et al. (1985) Dermal wound repair: role of collagen matrix implants and synthetic polymer dressings. J Am Dermatol 12: 409–419
3. Brown G et al. (1989) Enhancement of wound healing by topical treatment with epidermal growth factor. N Engl J Med 321: 76–79
4. Mayno G (1979) The story of the myofibroblasts. Am Surg Pathol 3: 535–542
5. Chvapil M, Kooperman CF (1982) Age and other factors regulating wound healing. Otolaryngol Clin North Am 15: 259

Possibilities for Application of High-Frequency Ultrasound in Clinical Research

K. Hoffmann, S. el-Gammal, T. Dirschka, K. Winkler, S. Feldmann, and P. Altmeyer

Due to the speed of innovation in microelectronics the ultrasound scanners now available in dermatology have decisive advantages over those available only 2 or 3 years ago [5, 7, 44, 45, 48, 55]. Today we have at our disposal not only the coloured high-frequency B-scan, but also abundant possibilities of image analysis [14, 26–29, 43, 49]. Direct computer-aided measurement (sonometry) of a structure (STOI) or region of interst (ROI) on the screen is no longer a problem. Amplitude measurements permit very precise determination of the echogenicity of preselected areas (densitometry). In addition, integrated (intelligent) computer systems offer a number of further possibilities [21]. Today we are also able to store the images in digital form on diskette or hard disk and to retrieve and process them at any time. It is thus only logical that we should think about whether ultrasonography might be of assistance to the dermatologist in clinical-experimental research. We will therefore discuss below some experimental applications of high-resolution ultrasound used by our working group.

Ultrasound Measurement of Skin Aging In Vivo

The literature contains little precise information on in vivo skin thickness in humans [18, 19, 23, 31, 56–58]. High-resolution ultrasound thus offers itself as a method of noninvasive measurement of skin thickness (sonometry). The availability of high-frequency scanners which permit B-mode imaging now also gives us the opportunity to examine larger populations [25].

We know from ultrassound examinations that the skin becomes thinner with increasing age [40]. The examinations on which this information is based were performed mainly with scanners only operating in A-mode [1, 10, 57]. Although these scanners permit evaluation of skin thickness they do not permit topographic orientation within the skin. Skin changes typical of actinic elastosis were thus not found [40].

Senile elastosis produces a characteristic reflex pattern on ultrasound examination [7, 17, 28, 50]. The physical phenomena which occur are a direct correlate of the morphological features of the elastotically transformed skin. It is thus important to look first at the structural changes in the skin.

Senile elastosis is a highly chronic aging process in the skin which results from exposure to UVB, UVA and also infrared radiation [32, 34]. In view of this aetiopathogenesis the term senile actinic elastosis is used [40]. The purpose of this term is to make a clear distinction between this extrinsic alteration of the skin and intrinsic aging of the skin not induced by external factors. The use of the word "senile" is intended to indicate that the changes appear decades after exposure and are thus characteristic of old age. However, ultrasound imaging of the skin shows that we can expect to find incipient elastosis from the age of 25 onwards [25, 50] so that it is better to restrict ourselves to the term *actinic elastosis*. Clinically we see pale yellowish, sometimes raised indurations in the exposed regions, especially the temples, the forehead and the back of the neck; the skin is wrinkled and lax, with variegated colouring and sometimes scaling [40]. Histologically the skin with chronic actinic damage shows a thinner epidermis, reduction of the subepidermal elastica plexus and fragmentation and clumping of collagen fibres in the upper dermis which stain like elastic fibres. The increase and alteration of this elastotic material is the correlate and indicator of elastosis as, on the one hand, it precedes and is more marked than all other elastotic changes and, on the other, indicates progression of the process [42, 51].

Ultrastructural examination shows that this elastotic material is a three-component system [11]. We find:

1. elastotic matrix, 2. microfibrils, and 3. electron-dense inclusions. We can assume that there is an active process of formation of the elastotic material with a tendency, as the elastotic fibre formation progresses, towards degenerative changes such as irregular fibre arrangement and later vacuolar disintegration. At the same time the production of collagen fibres declines. There is an excessive increase in proteoglycans and glycosaminoglycans. In the upper dermis, and less often also in the epidermis, we find a sparse inflammatory infiltrate [37]. This complex process of fibre restructuring ends in complete dermal metamorphosis which appears as a tangle of haphazardly arranged fibres and finally as an amorphous disorganized mass [34, 42].

Case Study. Figure 1 shows the ultrasound scan of the cheek of a 48-year-old woman. Below an entry echo running in a straight line and slightly thickened compared with control populations, we see an echo-poor (black) band with well-defined boundaries running in a longitudinal direction. Within this echo-poor band we see inhomogeneously distributed, strong internal reflexes. The reflex pattern of the underlying corium is normal for the patient's age. Below this we see the subcutis.

Figure 2 shows the ultrasound scan of the forehead of a 68-year-old woman. We again see a slightly thickened entry echo and below there is an echolucent band with marginally located, ill-defined internal echoes. The border with the underlying corium is irregular and "serrated". The border between the corium and the subcutis is also indistinct. At the bottom of the picture, forming the border of the subcutis, we see the galea and below it the skull bone.

In the B scan the actinic elastosis appears between the entry echo and the dermal reflexes as an echo-poor, frequently also echolucent, band containing inhomogeneously distributed, ill-defined internal reflexes. The borders with

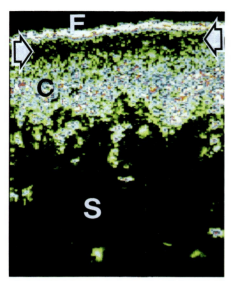 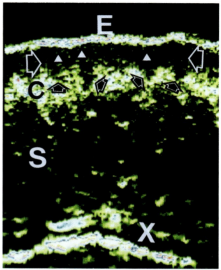

Fig. 1. Ultrasound scan[1] of the cheek (at the level of the zygomatic bone) of a 48-year-old woman. E, entry echo; *arrows*, echolucent band; C, corium; S, subcutis

Fig. 2. Ultrasound scan of the forehead of a 68-year-old woman. E, entry echo; *open arrows*, echolucent band; *arrowheads*, internal echoes; serrated *closed arrows*, serrated border of the corium; X, galea/skull bone

the entry echo is usually sharp. The basal border can be indistinct. In particular in severe elastosis the inferior margin of the echo-poor band is frequently "serrated" [7, 28, 29], in less severe elastosis the border is usually sharp. We refer to this as the echolucent band (ELB). The severity of the elastosis, i. e. the width of the zone of elastotic transformation in the upper dermis, can be measured directly on the ultrasound scan using a graticule which can be displayed on the screen. On account of the indistinct dorsal demarcation it is sometimes difficult to determine the depth of the band. In these cases the thickness of the band can be measured in a so-called "summated A-scan". Here all the reflex lines composing the B-scan are shown as a single averaged amplitude image. The simultaneous presentation of this summated A scan and the corresponding B scan permits highly accurate measurement of the visualized structures. As a rule the measurements show no inter-examiner variation when this procedure is used. The software integrated in the scanner permits densitometric quantification of the density and intensity of the echoes in particular areas.

---

[1] All the ultrasound scans presented in this paper were made with the DUB 20 (Taberna pro medium, Lüneburg, FRG). In principle, however, such results can also be obtained with the Dermascan C Cortex, Hadsund, DK or with other scanners.

That the ELB is the ultrasonic correlate of actinic elastosis is supported by the following evidence:
- The phenomenon of the echo-poor (to echolucent) band below the entry echo is found only in areas of the skin exposed to light (forehead, cheek, outer aspect of the forearm etc), but not on the buttocks or proximal thighs, i.e. in regions of the skin protected from sunlight. To date no ELB has ever been found in children.
- Knowledge of the micromorphology of actinic elastosis explains the development of the ELB in actinically damaged skin.
- The corial reflexes are produced mainly by the bundles of collagen fibres. As a result of the actinic exposure the subepidermal elastica plexus is destroyed and the upper and middle dermis are homogenised into an amorphous structure so that there is a depletion of interfaces in the dermis.
- The frequently found, sparse inflammatory infiltration is echo-poor [28].

The high-frequency B-scan permits exact quantification of the actinically damaged dermis and gives us a noninvasive means of determining the extent of damage. The ELB becomes wider and also less echogenic with increasing age. It is important not to confuse the ELB of actinic elastosis with similar phenomena produced by marked inflammatory infiltration of the skin (e.g. atopic dermatitis) or in the skin of a rosacea patient. It is also important that the skin is always examined under the same degree of tension as tautening of the skin also leads to an immediate increase in reflectivity in the ELB.

A combination of ultrasound measurement of the thickness of the echo-poor band and densitometric quantification of the internal echoes could conceivably be employed to observe the course of development in longitudinal studies. On the other hand exact quantification of treatment of this skin condition, e.g. with topically applied retinoids [33] or hyaluronic acid, might be possible. Unfortunately no conclusive data on this is yet available.

Measurement of Skin Thickness Under Corticoid Treatment

In addition to the many beneficial and desirable effects of topically applied corticoids these preparations also have a number of significant adverse effects on the skin. Here ultrasonography is a suitable method to quantify the morphological changes. Amongst the adverse effects, corticoids are known to cause the following morphological changes in the skin [2–4]:
- Inhibition of epidermal proliferation and regeneration
- Degeneration of collagen and destruction of elastic connective tissue
- Atrophy of adipose tissue

When using ultrasound to examine these adverse effects in clinical trials a number of fundamental principles must be observed. Not all parts of the body are equally suitable for ultrasound examination. In the corium of the back, for example, the basal border is difficult to identify. Further, the echoes are ill defined and there is no distinct basal demarcation. The thighs and the buttocks are also less suitable for such investigations as screening examinations have shown that projections and islands of fatty tissue in the corium are often found in these regions. The forearm, on the other hand, with its well-defined boundaries and good visualization of the thin corium is well suited for monitored testing using ultrasound. As far as possible, measurement of skin atrophy under corticoid treatment should be performed in healthy skin as this reduces the likelihood of measuring errors such as might, for example, be caused by inflammatory infiltration or oedema.

Up to now the echo texture of the test site "forearm" has not yet been described. However, knowledge of the echo pattern of healthy skin in this region is a precondition for exact evaluation of the ultrasound scans in all clinical-experimental undertakings. Thus, individual deviations of skin structure can only be evaluated in direct comparison with healthy skin. Concomitant examination of healthy skin is thus indispensable.

The skin on the volar side of the forearm shows a characteristic structure in the ultrasound scan. Entry echo, corium, subcutis and sometimes the muscle fascia can be readily distinguished. The corium in this skin area can be divided into an echo-poor (upper to middle corium) and an echo-rich (middle to lower corium) portion. Determination of the skin thickness by ultrasound is not a problem as the lower border of the corium is well defined. Men have thicker skin on the volar forearm than women. The mean thickness of 1254 µm in men is 23.87 % greater than that of 1012 µm in women. In our experience, when a highly potent steroid (clobetasol-17-propionate) is applied several times a day for 4 weeks the first identifiable skin changes in ultrasound can be seen from the 14th day onwards. The entry echo becomes narrower and the reflex pattern becomes less homogeneous than in the previous scans. The echo texture of the upper corium becomes looser. At this point the skin thickness is reduced by about 50 µm compared with the initial measurement. In the subsequent period the ultrasound image shows no additional changes apart from a further reduction in skin thickness of up to 20 % (max. 170 µm).

Other working groups have also shown clearly that ultrasound is currently the best noninvasive procedure for quantification of dermal atrophy [20, 24, 38].

Wound Healing Model Monitoring by Ultrasound

Although various wound healing models have been discussed for years, no model fulfilling all conditions has yet been able to assert itself. This is due to the complex variables influencing wound healing. A standardized in vivo model for wound healing in humans generally accepted in medicine has therefore not yet been defined. There are, moreover, no objective and noninvasive measuring systems available for quantification of wound healing processes in the deeper layers of the skin.

Cryosurgery, a wound healing model for the skin, is a therapeutic procedure which is particularly suitable for the treatment of malignant epithelial tumours, especially of basal cell carcinomas of the face. As a result of the high incidence of the basal cell carcinoma we can apply strict inclusion criteria and thus obtain a homogeneous patient sample. The required standardization of the wounds can also as a rule be achieved in cryosurgery: both the surface area and the depth of the defect can be controlled by the size of the probe, the freezing temperature and the number of freezing cycles [6, 39, 64]. Ultrasound has already often been used for monitoring the course of repair processes in the skin [13, 15, 63].

We used ultrasound to monitor the healing process in 75 patients who had undergone cryosurgery of basal cell carcinomas in the head and neck region in order to determine the extent to which ultrasound is able to provide additional information on wound healing in the skin.

Case Study. In a 69-year-old woman a solid basal cell carcinoma on the right cheek was confirmed by biopsy a few weeks previously (Fig. 3). The corresponding ultrasound scan (Fig. 4) shows an echolucent tumour area with sharply defined basal margins but no

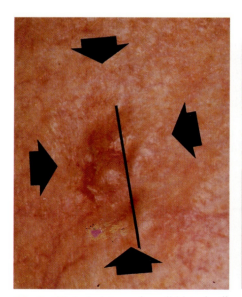
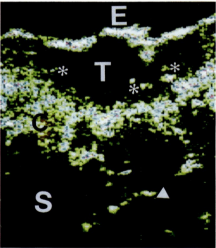

Fig. 3. Clinical picture of a solid basal cell carcinoma on the cheek of a 69-year-old woman. The ultrasound plane of section corresponds to the *marked line*. *Arrows* mark the clinically and sonographical determined tumour boundaries

Fig. 4. Ultrasound scan corresponding to the plane of section marked in Fig. 3. *E*, entry echo; *T*, tumour; *C*, corium; *S*, subcutis; asterisks, marginally situated, weak to strong internal reflexes; *arrowhead*, band of connective tissue in the subcutaneous fatty tissue

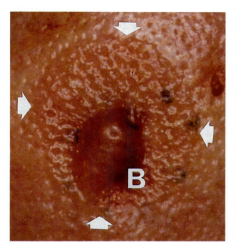
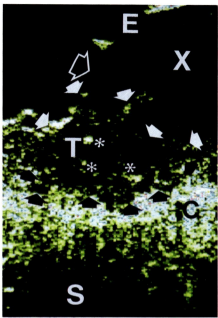

Fig. 5. Clinical picture 1 day after cryosurgery (20-mm probe, probe temperature −154 °C, tissue temperature −29 °C). *Arrows*, margins of defect; *B*, bulla

Fig. 6. Ultrasound scan recorded above the bulla. *E*, entry echo; *X*, lumen of the bulla; *open arrow*, loss of echoes due to scattering phenomena at the lateral ascending wall of the bulla; *T*, former tumour area; *closed arrows*, borders of the tumour area; *C*, corium; *S*, subcutis; *asterisks*, internal reflexes

distinguishable lateral demarcation. The entry echo is slightly thickened at the centre and interrupted in places due to scattering phenomena. Occasional marginally located, weak to strong internal reflexes can be seen within the echo-poor tumour area. The inferior border between the corium and the subcutis is irregular, but clearly distinguishable. The subcutis displays narrow reflex bands which correspond to bands of connective tissue. One day after cryosurgery of the basal cell carcinoma using a 20-mm probe a bulla developed within the region of the tumour (Fig. 5). The outline of the probe can be seen on the healthy peritumoral skin. The ultrasound scan (Fig. 6) depicts the bulla as a large echolucent area. The entry echo arising from the top of the blister is distinctly thinner and is interrupted at the lateral, ascending edges of the blister due to scattering phenomena. The necrotic tumour masses within the blister are shown as an echo-poor area containing ill-defined, inhomogeneously distributed internal reflexes. The border between the necrotic tumour area and the underlying corium is discernible. The inferior border between the corium and subcutis is indistinct on account of the development of an inflammatory infiltrate and oedema.

On day 21 (Fig. 7) the lesion is still covered in places by a fibrinous layer although most of it is already reepithelialized. The corresponding ultrasound image (Fig. 8) originates from the border of the lesion. Two entry echoes can be seen. The lower one can be interpreted as preformed epithelium below the more echogenic fibrinous layer. In the necrotic area strong internal reflexes can be seen. Its basal demarcation is indistinct. The border between the lower corium and the subcutis is still blurred. Three months after the cryosurgery (Fig. 9) the necrotic area has disappeared. On the former lesion we see the epithelial hyperplasia which

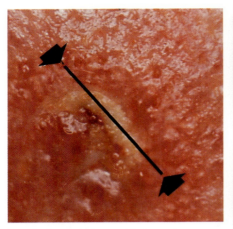

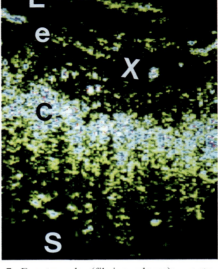

Fig. 7. Clinical picture 21 days after treatment *Line/arrows*, plane of section above the fibrinous layer

Fig. 8. Ultrasound scan corresponding to Fig. 7. *E*, entry echo (fibrinous layer); *e*, entry echo (necrotic area); *X*, necrotic area; *C*, corium; *S*, subcutis

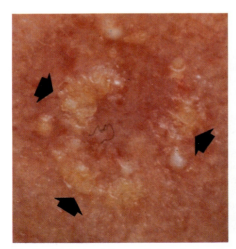

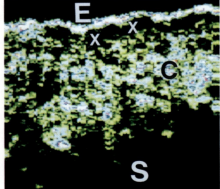

Fig. 9. Clinical picture of the lesion 3 months after cryosurgery. *Arrows*, fibrinous layer

Fig. 10. Ultrasound scan corresponding to Fig. 9. *E*, entry echo; *X*, scar area; *C*, corium; *S*, subcutis

often occurs after cryosurgical procedures and is also referred to as a "pseudorelapse". The ultrasound scan was made after removal of the hyperplasia. Below a now normal, slightly undulating entry echo the scar tissue appears as a narrow, echo-poor band. The image of the corium again shows approximately the same reflex pattern as that found in the initial scan (Fig. 10).

Sonometric measurement of the depth of tumour invasion is a particularly valuable aid in the standardization of cryolesions. Together with the superficial tumour area it permits us to calculate the tumour volume (Fig. 11). This corresponds approximately to the damage to be expected after cryosurgery [39, 64]. Taking this initial volume as the maximum expected damage the percentage wound healing on the subsequent days can readily be calculated.

Observation of cellular repair processes in the echo-poor necrotic area is limited by the resolution of the scanner. Thus, granulation tissue is not always exactly discernible on the 20-MHz sonogram. In some cases differentiation of granulation tissue and fresh scar tissue is possible, as both tissues appear equally echo-poor, by comparing sonograms recorded at different points in time. The follow-up examination is of particular importance as echo-poor internal echoes are found in the cryolesion at both the beginning and the end of the healing process. In the early phase after cryosurgery (days 2–4) the echo-poor internal echoes at the base of the ulcer can be interpreted on the basis of histological examinations as a conglomerate of remains of skin appendages and vessels occluded by fibrin-rich thrombi. On the other hand,

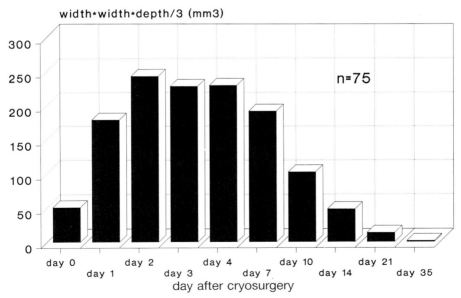

Fig. 11. Changes in the ultrasonically and clinically determined tumour volume over time. On the basis of our measurements, in later studies the volume should only be determined on days 0, 2, 10, 21 and around the 35th day

the most likely interpretation of the internal echoes present in the lesion at the end of the healing process is that they represent newly formed fine-fibrillary connective tissue which, on account of its irregular structure, forms interfaces for the ultrasound signal and thus gives rise to echoes.

The computer system integrated in the scanner permits continuous determination of the size of the echo-poor area of the lesion so that increases and decreases in size during the healing process can be accurately measured. We frequently find that, as already described by Lawrence and Shuster [37], it is difficult to distinguish between the inferior border of the corium and muscle fascia or subcutaneous bands of connective tissue and islands of fatty tissue, and that there is considerable oedematous enlargement of the corium. The absence of a discernible dermis-subcutis border, which often persists up to the 14th postoperative day, is not adequately explained by the persistence of the oedema and thus the continued expansion of the corium. It is also conceivable that we have here a phenomenon similar to that already reported by Brink[15] who describes thermic transformation of the originally echo-poor fatty tissue to echo-poor structures.

The reduced echogenicity is caused by a reduction of the interfaces in the more loosely structured exudative corium. On the other hand there is a considerable increase in absorption by the collagen bundles which have been pushed apart. In some cases disturbances of wound healing were reflected on the one hand in prolonged clinical phases of wound healing and on the other hand in persistence of reduced reflectivity in the region of the inflammatory infiltration on the ultrasound scan.

The exact determination of the depth of tumour invasion ensures correct choice of cryocycles, probe size and freezing temperature which are crucial for successful cryosurgery of basal cell carcinomas. In our sample the area and depth of the cryolesion were decisive for the duration and course of healing. We also found regional difference in the duration of wound healing in basal cell carcinomas of equal size. Basal cell carcinomas in the upper third of the face (forehead, temples) and the ear healed more slowly than basal cell carcinomas in the middle and lower thirds of the face (nose, lip, chin, neck). This is very probably due to the fact that the subcutaneous layer of fatty tissue in the temple/forehead region is only thin so that there is complete necrosis extending as far as the adjacent bony structures. Therefore we recommed that the tumour sites and sizes suitable for cryosurgery should be exactly defined in wound healing studies.

Quantification of Allergy Tests

In routine dermatological diagnosis type IV reactions are usually assessed visually and by determination of the diameter of palpable indurations.

The imprecision and subjective colouring of this simple method [62], which also neglects the important parameter of depth, has long been known. The search for a suitable method of quantification which also takes into account the depth of the reactions has not hitherto been very successful.

Measurement of skinfold thickness [58], which has also been used for evaluation of allergic reactions [37, 60, 61], proved to be too inexact in humans as the skinfold also contains subcutaneous tissue [18, 19, 23]. Radiographic methods [10] are not justifiable on account of the radiation exposure alone. Measurement of changes in blood flow velocity [8, 61] fails when it comes to differentiating very marked allergic reactions [54]. Ultrasound thus offers itself as measuring method [9, 12, 52, 53]. In allergic reactions the one-dimensional representation of the echoes in the A-scan is not suitable for the exact determination of the corium-subcutis border in regions with inflammatory infiltration or oedematous swelling. This has changed fundamentally with the advent of the latest generation of scanners as the modern, high-frequency B-mode scanners permit two-dimensional imaging of the type IV reaction and direct comparison with the histological section [22].

It is sometimes necessary to determine the functional status of cell-mediated immunoreactivity in patients [16, 30, 36, 41, 46, 59]. For this purpose a test system in the form of a stamp for intradermal administration of recall antigens has been developed (Multitest Mérieux) [35]. The antigens are applied to the volar surface of the forearm and the reaction evaluated 48 h later. The indurations which develop consist mainly of lymphocytic infiltrates [47]. However, they also contain an oedematous component. For quantification of type IV reactions to recall antigens, however, only the lymphocytic infiltrates are relevant. The oedema distorts the exact quantification of the reaction.

Case study. Figure 12 shows the ultrasound scan of the healthy right forearm (ventral aspect) of a 45-year-old healthy man before administration of a recall antigen test (the subsequent ultrasound scans originate from the identical site). Below the entry echo the two-layered corium consisting of an echo-poor and an echo-rich layer can be seen. The demarcation between the echo-rich layer and the subcutis is sharp throughout. The underlying subcutis is interspersed with bands of connective tissue. The scan obtained 24 h later (Fig. 13) already shows a marked reaction. The upper and lower boundaries of the resulting skin induration are evident. The corium shows a considerably looser structure in the reaction area which can be attributed mainly to the presence of oedema. Above the entry echo we see an echo-rich spot of a vellus hair. After 48 h (Fig. 14) the inflammatory infiltration of the corium has caused further thickening of the skin and the border to the subcutis has become indistinct at the lower pole of the reaction area. After 72 h (Fig. 15) some of the infiltration has subsided. This is indicated by an increase in the echogenicity of the reaction area and a reduction in skin thickness.

Indurations display some characteristic features in ultrasound. We almost regularly find convex bulging of the skin surface. The entire corium increases in thickness and becomes more loosely structured. The altered reflex pattern is seen particularly clearly in the echo-poor layer of the corium in the form of diminished echogenicity. Here we sometimes find almost completely echolucent areas. The underlying echo-rich corium also undergoes important changes. While in the healthy skin it forms a clear,

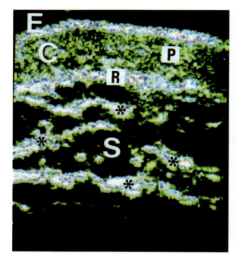

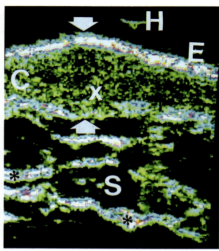

Fig. 12. Ultrasound scan of the healthy right forearm (volar surface) of a 45-year-old man. *E*, entry echo; *C*, corium; *R*, echo-rich corium; *P*, echo-rich corium; *asterisks*, bands of connective tissue in the subcutaneous fatty tissue; *S*, subcutis

Fig. 13. Ultrasound scan of exactly the same site as in Fig. 11 24 h after administration of the Multitest Merieux. *H*, hair; *X*, reaction area; *E*, entry echo; *C*, corium; *S*, subcutis; *arrows*, maximum limits of the reaction *asterisk*, bands of connective tissue

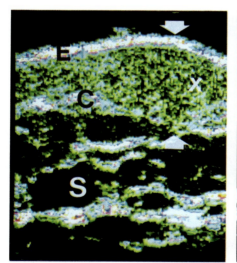

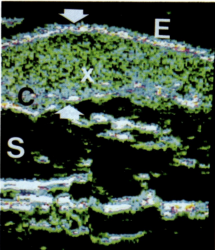

Fig. 14. Ultrasound scan 48 h after administration of Multitest Merieux (identical area to Fig. 12). *Arrows*, maximum limits of the reaction; *X*, reaction area (distinctly enlarged); *S*, subcutis

Fig. 15. Ultrasound scan 72 h after administration of Multitest Merieux (identical area to Fig. 13). *Arrows*, maximum limits of the reaction which has now subsided; *X*, reaction area (distinctly smaller); *S*, subcutis; *E*, entry echo; *C*, corium

highly echogenic, largely straight border with the subcutis, in the indurations it usually bulges into the subcutis and as a rule is loosely structured. In some cases the reflexes of the echo-rich area have partially – and in particularly strong reactions completely – disappeared. This explains why the A-scan is inadequate for determination and quantification of changes in the reflex pattern.

Indurations are not necessarily associated with convex bulging of the skin surface; the reaction can also manifest solely as a convex protrusion of the lower corium into the subcutis. When evaluating the induration it is therefore important to pay particular attention to the changes in the lower corium, which is accessible sonographically but not clinically. Even in test areas which do not react with a clinically palpable induration, in the majority of cases the ultrasound examination is able to detect an, albeit less marked, increase in skin thickness.

A reliable distinction between infiltrate and oedema is not possible with 20-MHz ultrasound even in B-mode. It must, however, be borne in mind that the histological section usually does not show an exact distinction between zones of infiltration and oedema either, but that both changes are closely interwoven and cannot be spatially separated from each other.

In summary we can say that 20-MHz B-mode ultrasound permits exact and objective assessment of type IV reactions. Use of 20-MHz ultrasound for routine diagnosis is justified and is to be recommended particularly in the case of doubtful reactions which are difficult to evaluate clinically. In addition, the method presented here can be used to develop models for testing local treatments of allergic skin diseases.

References

1. Alexander H, Miller DL (1979) Determining skin thickness with pulsed ultrasound. J Invest Dermatol 72: 17–19
2. Altmeyer P, Zaun H (1976) Ergebnisse reflexionsphotometrischer Bestimmungen der Vasokonstriktion nach topischer Steroidapplikation. Arch Dermatol Res 255: 51–56
3. Altmeyer (1977) Ein Beitrag zur Histologie der von Kortikoidexterna verursachten Hautveränderungen. Hautarzt 28: 83–88
4. Altmeyer P (1980) Die Beeinflussung der epidermalen und bindegewebigen Anteile der Kutis durch moderne Kortikoidexterna. Aktuel Dermatol 6: 63–66
5. Altmeyer P (1989) Dermatologische Ultraschalldiagnostik – gegenwärtiger Stand und Perspektiven. (editorial) Z Hautkr 64: 727–728
6. Altmeyer P, Luther H (1989) Die dermatologische Kryochirurgie. Aktuel Dermatol 15: 303–311
7. Altmeyer P, Hoffmann K, el-Gammal S (1990) Sonographie der Haut. Münch Med Wochenschr (18): 14–22
8. Andersen KE, Staberg B (1985) Quantification of contact allergy in guinea pigs by measuring changes in skin blood flow and skin fold thickness. Acta Derm Venereol (Stockh) 65: 37–42
9. Beck S, Spence VA, Lowe JG, Gibbs JH (1986) Measurement of skin swelling in the tuberculin test by ultrasonography. J Immunol Methods 86: 125–130

10. Black MM (1969) A modified radiographic method for measuring skin thickness. Br J Dermatol 81: 661–666
11. Braun-Falco O (1969) Die Morphogene der senil aktinischen Elastose. Arch Klin Exp Dermatol 235: 138–160
12. Brazier S, Shaw S (1986) High-frequency ultrasound measurement of patch test reactions. Contact Dermatitis 15: 199–201
13. Breitbart EW, Hicks R (1986) Wundheilung: objektive Kontrolle durch Ultraschall Zentralbl Hautkr 152: 559
14. Breitbart EW, Müller CH, Hicks R, Vielauf D (1989) Neue Entwicklungen der Ultraschalldiagnostik in der Dermatologie. Aktuel Dermatol 15: 57–61
15. Brink JA, Paul W, Sheets PW, Dines KA, Etchison MR, Hanke CW, Sadove AW (1986) Quantitative assessment of burn injury in porcine skin with high-frequency ultrasonic imaging. Invest Radiol 21: 645–651
16. Delbrück H, Schwarze G, Scharding B (1982) Cutaneous tests with recall antigens in tumour patients and healthy subjects. Experience with a new Multitest system. Tumordiagnostik 3: 18–24
17. Dines KA, Sheets PW, Brink JA, Hanke CW, Condra KA, Clendenon JL, Goss SA, Smith SS, Franklin TD (1984) High frequency ultrasonic imaging of the skin: experimental results. Ultrason Imaging 6: 408–434
18. Dykes PJ, Marks R (1976) Measurement of dermal thickness with the Harpenden skinfold caliper. Arch Dermatol Res 256: 261–263
19. Dykes PJ, Mark R (1976) Measurement of skin thickness: a comparison of two in vivo techniques with a conventional histometric method. J Invest Dermatol 21: 418–429
20. Dykes PJ, Hill S, Marks R (1988) Assessment of the atrophogenicity potential of corticosteroids by ultrasound and by epidermal biopsy under occlusive and nonocclusive conditions. In: Christophers E et al. (eds) Topical corticosteroid therapy. Raven, New York, pp 111–117
21. El-Gammal S (1990) Experimental approaches and new developments with high frequency ultrasound in dermatology. Zentralbl Hautkr 157: 327
22. Feldmann S, Hoffmann K, el-Gammal S, Altmeyer P (1990) Sonographic quantification of the tuberculin-type reaction, Zentralbl Hautkr 157: 320–321
23. Fornage DW, Deshaynes JL (1986) Ultrasound of normal skin. J Clin Ultrasound 14: 619–622
24. Gomez EC, Berman B, Miller DL (1982) Ultrasonic assessment of cutaneous atrophy caused by intradermal corticosteroids. J Dermatol Surg Oncol 8: 1071–1074
25. Görtz S, Hoffmann K, el-Gammal S, Altmeyer P (1990) High frequency b-scan sonography and skin-thickness measurement of normal skin. Zentralbl Hautkr 157: 319–320
26. Hoffmann K, el-Gammal S, Altmeyer P (1989) 20 MHz B-scan Sonographie an Händen und Füßen. In: Altmeyer P et al. (eds) Handsymposium: Dermatologische Erkrankungen der Hände und Füße, Roche, Basel, pp 285–300
27. Hoffmann K, el-Gammal S, Matthes U, Altmeyer P (1989) 20 MHz Sonographie der Haut in der präoperativen Diagnostik. Z Hautkr 64: 851–858
28. Hoffmann K, Stücker M, el-Gammal S, Altmeyer P (1990) Digitale 20- MHz-Sonographie des Basalioms in b-scan. Hautarzt 41: 333–339
29. Hoffmann K, el-Gammal S, Altmeyer P (1990) B-scan Sonographie in der Dermatologie. Hautarzt 41: W7–W16
30. Kerman RH, Floyd M, Van Buren CT (1980) Improved allograft survival of strong immune responder high risk recipients with adjuvant antithymocyte globulin therapy. Transplantation 30: 450–454
31. Kirsch JM, Hanson ME, Gibson JR (1984) The determinatin of skin-thickness using conventional ultrasound equipment. Clin Exp Dermatol 9: 280–285
32. Kligmann AM (1969) Early destuctive effect of sunlight on human skin. JAMA 210: 2377–2380
33. Kligman AM, Kligmann LH (1988) The treatment of photoaged skin with topical retinoic acid. Perspect Plastic Surg 2: 63–86

34. Kligmann LH (1986) Photoaging. Manifestation, prevention and treatment. Dermatol Clin 4: 517–528
35. Kniker WT, Anderson CT, Roumiantzeff M (1979) The Multitest system: a standardised approach to evaluation of delayed hypersensitivity and cellmediated immunity. Ann Allery 43: 73–79
36. Kune GA (1978) Lifethreatening surgical infection: its development and predication. Ann Coll Surg Engl 60: 92–98
37. Lawrence CM, Shuster S (1985) Comparison of ultrasound and caliper measurements of normal and inflamed skin thickness. J Dermatol 112: 195–200
38. Lubach D, Grüter M (1988) Vergleichende Untersuchung über die hautverdünnende Wirkung vom Amcinoid und Prednicarbat an unterschiedlichen Körperregionen des Menschen. Aktuel Dermatol 14: 197–200
39. Luther H, Banas J, Darwecke-Pickardt G, Hoffmann K, Fabry H, Altmeyer P (1989) Die Kryochirurgie des Basalioms. Z Hautkr 64: 748–755
40. Marks R (1990) Hauterkrankungen beim älteren Menschen. Deutscher Ärzte Verlag, Cologne
41. Martini GA, Sodomann CP (1976) Cellular immune response in chronic hepatitis. Proceedings International Symposium. Montecatini, pp 100–106. Karger
42. Mera SL, Davies JD (1987) Progress in the histochemistry of elasic fibres. Med Lab Sci 44: 237–242
43. Murikami S, Miki Y (1989) Human skin histology using high-resolution echography. J Clin Ultrasound 17: 77–82
44. Payne PA (1983) Non-invasive skin measurement by ultrasound. RNM Images 13: 24–26
45. Payne PA (1985) Medical and industrial applications of high resolution ultrasound. J Phys E Sci Instrum 18: 465–473
46. Petit JC, Klein T, Haegele P (1978) Apport des tests immunologiques pur l'établissement du pronostic des tumeurs malignes solides. Sem Hop Paris 54: 1144–1148
47. Poulter LW, Duke SO, Janossy G, Panayi G (1982) Immunohistological analysis of delayed-type hypersensitivity in man. Cell Immunol 74: 358–369
48. Price R, Jones TB, Goddard J Jr., James AE (1980) Basic concepts of ultrasonic tissue characterization. Radiol Clin North Am 18: 21–30
49. Querleux B, Léveque JL, de Rigal J (1988) In vivo cross-sectional ultrasonic imaging of human skin. Dermatologica 177: 332–337
50. Rigal J, Escoffier C, Querleux B, Faivre B, Agache P, Leveque JL (1989) Assessment of aging of the human skin by in vivo ultrasonic imaging. J Invest Dermatol 93: 621–625
51. Schuster S, Black MM, McVitie E (1975) The influence of age and sex on skin thickness, skin collagen and density. Br J Dermatol 93: 639–643
52. Serup J, Staberg B, Klemp P (1984) Quantification of cutaneous oedema in patch test reactions by measurement of skin thickness with high frequency pulsed ultrasound. Contact Dermatitits 10: 88–93
53. Sondergaard J, Serup J, Tikjob G (1985) Ultrasonic a- and b-scanning in clinical and experimental dermatology. Acta Dermato Venereol 65 [Suppl 120]: 76–82
54. Staberg B, Klemp P, Serup J (1984) Patch test responses evaluated by cutaneous blood flow measurements. Arch Dermatol 120: 741–743
55. Strasser W, Vanscheidt W, Hagedorn M, Wokalek H (1986) B-scan Ultraschall in der Dermatologie. Fortschr Med 25: 495–498
56. Tan CY, Marks R, Payne P (1981) Comparison of xeroradiographic and ultrasound detection of corticosteroid induced dermal thinning. J Invest Dermatol 76: 126–128
57. Tan CY, Statham B, Marks R, Payne PA (1982) Skin thickness measurement by pulsed ultrasound: its reproducibility, validation and variability. Br J Dermatol 106: 657–667
58. Tanner JM, Whitehouse RH (1955) The harpenden skinfold caliper. Am J Phys Anthropol 13: 743–746

59. Vogt M (1983) Erworbenes Immundefektsyndrom (AIDS). Dtsch Med Wochenschr 108 (50): 1927–1933
60. Wahlberg JE (1983) Assessment of skin irritancy: measurement of skin fold thickness. Contact Dermatitis, 9: 21–26
61. Wahlberg JE, Nilsson G (1984) Skin irritancy from propylene glycol. Acta Derm Venereol (Stockh) 64: 286–290
62. Weil CS, Scala RA (1987) Study of intra-interlaboratory variability in the result of rabbit eye and skin irritation tests. Toxicol Appl Pharmacol 19: 276–360
63. Winkler K, Hoffmann K, el-Gammal S, Altmeyer P (1990) The repair process of a wound healing model under sonographic control. Zentralbl Hautkr 157: 327–328
64. Zacarian SA (1985) Cryosurgery for skin cancer and cutaneous Disorders, 1st edn. Mosby, St Louis

Intravascular Ultrasound

R. Hammentgen, V. Godder, S. el-Gammal, M. Meine, M. Bergbauer, and D. Ricken

Introduction

Intravascular ultrasound (IVUS) requires special catheters with miniaturized ultrasound detectors on the tip. Morphology and pathology of blood vessels and blood flow velocities can be examined. In conventional angiography dye is injected through a catheter into the vessel of interest. The contrasting material provides a two-dimensional negative staining cast of the three-dimensional inner surface of the vessel. The angiologic morphology therefore is studied therefore indirectly, whereas ultrasound detectors directly visualized the vessel wall [8]. With the exception of video densitometry common angiography allows only qualitative statements concerning the blood flow pattern. In contrast, intravascular Doppler ultrasound methods enable a quantification of flow [6, 9, 10, 12].

We used the following technical instrumentation: Hemodynamic measurements were accomplished with a velocimeter (Millar) connected to a 4F Doppler catheter (Fig. 1). The Doppler crystal mounted at the tip of the catheter operated in pulse-echo mode. The gate position could be varied in a distance from 1–10 mm to the crystal. The reflected signals were evaluated with a special spectral analytical method called zero crossing. Precise positioning of the catheter under angiographic control is facilitated by a steerable guide wire. Furthermore, the guide wire stabilizes the catheter which especially affects the axial orientation of the ultrasound beam.

Intravascular Flow Measurement

Intravascular flow measurement was validated by in vitro experiments. The Doppler catheter was introduced into a closed system of tubes with a known cross-sectional area and was floated in a fluid stream which was injected in a pulsatile mode. Different fluids were injected at various flow velocities:
1. physiological saline, 2. lipoid solution, 3. Echovist, and 4. heparinized blood.

Phasic and mean flow velocities were measured using the zero crossing method (Fig. 1). Flow volume was calculated by multiplying the cross-sectional area (CSA) with the velocity-time integral (VTI) (Fig. 2).

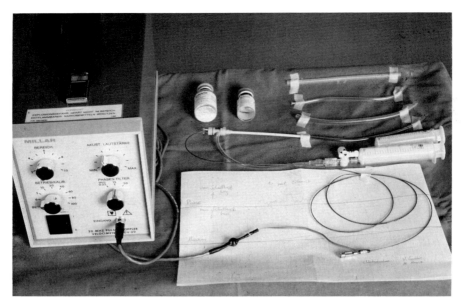

Fig. 1. Doppler velocimeter connected with a 4F Doppler catheter (20 MHz), tube system and flow registration (zero crossing)

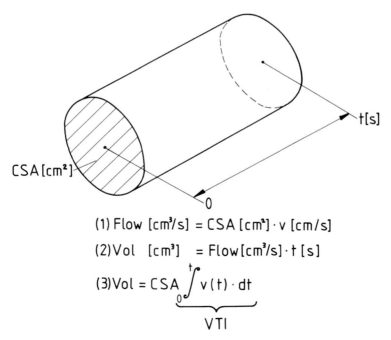

(1) Flow $[cm^3/s]$ = CSA $[cm^2] \cdot v$ $[cm/s]$

(2) Vol $[cm^3]$ = Flow$[cm^3/s] \cdot t$ $[s]$

(3) Vol = CSA $\underbrace{\int_0^t v(t) \cdot dt}_{VTI}$

Fig. 2. Velocity-time integral (*VTI*); calculation of flow volume (*Vol*)

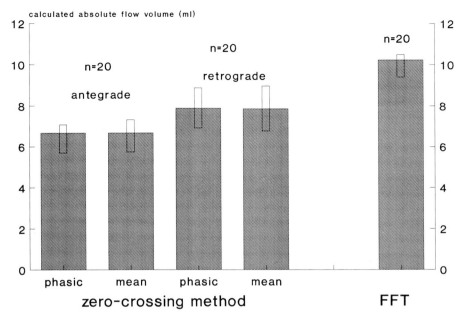

Fig. 3. Results of different methods of intravascular Doppler flow measurement after injection of 10 ml Echovist into a tube system 3 mm in diameter. A retrograde flow moves towards and antegrade flow moves away from the transducer. Zero crossing (*left*); fast Fourier Transforms (*FFT; right*)

Obviously the fluid echogenicity contributed directly to the quantity of reflected signals. Reflecting structures which lead to acoustic impedance shifts are a prerequisite for Doppler flow measurements. Although micelles form adequate interfaces, lipoid emulsions give an insufficient reflection. The strongest reflection signal was observed using the contrast medium Echovist, which contains air bubbles of definite size (7 μm diameter). Nevertheless, even when Echovist was injected into the tube system, the flow volume was systematically underestimated by 20%–30%. Using mean or phasic flow velocities revealed similar results (Fig. 3).

In the next step we used a more precise form of spectral analysis. After transforming the analog Doppler signal into a discrete sampled digital set of points, spectral analysis was calculated by Fast Fourier transforms (FFT; (Fig. 4). For this purpose we modified software (MDV) known to be adequate. Using the same experimental setup we were then able to determine flow volumes more precisely. The product of FFT mean VTI and CSA seems to be better method to measure the absolute flow volumes. In our trial the CSA was known. In vivo CSAs of coronary or peripheral arteries have to be determined from several angiographic planes if ultrasound imaging systems are not available.

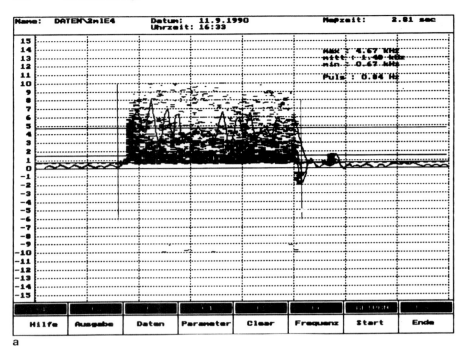

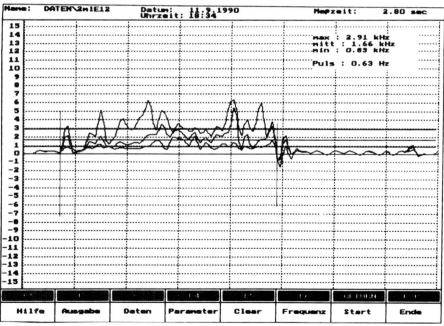

Fig. 4a, b. FFT spectral analysis of intravascular signals. **a** Gray scale display. **b** Maximum, mean, and minimum flow velocities

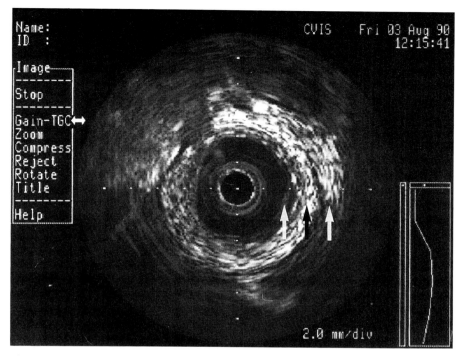

Fig. 5. Intravascular ultrasound image. Peripheral artery with typical lamination: intima, media, adventitia (*arrows*)

Intravascular Two-Dimensional Imaging

Today two-dimensional intravascular ultrasound transducers supply B-scan images of vessels comparable to transverse sections in pathology [13, 14]. The wall lamination of peripheral arteries in intima, media, and adventitia can be differentiated easily (Fig. 5). This catheter has an incorporated 20-MHz crystal transducer, which is rotated by a flexible shaft and registers a 360° view like a radar system.

The ultrasound images provide a clear distinction of vessel wall structures, sclerosis, or thrombosis.

Future Developments

The efficacy of interventional procedures like percutaneous transluminal coronary angioplasty, laser treatment, or direct atherectomy depends on correct information about the orientation, location and size of the vascular occlusion [1, 2, 4, 7]. We therefore need an ultrasound scanner oriented along the catheter axis. Furthermore combined catheters are necessary to view the flow and the two-dimensional structure morphology simultaneously [8]. Absolute volume and reserve of coronary flow [3, 5, 11] would then be measured during the same procedure. Vascular resistance and its reactions on pharmacological interventions could be determined in connection with arterial pressure.

The major fields of application of intravascular ultrasound are in cardiology and peripheral angiology. Indications in phlebology are to be expected soon.

References

1. Altobell SA, Nerem RM (1985) An experimental study of coronary artery fluid mechanics. J Bio Mech 107: 16–23
2. Gould KL (1985) Quantification of coronary artery stenosis in vivo. Circ Res 57: 341–353
3. Hoffman JIE (1984) Maximal coronary flow and the concept of coronary vascular reserve. Circulation 70: 153–159
4. Johnson EL, Yock PG, Hargrave VK, Srebo JP, Manubens SM, Seitz W, Ports TA (1989) Assessment of severity of coronary stenoses using a Doppler catheter. Circulation 80: 625–635
5. Klocke FJ (1987) Measurements of coronary flow reserve: defining pathophysiology versus making decisions about patient care. Circulation 76: 1183–1189
6. Sako Y (1984) Clinical use of blood flowmeters. Angiology X: 206–213
7. Serruys PW, Juilliere Y, Zijlstra F, Beatt K, De Feyter PJ, Suryappranata H, Van Den Brand M, Roelandt J (1988) Coronary blood flow velocity during percutaneous transluminal coronary angioplasty as a guide for asessment of the functional result. Am J Cardiol 61: 253–259
8. White MW, Yock PG (1989) Intravascular ultrasound: Catheter-based Doppler and two-dimensional imaging. Card Clin 7: 525–536
9. White CW, Wilson RF, Marcus ML (1988) Methods of measuring myocardial blood flow in humans. Prog Cardvasc Dis 31: 79–94
10. Wilson RF, White CW (1987) Doppler echocardiography in aortic, coronary and myocardial disease as well as congenital lesions. Herz 12: 163–176
11. Wilson RF, Laughlin DE, Ackell PH, Chilian WM, Holida MD, Hartley CJ, Armstrong ML, Marcus ML, White CW (1985) Transluminal, subselective measurement of coronary artery blood flow velocity and vasodilator reserve in man. Circulation 72: 82–92
12. Yock PG, Johnson EL, Linker DT (1988) Intravascular ultrasound: Development and clinical potential. Am J Card Im 2: 185–193
13. Yock PG, Linker DT, Angelson BAJ (1989) Two-dimensional intravascular ultrasound: Technical development and initial clinical experience. J Am Soc Echo 2: 296–304
14. Yock PG, Linker DT, Arenson J, Thapliyal H, Saether O, White N, Angelson B (1989) Intravascular two-dimensional catheter ultrasound: clinicaal studies in the periphery. Cath Sens Im Tech 1068: 150–156

50 MHz Ultrasound

A 50-MHz High-Resolution Ultrasound Imaging System for Dermatology*

S. EL-GAMMAL, K. HOFFMANN, T. AUER, M. KORTEN,
P. ATLMEYER, A. HÖSS, and H. ERMERT

Introduction

In the fields of internal medicine and surgery, diagnostic imaging methods have found wide application. This is, among other reasons, due to the fact that organ systems are studied and treated in internal medicine, which are not directly accessible to the doctor. Of all available imaging methods ultrasound, particularly, has gained a larger impetus because this method is harmless to the patient and can be repeated as many times as necessary.

Since the structures studied are localized several centimeters under the skin, only macroscopic enlargements are necessary. Machines working in the frequency range between 2.5 and 7.5 MHz are commonly used because the in-depth signal penetration is inversely proportional to the frequency of the ultrasonic probe. However, the resolution of the ultrasound machines (including CT and NMR) are completely insufficient, only resolving down to about 1 mm, for the study of dermatological structures like hair appendages which are typically only 2 mm thick.

The dermatologist, on the other hand, showed little interest for these techniques, since his organ of interest the skin, is easily accessible. He can directly study the skin lesions in their body distribution, shape and palpable consistency. It is therefore a widely spread opinion that ultrasound can only deliver additional information about their in-depth extension.

Because of the limits of existing ultrasound systems, new, high-resolution imaging methods had to be developed for dermatology. In finding noninvasive methods which are acceptable to the patient, it was logical to develop high-frequency ultrasound imaging systems, since by increasing the frequency, the resolution increases. However, due to frequency-dependent signal attenuation in biological tissues, in-depth signal penetration is reciprocally proportional to the frequency. Fortunately the structures of interest in the skin lie only a few millimeters beneath the skin surface. Frequencies between 20 and 100 MHz should consequently be of interest in dermatology.

---

* This work was supported by the Deutsche Forschungsgemeinschaft. Essential parts of this publication are part of the dissertation of Mr. Auer (inflammatory diseases) and of Mr. Korten (tumours).

Already today 20-MHz ultrasound imaging systems promise additional preoperative information about the extension of tumorous and inflammatory diseases below the skin's surface [4, 12]. However, since very subtle infiltrates are of interest, a special effort has to be made to further improve the resolution and objectify the physician's palpatory sense. It will be shown that the resolution of the 20-MHz ultrasound imaging systems on the market is insufficient to study epidermal processes or fine infiltrates in the corium.

On the other hand, we should bear in mind that ultrasound images can be understood as the interference of different ultrasound phenomena, e.g. scattering, absorption and reflection. The interference of these different phenomena can cause nonexisting structures to appear. This is why at the present state of technology it is hazardous to extract singular structures from an ultrasound image without histological confirmation of the results.

We designed and constructed a digital 50-MHz ultrasound imaging system, reaching today's limits in the study of *in vivo* skin structures.

The present study addresses the following questions:
1. Is this new technology able to resolve epidermal structures?
2. Can the image be correlated to the different structures seen at histological examination?

Additionally, this high-resolution imaging method will be used to investigate different inflammatory diseases and skin tumours.

Materials and Methods

The Transducer

Because of the high signal attenuation in biological tissue (about 1 dB MHz^{-1} cm^{-1}) only the pulse echo mode can be used. We used a point-focused ultrasound transducer built on a polymer basis (polyvenylidendifluoride). This new active transducer has incorporated a wideband transmitter and a receiver preamplifier. The main disadvantage of this construction is that the shape of the transmitted pulse cannot be manipulated (inverse or optimal prefiltering of the transmitter pulse are therefore not possible). On the other hand, the necessary external electronic parts are minimized, only a trigger signal is required.

The ultrasound transducer element has a diameter of 3 mm, a radius of curvature of 12 mm and a focal point approximately 11.5 mm in water. As coupling medium between transducer and skin a water path without membrane or contact gel is used. The ultrasound beam width in the focus area is about 125 µm (lateral resolution) and the axial resolution 37.5 µm.

The Applicator

To record a two-dimensional B-scan image, the transducer, which is axially oriented (z-axis), is moved laterally in a water bath used, as coupling medium. In our case, two stepper motors were mounted perpendicularly in the applicator to move the transducer in the direction of the x- or y-axis (Fig. 1a, b). To ensure that no air bubbles are trapped under the concave surface of the transducer, a small sponge has been mounted in the applicator lateral from the scanning window to wipe them off (Fig. 1c).

Technical Design

Figure 2a shows a block diagram of the 50-MHz ultrasound computer imaging system and Fig. 2b the actual equipment. To register an A-scan, the transmitter is initially triggered and the returning echo is preamplified (Fig. 2a). The strong signal attenuation in biological tissues makes use of a time-gain-control (TGC) amplifier necessary to amplify the backscattered echoes by 8 dB, according to the time elapse (assuming 1600 m/s) over a distance of about 4 mm. The single A-scans are then sampled with a transient recorder (Type Sony Tektronix RTD 710) with 1024 quantization levels (10 bits[1]) and a sampling frequency of 200 MHz.

Alternatively, we used a coherent quadrature demodulation to enhance the signal-to-noise ratio by reducing the sampling frequency [14]; synchronous twochannel sampling was then accomplished in the transient recorder. This recorder can also average several A-scans at a single transducer position to improve the signal-to-noise ratio. For optimal signal amplification within the quantization limits of the transient recorder, single A-scans could be viewed on an oscilloscope. The 1024 digitized sampling points of the A-scan were the collected by an IBM Model 80 using an IEC databus (Fig. 2a) and stored line by line as a radio-frequency image (RF image). This was then demodulated using envelope detection to calculate the 255 grey-scale levels on the low-frequency (LF) image. We used a false-colour codation to make the dynamic range of all 256 quantization levels visible. The colour palette was adjusted to the 20-MHz ultrasound imaging system DUB20 (Taberna pro Medicum, Lüneburg, FRG) standard colour table [13].

Histology and Ultrasound Images

In ultrasound, impedance changes are responsible for different reflection phenomena seen on the images. Histological correlation is imperative for structure recognition.

We have to bear in mind that the ultrasound beam has a focal area of 125 μm diameter. On the other hand the transducer is moved over a distance of about 10 mm laterally. It can easily be seen that small variations in the

---

[1] **binary digit** (bit); basic element of every computer memory. This element can only have one of two states: 0 or 1 (binary system).

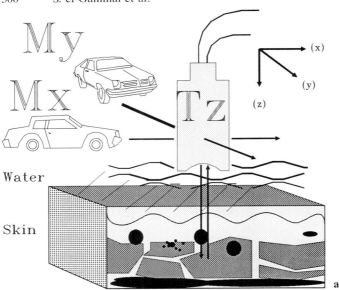
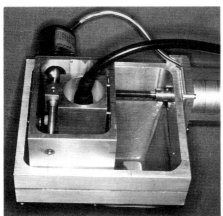
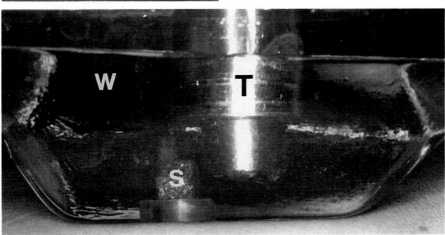

Fig. 1a–c. The applicator. **a** The orientation of the three axes of the orthogonal coordinate system in the applicator. **b** Photographic top view of the applicator showing the transducer and the perpendicularly oriented stepper motors **c** After gently pressing the applicator to the skin, it is filled with water (*W*). A sponge (*S*) fixed at the bottom of the applicator is used to strip off the air bubble beneath the concave surface of the transducer (*T*)

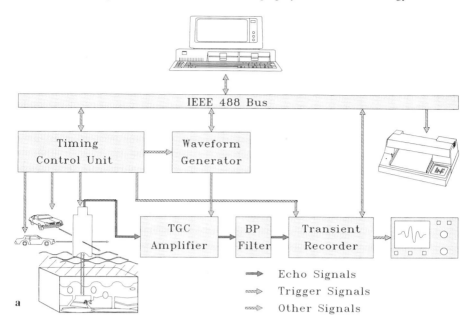

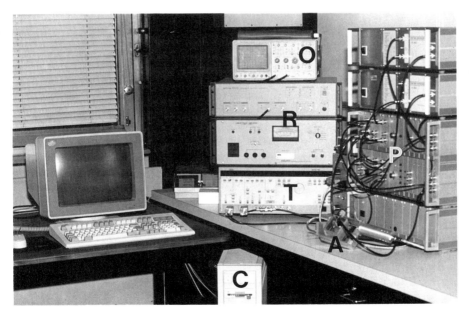

Fig. 2a, b. The technical setup. **a** Data processing block diagram with the different units of the 50-MHz ultrasound computer imaging system. **b** The different components of the 50-MHz system. *C*, computer; *A*, applicator; *P*, preamplifier; *T*, TGC amplifier; *R*, transient recorder; *O*, oscilloscope

tilting of the knife biopsy, tissue distortion or unequal shrinkage during the fixation process can show completely different structures at histological examination than were seen in sonography. Special care has to be taken therefore to gain truely comparable images.

In a first step the B-scan section plane has to be marked on the skin with a thin water- and wipe-proof pen. If necessary, the skin should be degreased before hand. After anaesthesia the first cut is placed directly on the demarcation line to reduce traction and tension forces. Only knife biopsies are sufficiently exact for this procedure. The region of interest is then excised spindle-shaped. The two section surfaces along the demarcation line are separated, placed on a sheet of cardboard and unpleated. If necessary, liquid correction fluid such as Tipp-Ex (which withstands formalin) can be used to mark the section border. During histological serial sectioning special care is necessary to cut the biopsy exactly parallel and tangential to the demarcation line.

However, differences between histological results and ultrasound images are not only caused by imprecise positioning or oblique sectioning. It has to be emphasized that our 50-MHz transducer has a lateral resolution of 125 µm in the focal area, which means that the ultrasound image shows superimposed structures of a section 125 µm thick. In histology, however, 6- to 8-µm-thick sections are standard.

Results

Ultrasound Image Processing and Layout

In order to compare 50-MHz images with the results of 20-MHz ultrasound images, a few factors have to be taken into account:
1. On the computer monitor the lateral compression of the ultrasound image in the 50-MHz machine is 1.5 times that of the axial direction, while the 20-MHz images are compressed 3 times.
2. The usable in-depth signal penetration of the 50-MHz machine is 4 mm. This value describes the skin thickness range from where the image signal is well above the noise level. The 20-MHz machines presently available on the market resolve structures up to a depth of 8 mm.
3. The better resolution of the 50-MHz ultrasound imaging system should allow a clearer and finer resolution of tissue structures.

To compare the 20- and 50-MHz ultrasound images, we recorded an radiofrequency (RF) image with an ordinary 20-MHz machine (DUB20, Taberna pro Medicum, FRG). Afterwards, the RF-image datafile was read into the computer program of the 50-MHz machine and demodulated (LF image).

Assuming a mean sound speed of 1600 m/s in the skin, the coarse scale along the borders of the image is 1 mm, while the fine scale is 100 µm (e.g. Fig. 3b, c).

Figures 3a-d show ultrasound images of normal skin of the forearm of a male. Figure 3a was photographed from the monitor of the DUB20 whereas Fig. 3b shows the image after being read and processed by our computer programm.

To correct for the different lateral compression of the 50- and 20-MHz images the 20-MHz ultrasound picture was stretched laterally by a factor of two. To correct for the smaller signal in-depth penetration of the 50-MHz equipment only the upper 4 mm of the 20 MHz image were visualised. An echolucent region ("W") is seen in the top region of the image; this is demarked by an echo-rich line ("E"). Following this, a intensely spotted texture with apparently randomly scattered echoes is seen ("C"). "H" denotes an ill-defined echo-poor structure, which leaves obliquely from the echo-rich band down through the intensely spotted echo texture. This longitudinal structure is difficult to follow at its lower border. Beneath the intensely spotted echo texture "C" a nearly echolucent region ("F") follows, which sometimes exhibits sparse, linear reflex stripes, depending on the body region studied.

Figure 3c shows the same section of skin recorded with our 50-MHz ultrasound imaging system. Note the much thinner echo line "E" in comparison to Fig. 3c. Beneath, the intensely spotted echo texture ("C") seems to be more structured. A quite sharply defined, echo-poor structure "H" leaves in an angle of about 50° from the echo-rich line "E" downwards through the intensely spotted echo texture. Its structure is sharply delimited at its lower border. As in the 20-MHz image, beneath "C" a nearly echolucent region ("F") follows.

Figure 3d compares the frequency spectrum of a single A-scan in the 20-MHz and 50-MHz image. Note that in biological tissue such as skin, the centre frequency of the transducer is reduced in comparison to the curves registered on metal plates or point sources used by the manufacturers.

Correlating histology shows that the above-described areas correspond to the water path ("W"), the corium ("C") and the subcutaneous fatty tissue ("F"). Between the water path and the corium lies an echo-rich line ("E"). From an anatomical point of view, one would expect that this echodense structure corresponds to some part(s) of the epidermis. We will therefore concentrate on this structure.

The Epidermis

Because the skin on the palms and soles is very thick, this localization is well suited for further examinations. Figure 4 shows an epiluminescent image of the studied skin region at a magnification x50. Note the ridge pattern of the palm. Evey one of the regularly arranged white dots on the ridges represents the orifice of an eccrine gland duct. It is easy to understand that the shape of the skin on the ultrasound image is greatly influenced by its orientation according to the ridges. The examination begins by studying the ridges in longitudinal direction along the ridge crest (Fig. 5a). To eliminate overmo-

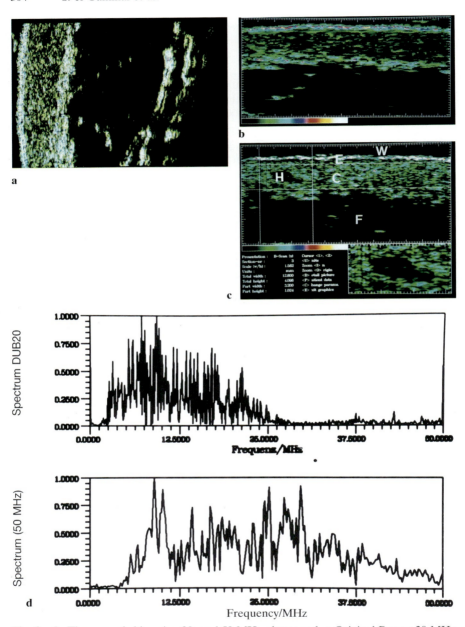

Fig. 3a–d. The normal skin using 20- and 50-MHz ultrasound. **a** Original B-scan 20-MHz image (DUB20) **b** 20-MHz image data read into the 50-MHz equipment. The image has been stretched by 2 in lateral and axial directions. The ruler at the borders is divided in 1/10 mm, the distance between two *longer bars* is 1 mm. **c** 50-MHz B-scan from the same skin region using the same dimensions as *b*. **d** Frequency spectrum of a single A-scan registered with the 20-MHz and 50-MHz transducer. *W*, water path; *E*, entry echo; *C*, corium; *F*, subcutaneous fatty tissue; *H*, hair follicle

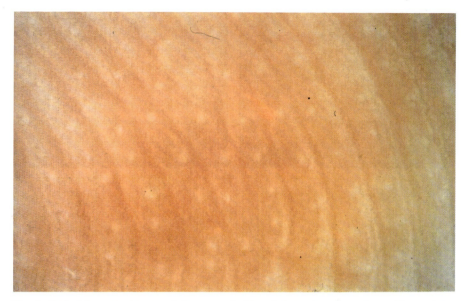

Fig. 4. Epiluminescent image of the normal skin of the palm. Note the orifices of the eccrine ducts on the crest of the ridges, × 50

dulation of the echoes from the echo-rich line "E", the A-scan signal amplification was further reduced.

The line "E" then breaks into several layers (Fig. 5b): A fine echo-rich linear line is followed by a fairly echo-poor layer. Beneath this a reflex-rich line delimits the echo-poor layer. As expected, the echo texture of the corium disappears at this amplification. In Fig. 5 the upper fine echo line is 120 μm, the medial echolucent layer 180 μm and the lower fine echo line 60 μm thick (Fig. 5c).

When the ultrasound image dissects the ridges perpendicularly (Fig. 6a) three interrupted, disconnected, fine echo lines beneath each other alternate with a shifted echo line (Fig. 6b). The alternating lines are about 250 μm wide, i.e. the mean distance between neighbouring ridge crests is 0.5 mm on the palms.

Experimental Approaches

To correlate the ultrasound images with known anatomical structures of the epidermis, the upper, echo-rich band must be identified with respect to the skin surface. For this purpose small amounts of copper powder were applied to the skin surface. The result is shown in Fig. 7a. The schematic drawing (Fig. 7b) compares the histological and ultrasound findings. It is evident that

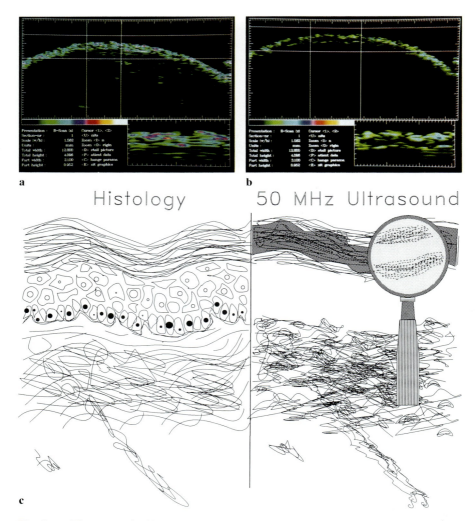

Fig. 5a–c. The normal skin of the palm in ridge direction using different analog amplification factors. **a** x1; note the wide skin entry echo. **b** x0.5 the skin entry echo desintegrates into several layers. **c** Schematic drawing of the different sonographic layers of the longitudinally sectioned ridged skin and their histological correlate. By reducing the amplification (*magnifying glass*) the skin entry echo breaks into two echo-rich lines with an echolucent line in between, using 50 MHz

the powder has filled the holes in the entry echo. No further echo lines become visible; the entry echo is just completed and enhanced.

We can conclude for normal ridged skin (Fig. 6) that only the crest and the valley of the ridges are seen as singular fine echo lines. In the region between the two the ultrasound beam is reflected in such a way to the side that no signal reaches the transducer.

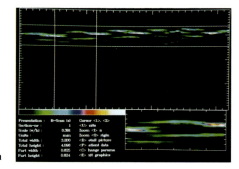
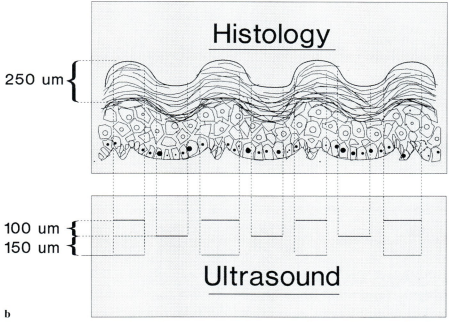

Fig. 6a, b. The normal skin of the palms perpendicular to the ridges. **a** Two echo-rich lines 250 μm beneath each other are shifted periodically up and down. The period is about 0.5 mm. The *four white lines* delimit a rectangle within the picture, which has been further enlarged in the *inset*. **b** Schematic drawing comparing histology and ultrasound. The upper echo-rich line segments correspond to the water/stratum corneum interface, the echo-rich line segments beneath originate from the stratum corneum/stratum malpigii interface. The mean difference in height between the ridge crest and valley is about 100 μm

Inflammatory Diseases

We studied several other inflammatory dermatoses such as psoriasis vulgaris, lichen planus, chronic eczema, and mycosis fungoides with the 50-MHz equipment. All these dermatoses show an echolucent band (ELB) in the

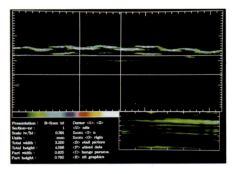

Fig. 7a, b. The normal skin of the palms perpendicular to the ridges after copper powder application. **a** No new echo lines have appeared. Only the slopes of the undulating upper echo-rich line are filled up by the copper powder. Further signal amplification exhibits the border between corium and epidermis (*inset*). Note the 1/10 mm ruler at the borders showing that the images have been zoomed digitally. **b** This finding suggests that the upper echo-rich undulating line corresponds to the water/stratum corneum interface (schematic drawing)

upper corium, sometimes bordered by an area of multiple undulating green reflex lines. The spindle-shaped knife biopsies were taken from the same skin region with exactly the same orientation as the ultrasound images. As we are interested in studying structures in the corium, the signal from the epidermis has to be overamplified. We therefore use the term *skin entry echo*, thereby indicating that the above-mentioned layers (Figs. 5, 6) have joined to form a single wide echo line.

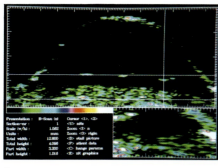 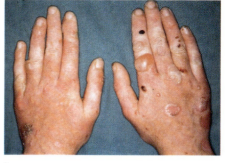

a b

Fig. 8a, b. Epidermolysis bullosa (50 MHz). **a** The macroscopic foto exhibits multiple bullae, partly haemorrhagic. **b** The ultrasound image of a dome-shaped clear bulla. Due to angular reflection phenomena, the diagonal slopes of the skin entry echo cannot be seen. Note the interrupted echo-rich line *(white horizontal line)* at the lower part of the echolucent dome-shaped region beneath the skin entry echo

Epidermolysis Bullosa Hereditaria

A 9-year-old girl was examined. Macroscopically polymorphous skin lesions were observed (Fig. 8a) consisting of bullae of variable size and partly pigmented cicatrices. The lesions were nearly exclusively located in the distal parts of the extremities, and the skin was rather thick on palpation.

The sonogram of a bulla on the back of the left hand shows an echo-poor protruding region which is vertically delimited by a dome-shaped reflex-rich echo border (Fig. 8b). Note that the echo signal of the diagonally oriented slopes of the skin is attenuated due to its angular orientation in relation to the transducer. In the lower region of the echolucent area a few horizontal reflex lines are seen which divide the area into two parts. Beneath this echo-poor region an area follows which has an echo texture characteristic for the corium.

Psoriasis Vulgaris

Figure 9a shows an epiluminescent microscopic image of the skin lesion at a magnification x50. Multiple dilatated capillary trees are observed, which are responsible for the reddish colour of the psoriasis plaque. Figure 9b reveals an irregular skin entry echo with focal reflex enhancements above. This is followed by a wide, nearly completely echolucent band (ELB) beneath. Note the two distinct echo shadows, which are possibly due to hyperkeratoses. In fact, the 50-MHz machine allows us to zoom and amplify an image section (see inset in Fig. 9b) to further analyze the skin entry echo. Figure 9c shows the corresponding histological section, which is characterized by hyperkeratosis, focal parakeratosis and regular elongation of the rete ridges.

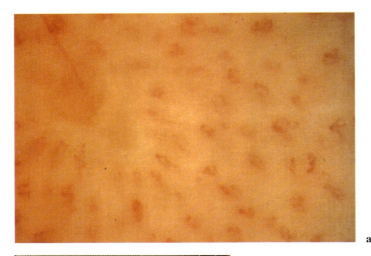

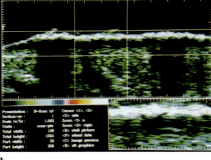

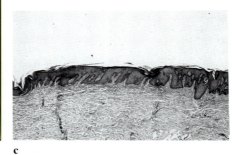

Fig. 9a–c. Psoriasis vulgaris. **a** Epiluminescent image showing the fine enlarged capillary loops in a psoriasis plaque. **b** The ultrasound image (50 MHz) exhibits an irregularly thickened skin entry echo with echo-rich lamellae protruding into the water path. Note the echo shadows emanating beneath the skin entry echo. In the upper corium an echo-poor band is seen. **c** The histological section exhibits hyperkeratosis, focal parakeratosis, and a regular elongation of the rete ridges. In the upper corium and dermal papillae a perivascular infiltrate is observed

In the stratum corneum small aggregations of neutrophilic granulocytes are seen. Perivascular lymphocytic infiltrate was noted in the upper corium and the dermal papillae.

Lichen Planus

The ultrasound image of lichen planus (Fig. 10a) exhibits an irregular skin entry echo. The corresponding histology (Fig. 10b) reveals an irregular hyperkeratosis and acanthosis. Contrary to the psoriasis (Fig. 9c), the dermal

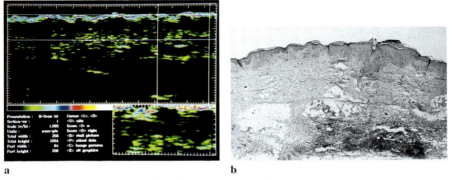

Fig. 10a, b. Lichen planus. **a** The ultrasound image (50 MHz) exhibits an undulating skin entry echo varying in thickness. In the upper corium an echo-poor bandlike zone with a few stronger reflexes is observed. The *inset* shows that this echolucent band (ELB) consists of smaller spotted, confluent, echo-poor areas. **b** Histology exhibits irregular hyperkeratosis and acanthosis. In the upper corium a spotted bandlike infiltrate is seen

papillae are not elongated. In the upper corium a diffusely spotted bandlike infiltrate is observed. Sonography exhibits a blurred, band-shaped, echo-poor to echolucent band (ELB) with a few stronger reflexes in the upper corium. At higher magnification multiple undulating reflex lines are seen at the borders of this region.

Mycosis Fungoides

A 62-year-old patient exhibited multiple, large, red, elevated and infiltrated skin lesions. The sonogram (Fig. 11a) shows a wide echolucent band (ELB)

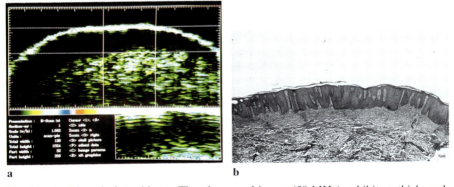

Fig. 11a, b. Mycosis fungoides. **a** The ultrasound image (50 MHz) exhibits a thickened, echo-rich skin entry echo with a wide, echo-poor, band-shaped zone in the upper corium. Note the fine undulating lines in the *inset* at the upper and lower border of the echo-poor zone. **b** Histology exhibits acanthosis, parakeratosis and an elongation of the dermal papillae accompanied by a dense, subepidermal infiltrate

beneath the skin entry echo. The corresponding histology (Fig. 11b) exhibits acanthosis, parakeratosis and an elongation of the dermal papillae accompanied by a dense, subepidermal infitrate which was sharply delimited towards the corium. For further analysis, this region of interest was enlarged and amplified in the ultrasound image (Fig. 11a insert). The formerly echolucent band shows foci of multiple horizontally oriented, undulating echo lines, especially in its lower and upper parts.

Skin Tumours

Of all skin conditions, tumours have received the most attention from the different research groups using high-resolution ultrasound. We shall therefore concentrate on the ultrasound image of some of the tumours in the clinical differential diagnosis of the malignant melanoma.

Seborrhoeic Keratoses

The histological section (Fig. 12b) shows a seborrhoeic keratosis of acanthotic type with a few horny invaginations, which appear in cross sections as pseudocysts. The sonogram (Fig. 12a) exhibits an irregularly enlarged skin entry echo with a few echo-rich spots. Beneath, the echo signal is attenuated, displaying a wide echo shadow below in the entire corium. Furthermore an echo-poor to echolucent spindle-shaped area (ELA) is apparent in the upper region of the corium.

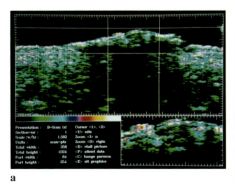
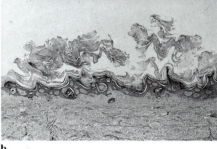

a   b

Fig. 12a, b. Seborrhoeic keratosis. **a** The ultrasound image (50 MHz) shows an about 500 μm enlarged, irregular skin entry echo. Beneath, an echo shadow makes the corial structures apparently disappear. Furthermore, an echolucent spindle-shaped zone is seen in the upper corium. **b** Histology exhibits an seborrhoeic keratosis of the acanthotic type with a few horny invaginations

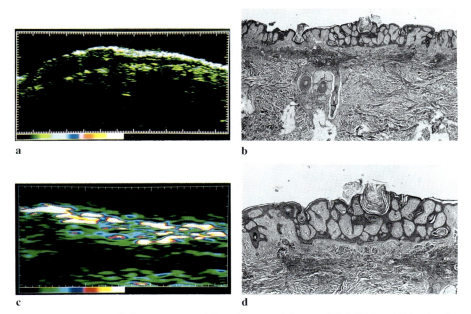

Fig. 13a–d. Naevocellular naevus. **a** The ultrasound image (50 MHz) exhibits in the overview a focally widened skin entry echo. Beneath, an echo-poor to echolucent area (ELA) with a few stronger linear reflexes is seen. This echo-poor area includes the region just beneath the skin entry echo in the *left* part of the picture. **b** The corresponding histology exhibits a net-shaped acanthotic epithelium with inclusions of fine-fibrillary connective tissue. At the left border only fine-fibrillary connective tissue is seen. **d** Close-up of the tumour region. The horny cysts and net-shaped acanthotic epithelium is summed up to an reflex-intense wide skin entry echo. At the left border, the fine-fibrillary connective tissue is echo-poor with a few dark-green reflexes

Naevocellular Naevus

The sonogram (Fig. 13a) exhibits a large inhomogenous skin entry echo. Next to reflex-rich, point-shaped and linear parts, low-reflex regions and dispersed zones were also seen. Beneath this an echolucent area (ELA) is present which runs roughly parallel to the skin entry echo and is often spindle-shaped. Below this a green intensely spotted reflex-rich zone, with a typical corial texture, is seen. The histological section (Fig. 13b) shows a net-shaped acanthotic epithelium with inclusions of fine-fibrillary connective tissue. This epithelium includes keratotic cores and a proliferation of rete ridges. In the upper and middle corium ovaloid nests and conglomerations of naevocellular cells were apparent. Tangential hair follicle sections with their appendages were also observed.

At higher magnification the inhomogenous skin entry echo and the undulating green reflex-intense lines can be studied (Fig. 13c, d). Note the echo-rich irregularly configured layer beneath the entry echo which corresponds to the tumour masses in histology.

Basal Cell Carcinoma

The sonogram exhibits a skin entry echo of variable echogenicity. Beneath the skin surface a echolucent area is seen, which is irregularly delimited at its lower border (Fig. 14a). Histological examination of a superficial basal cell carcinoma (Fig. 14b) shows that these areas correspond to finger-, or burgeonlike solid proliferations of basophilic basaloid cells. Around the basal cell conglomerates, sparse inflammatory stroma reaction which is shaped like a glove is seen. These echolucent burgeons penetrate the upper corium structures (Fig. 14c, d).

Malignant Melanoma

Figure 15b shows a histological section of a partly pigmented, partly unpigmented malignant melanoma in the upper and middle corium. Note the

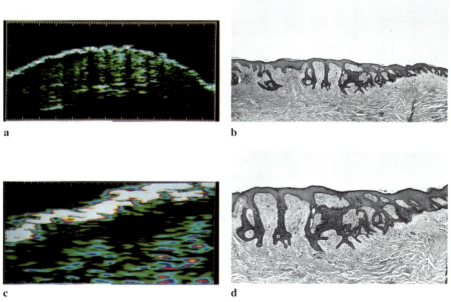

Fig. 14a–d. Superficial basal cell carcinoma. **a** The ultrasound image (50 MHz) overview exhibits a skin entry echo with a variable echogenicity. The echolucent area (ELA) beneath is irregularly delimited at its lower border. **b** Multiple finger- and burgeonlike solid proliferations of basophil basaloid cells are seen. Around the basal cell conglomerates a glove-shaped sparse inflammatory stroma reaction is seen. **c** At higher magnification, the interdigitation of the echo-poor burgeons with the texture of the corium is exhibited. **d** Corresponding histology

A 50-MHz High-Resolution Ultrasound Imaging System for Dermatology

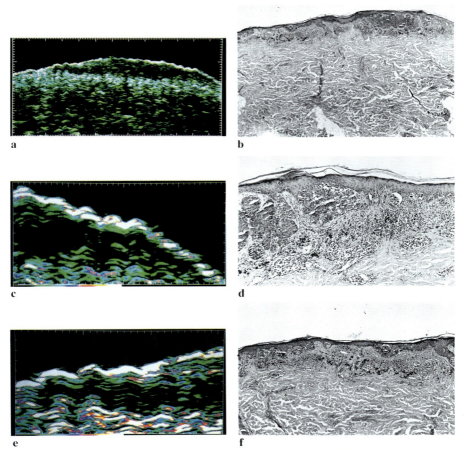

Abb. 15a–f. Malignant melanoma. **a** The ultrasound image (50 MHz) exhibits a spindle-shaped echolucent area (ELA) in the upper corium. **b** The corresponding histology exhibits large tumor cell conglomerates in the upper corium and intraepidermally. **c** Detailed enlargement of the right region. Note the echo-poor ovaloid area surrounded by undulating echolines. **d** The corresponding histology exhibits tumour cell conglomerates surrounded by an infiltrate. **e + f** Detailed enlargement of the left border of the tumour. Multiple, fine, undulating reflex-rich lines are seen in the formerly spindle-shaped region (*e*). The small scattered tumour nests seen in histology (*f*) cannot be resolved

large tumour cell conglomerates in the upper corium and the junctional zone. The corresponding sonogram exhibits a spindlelike echolucent area in first approximation beneath a thin skin entry echo (Fig. 15a). At the borders of this region irregularly shaped areas of fine undulating echo-rich reflex lines are seen. Below this region the echo texture of the corium is observed. The demarcation towards the echolucent area at the lower border is not sharp.

A detailed enlargment of the right region of the tumour shows large tumour-cell conglomerates with spindlelike cells (Fig. 15c). Within the connective tissue, between and below the tumour cell nests, an inflammatory infiltrate is visible. The sonogram, which was also amplified (x1.2), exhibits echolucent regions within zones of undulating reflex-rich lines in the formerly homogenous spindle-shaped area. Note the zones of fine green undulating lines beneath the skin entry echo. In the lower third of the figure the texture of the corium can be observed.

The left border of the spindle-shaped, echo-poor area is shown in Figs. 15e, f. The histological section exhibits a peritumoral inflammatory infiltrate with small scarce solitary tumour nests. The sonogram shows a zone of densely packed green undulating echo-rich lines beneath the skin entry echo corresponding to the infiltrate region in histology.

Discussion

Technical Equipment

A new polyvenylidendifluoride (PVDF) transducer technology enabled us to develop an ultrasound transmitter/receiver which is not much bigger than the 20-MHz ceramic transducers commercially available, but has much better lateral and axial resolution. We measured a lateral and axial resolution of 125-µm and 37.5 µm in biological tissue. The resolution of the 50-MHz machine is therefore about two times better than the resolution of the 40-MHz ultrasound equipment used by Murakami and Miki [18]. Note that our PVDF transducer did not itself reduce the image quality due to technical problems. Commenting upon his 50-MHz PVDF transducer, Dines [6] observed no advantage in employing higher frequencies for ultrasound diagnostics because of transducer image interference effects. We have found, that improving the system in the four following ways enhances image interpretation markedly:

1. To analyze epidermal substructures, low analog signal amplifications are necessary, thereby reducing signal depth. To study the corium and other deeper-lying structures, high signal amplifications are needed. To correct for these different analog signal amplifications, a digital image amplification must also be implemented. This software tool is necessary to study different skin layers (e.g. epidermis, corium) sequentially just by using different analog signal amplifications without having to exchange the transducer. Our method is superior to the exchange of the 25- and 40-MHz transducer [18].
2. By reducing the sampling distance down to 25 µm (oversampling), the resolution of the transducer can be optimized. In consequence the quality of the mechanical parts becomes increasingly important. Today's commercial high-frequency ultrasound imaging systems for in vivo skin studies use sampling steps of only 100 µm laterally.

3. Correct computer image processing is time consuming but necessary. The radio-frequency (RF) images are demodulated using envelope detection. This intermediate step reduces noise in comparison to the simple signal rectification and smoothing applied on ultrasound images from other equipment.
4. The lateral compression of the ultrasound images in comparison to histology has to be reduced from 3 (e.g. DUB 20) to 1.5. This lateral expansion has several advantages: the structures are more easily recognized and can be readily compared with histology, since they have a shape closer to reality.

The Epidermis

The first high frequent (HF) ultrasound examinations of the human skin used an unfocused 15-MHz transducer [2]. Later skin atrophy under topical corticosteroids was also characterized using this method [23]. By analyzing the A-scan signal, these research groups differentiated three structures: the dermis, the fatty tissue compartment and the muscular layer. In 1981, Cole et al. [5] measured the epidermis thickness using a 10-MHz transducer and found values between 1 and 3 mm. They pointed out that B-scan images are superior to single A scans since the two-dimensional images are comparable to histology. Other authors [9, 11] preferred to consider the skin as the summation of epidermis and dermis and were satisfied with simple thickness measurements of the cutis and the subcutaneous fatty tissue. As a matter of fact, the rarity of HF machines and the difficulty in resolving smaller structures hindered the further spreading of this new diagnostic tool.

The 50-MHz equipment can close this gap; it enables the study of gross epidermal and fine corial structures. Using a comparable echo signal amplification level the skin entry echo is only half as wide as in the lower-frequency 20-MHz machines (Figs. 3c, d). With 50 MHz the skin entry echo is comparable with thickness measurements obtained in histology.

Even very small structures lying above the epidermis (Fig. 9b) such as horn squamae, hairs or skin ridges (Fig. 6a) can be followed with great detail. A simple reduction of the analog signal amplification exhibits on the palms and the soles, and with certain restrictions, for the first time, also on the back of the patient, that the skin entry echo is composed of several layers (Fig. 3a, b). The skin entry echo ceases to be an illdefined, echo-rich line [16, 19, 20].

It is interesting to notice that the acoustic microscope has revealed two layers of different echogenic behaviour within the epidermis (U. Matthes et al., this volume). Our findings in vivo are in accordance with acoustic microscopy. Fine-granular structures like metal powder only increase the entry signal and make the slopes of the ridged skin apparent. Since the previously apparent structures were just confirmed and completed and no new structures became visible (Fig 6a, 7a), we could show that the upper border of the first layer (see Fig. 5) corresponds to the border between water and stratum corneum. By comparing our thickness measurements on the palms with histology we can show the upper echolucent layer corresponds to the stratum corneum. The border between the stratum corneum and stratum Malpighii produces a fine echo-rich line. Beneath, the stratum spinosum is echolucent.

By accepting this interpretation we can easily classify the echo-rich structure above the epidermis in psoriasis as hyperkeratotic zones and squamae. The comparison with histology shows us that our assumption was right. Furthermore focal epidermal hyperkeratoses produce a stronger focal echo-rich signal.

In psoriasis the lower border of the skin entry echo is irregular in the regions where the histological section shows elongated and enlarged psoriatric dermal papillae. The focal hyperkeratotic zones we had discussed before also produce signal attenuation (echo shadow) of the deeper skin layers.

In normal sonograms the echo signal is strongly amplified to view structures in depth, thereby merging this structures with a *wide skin entry echo*. It is remarkable that the hyperkeratosis is observed as an echo-rich structure and that focal epidermis strips show a focal echo-rich signal.

The Corium

The corium shows a homogenous, apparently randomly scattered mixture of multiple ovaloid echo-rich structures oriented preferentially horizontally. It can be clearly delimited from the echo-poor to echolucent fatty tissue region. It has been observed that in scleroderma the corium may become thicker and shows more pronounced echo reflexes [1, 21]. The good resolution of the 50-MHz equipment exhibits small anatomical structures within the corium such as hair follicles (Fig. 3c). It is therefore possible to analyse successful the hair follicle and the sebaceous gland [8].

The Subcutaneous Fatty Tissue

The 50-MHz technology is presently not well suited to study of subcutaneous fatty tissue, since in-depth echo signal reception is restricted to about 4 mm in the human skin. The fatty tissue is echolucent. In this region a few elongated echo-rich structures diagonal or parallel to the skin surface can often be seen. The correlationg histological section shows that these structures correspond to connective tissue septa, with nerve and vessel routes. Note that the skin thickness and anatomy differs greatly in different body regions [10].

Inflammatory Diseases

The use of low-frequency ultrasound machines (e.g. 15–20 MHz) in inflammatory diseases is limited due to two ultrasound phenomena:

1. Echo-poor zones within the inflammatory infiltrate do not show any sonographic differences from tumorous processes.
2. In the region of the dermal papillae a discrete inflammatory infiltrate produces a rather uniform, echolucent band (ELB), a situation which makes differential diagnosis from neoplastic diseases difficult. As has been put forward by Murakami and Miki [18], "dense inflammatory infiltrates, hypertrophic sebaceous glands and epithelial or mesenchymal tumour cell nests within the dermis were clearly demonstrated as echolucent masses or zones within a relatively dense dermal echo. However, they all looked alike".

For this reason we focused on the echolucent band of inflammatory infiltrate. Figures 9, 10 and 11 show that with further amplification this transitional zone between epidermis and corium is no longer echo-poor, but shows areas of multiple undulating fine echo lines. In all diseases examined in the present study, the gross sonographic texture of the infiltrate remained the same. However, the density of the infiltrate, as observed in histology, influenced the number and distribution of the fine undulating echo lines.

For diagnostic purposes it is interesting to know whether an intraepidermal bulla can be differentiated from a subepidermal bulla sonographically. We have to say that at the present stage of our knowledge, the 50-MHz equipment can only partly give an answer [3]. At the lateral border of the bulla the total skin entry echo has lifted itself from the underlying corium. This could be interpreted as a subepidermal bulla. From a theoretical point of view, however, a intraepidermal bulla should not be distinguished since an echo-poor structure would be apparent in a echolucent stratum spinosum. In practice this is only partly true, since the bottom of the bulla is demarcated by horizontal lines, a situation that corresponds histologically to focal reepithelization zones.

Skin Tumours

The malignant melanoma is in a first approximation a homogenous, spindle-shaped, echo-poor tumour [4, 16, 17]. Recent publications have stated that tumour masses and surrounding infiltrate look alike in ultrasound [12, 18]. Using 50 MHz and a higher magnification and amplification (Fig. 15c–f) one observes, however, that this is not true any longer. We can now observe solitary, round, nearly echolucent regions, which can be correlated to the tumour convolutes in the histological section. The peri- and subtumoral inflammatory infiltrate corresponds to zones of multiple undulating, reflex-rich green lines. Similar phenomena were also observed in the left part of the sonogram where the infiltrate predominated (Fig. 15e). The amplification we chose in the present example to differentiate between tumour and infiltrate poses immediately a new problem. Since at present no generally accepted amplification values are available, the results are therefore not reproducible on different machines, especially when their analog amplifiers do not function linearly. Different authors therefore argue quite logically [12, 18] that tumour parenchyma and infiltrate cannot be differentiated in the 20-MHz machines. In our experience very dense infiltrates and tumour masses melt together also on our 50-MHz sonograms. Since it is known from acoustic microscopy (U. Matthes et al., this volume) that infiltrate cells diffusely scatter the echo signal, it should be possible to use higher frequency transducers, combined with image processing methods, to make tissue differentiation easier. Murakami and Miki [18] used a 40-MHz sector scanner in dermatology and claimed that they were not able to differentiate between any kind of infiltrate and greater tumour conglomerates of the skin. It should be noted, however, that this particular publication is devoid of a technical description of the amplifier and transient recorder used. The sampling frequency and how many quantization levels were used for the returning echo signal are neither mentioned. Possibly the use of a membrane and sector scanner further deteriorated the image by filtering out the high frequency elements of the image.

The naevocellular naevus is an important benign tumour in the differential diagnosis of malignant melanoma. The skin entry echo over the spindle-shaped, echo-poor region corresponding to the tumour parenchyma is irregular, thickened and inhomogenous. By studying the corresponding histological section, a netlike acanthotic epithelium with fine-fibrillary connective tissue is seen. Multiple horny cores are also present. The sonogram cannot resolve this region exactly (Fig. 13), because it sums these structures up to a inhomogenous wide skin entry echo. Presently it remains unclear whether the horny cores of the papillomatous dermal naevocellular naevus seen in histology eclipse the connective tissue in the sonogram. We would like to emphazise that the 50-MHz equipment is presently not able to differentiate between the tumour parenchyma of the naevocellular naevus and malignant melanoma. Other authors have made similar statements using 20- to 40-MHz equipment [16, 18].

Lateral dissemination is of great interest in basal cell carcinoma. This holds especially for the sclerodermiform type. Circular oriented punch biopsies and a control of the borders of the excised tissue are a generally accepted procedure. With 20-MHz sonography tumour parenchyma, stroma and infiltrate can be differentiated from the surrounding tissue, as long as no actinic elastosis is present [4, 22]. As stated earlier, the 20-MHz machine, however, cannot discriminate between infiltrate and tumour masses since both structures are summed into an echolucent area [21].

Although the image resolution should still be further improved, different epidermal layers can be demonstrated at frequencies well below 300 MHz, as has been extrapolated by Breitbart and Rehpennig [4]. Medium resolution ultrasound equipment for dermatology, including 20 MHz (e.g. DUB20, Dermascan C), can be used successfully to study structures 2–8 mm beneath the skin surface. Epidermal and upper corial processes should, however, be studied at higher frequencies; 50 to 80 MHz ultrasound equipment is well suited to study these structures.

New Perspectives

We are in the process of compiling the sonographical characteristics of the inflammatory infiltrate using 50 MHz. Furthermore, image analytical concepts are being developed which enable us to compare the texture in different images within a interactively defined "region of interest". These findings could perhaps make differentiation of tumorous processes easier.

Conclusion

High resolution ultrasound imaging methods enable us to study epidermal and corial structures. For this purpose we developed a 50 MHz system with an axial resolution of 37.5 µm and a lateral resolution of 125 µm in biological tissue. To interpret the sonographic pictures, correlating histology is essential.

By reducing the preamplification of the analog echo signal prior to digitization, we could show that the so-called "skin entry echo" on the palms and the soles breaks into several layers. Metal powder experiments and the correlation with histology suggest that the upper echorich layer corresponds to the interface between the water path and the str. corneum and the second, echorich layer corresponds to the interface between the str. corneum and str. Malpighii. The anatomical nature of the third, echolucent layer beneath the second, echo rich layer on the palms and soles remains open for speculation. From its localisation it should correspond to the stratum Malpighii, which is delimited by the intensely scattered echo-texture of the corium beneath.

Supraepidermal keratotic material such as squamae are observed as echorich structures. Focal hyperkeratosis is often accompanied by an in-depth signal attenuation (e.g. seborrheic keratosis, Psoriasis vulgaris).

The corium exhibits multiple, apparently randomly scattered ovaloid reflexes, the subcutaneous fatty tissue is echolucent. Connective tissue septa with blood vessel routes are seen as linear echorich structures, forming a subcutaneous network which interconnects in a diagonal direction with the corium and the fascia by passing through the echopoor subcutaneous fatty tissue.

The inflammatory infiltrate typically shows a texture of fine undulating echo lines, thereby making it often possible to differentiate between the echolucent tumour areas and regions of scattered infiltrate. Presently it is not possible to differentiate between the sonographic texture of different skin tumours and/or between tumours and dense inflammatory infiltrate.

References

1. Akesson A, Forsberg L, Hederström E, Wollheim E (1986) Ultrasound examination of skin thickness in patients with progressive systemic sclerosis (sclerodorma). Acta Radiol Diagn 27: 91–94

2. Alexander H, Miller DL (1979) Determining skin thickness with pulsed ultrasound. J Invest Dermatol 72: 17–19
3. Auer T, el-Gammal S, Hoffmann K, Altmeyer P, Höss A, Ermert H (1990) A 50 MHz ultrasonic imaging system for dermatology: inflammatory diseases. Zentralbl Haut-Geschlechtskr 157:321
4. Breitbart EW, Rehpennig W (1983) Möglichkeiten und Grenzen der Ultraschalldiagnostik zur in vivo Bestimmung der Invasionstiefe des malignen Melanoms. Z Hautkr 58: 975–987
5. Cole GW, Handler SJ, Burnett K (1981) The ultrasonic evaluation of skin thickness in scleroderma. J Clin Ultrasound 9: 501–503
6. Dines KA (1984) High frequency ultrasound imaging of the skin, experimental results. Ultrasound Imaging 6: 408–434
7. el-Gammal S (1990) Experimental approaches and new developments with high frequency ultrasound in dermatology. Zentralbl Haut- Geschlechtskr 157: 327
8. el-Gammal S, Kenkmann J, Hoffmann K, Altmeyer P, Höß A, Ermert H (1990) The 3D architecture of human skin appendages in-vivo. In: Elsner N, Roth G (eds) Brain–perception–cognition. Thieme Stuttgart p 532
9. Fornage BD, Deshayes JL (1986) Ultasound of normal skin. J Clin Ultrasound 14: 619–622
10. Görtz S, Hoffmann K, el-Gammal S, Altmeyer P (1990) High frequency B-scan sonography and skin thickness measurements of normal skin. Zentralbl Haut-Geschlechtskr 157: 319
11. Hansen WE, Kehrer H (1987) Assessment of cutaneous fat and body fat by ultasound. Klin Wochenschr 65: 407–410
12. Hoffmann K, el-Gammal S, Matthes, U, Altmeyer P (1989) Digitale 20 MHz Sonographie der Haut in der präoperativen Diagnostik. Z Hautkr 64: 851–858
13. Höss A, Ermert H, el-Gammal S, Altmeyer P (1989) A 50 MHz ultrasonic imaging system for dermatologic application. IEEE Ultrason Symp Proc, pp 849–852
14. Höss A, Ermert H, el-Gammal S, Altmeyer P (1989) Hochauflösendes Ultraschallsystem für die Untersuchung von Hautkrankheiten und zur Tumordiagnostik in der Dermatologie. Tagung der Deutschen Gesellschaft für Biomedizinische Technik, Kiel 1989
15. Korten M, el-Gammal S, Hoffmann K, Altmeyer P, Höss A, Ermert H (1990) A 50 MHz ultrasonic imaging system for dermatology: skin tumours. Zentralbl Haut-Geschlechtskr 157: 326
16. Kraus W, Nake-Elias A, Schramm P (1985) Diagnostische Fortschritte bei malignen Melanomen durch die hochauflösende Real-time-Sonographie. Hautarzt 36: 386–392
17. Miyauchi S, Tada M, Miky Y (1983) Echographic evaluation of nodular lesions of the skin. J Dermatol 10: 221–227
18. Murakami S, Miki Y (1989) Human skin histology using high-resolution echography. J Clin Ultrasound 17: 77–82
19. Querleux B, Leveque JL, de Rigal J (1988) In vivo cross-sectional ultrasonic imaging of human skin. Dermatologica 177: 332–337
20. Schwaighofer B, Pohl-Markl H, Frühwald F, Stiglbauer R, Kokoschka EM (1987) Diagnostic value of sonography in malignant melanoma. Forschr Röntgenstr 146 (4): 409–411
21. Serup S (1984) Localized scleroderma (morphoea): thickness of sclerotic plaques as measured by 15 MHz pulsed ultrasound. Acta Derm Venereol (Stockh) 64: 214–219
22. Stücker M, Hoffmann K, el-Gammal S, Altmeyer P (1990) Digitale 20 MHz Sonographie des Basalioms im b-scan. Hautarzt 41: 333–339
23. Tan CY, Marks R, Payne P (1981) Comparison of xeroradiographic and ultrasound detection of corticosteroid inducted dermal thinning. J Invest Dermatol 71: 126–128

GHz Ultrasound Microscopy and Ultrastructure

Scanning Acoustic Microscopy: A New Procedure to Examine Skin Sections

N. Buhles, P. Altmeyer, and J. Bereiter-Hahn

Introduction

This study evaluates the possibilities of scanning acoustic microscopy (SAM)) in histopathology. The Ernst Leitz scanning acoustic microscope (ELSAM) was originally employed in material research. In this study ELSAM has been applied on sections of snap-frozen biological material.

Materials and Methods

Tissue specimens of melanocytic nevi, malignant melanomas, blue nevi and solid basal cell carcinomas were examined.

The biopsies were divided into two equal parts: one part was fixed with formaldehyde and embedded in paraffin for routine diagnostic examination. The other part was snap-frozen in liquid nitrogen and stored at −70 °C until use. Cryostat sections of 5 µm were alternately mounted on two glass slides. One glass slide was used for ultrasound examination; the other slide was stained with haematoxylin-eosin. The sections examined by light microscope can then be compared to the structures observed in SAM. Ultrasound microscopy was performed with a SAM developed by Ernst Leitz (Wetzlar, FRG). Water served as a coupling medium between the acoustic lens and the specimen, thus resulting in a lateral resolution of 1.2 µm at 1.0 GHz [1].

The reflection signals were registered by a detector, transformed to voltage oscillations and visualized as brightness modulation on a video monitor. For any focal plane chosen, the specimen was scanned line by line to produce a complete acoustic image. A „line scan mode" reveals the amplitudes of the reflected ultrasound, thus the overall reflection and resorption properties of each structure can be measured. Zones of high echo intensity appear as bright areas.

In order to obtain comparable results, the surface of the glass slide was focussed in all examinations (focal plane) and defined as total reflection.

Results

The ultrasound image reveals the following stratification of the epidermis: the stratum corneum and the stratum granulosum appear dark (low echo intensity). From stratum spinosum towards the stratum basale we found an increase in brightness. The collagen fibres of the corial connective tissue appear dark. The bright zones in the corium were due to tissue-free freezing artefacts, where the echo intensity of the glass slide was measured.

The examined skin tumors differ in their echo signals: The tumor parenchyma of malignant melanoma is characterized by a high echo intensity.

Melanocytic nevi are clearly delineated from the surrounding tissue, but are definitively more inhomogeneous than the malignant melanoma. Bright zones of high echo intensity alternate with grey zones (lower echo intensity).

The appearance of the solid basal cell carcinomas examined is different from that of the melanomas and melanocytic nevi. The echo intensity of the tumor parenchyma is similar to the overlying epithelium. The zone of low echo intensity in the basal cell carcinoma corresponds to tumor cells arranged in palisades, which are characteristic for basal cell carcinomas.

Compared to these tumors the echo intensity in blue nevi is reduced.

Discussion

Using SAM, the physical properties of biological material may be investigated at microscopic dimensions. Our observations show that the SAM images of unstained frozen sections can be correlated to the structure of light microscopy.

The homogeneous echo intensity of the malignant melanoma was not unexpected, as in vivo examinations show similar results [2, 3]. The reasons for this phenomenon have not yet been clearly understood.

Interestingly basal cell carcinomas have the same echo intensity as the epidermis. However, the inhomogeneous arrangement of the tumour cells allows physiological and pathological epithelial structures to be distinguished. Here, SAM ist superior to classical in vivo ultrasound methods.

The low echo intensity of the stratum corneum can be caused by:
1. Echo signals being absorbed by the stratum corneum
2. Diffuse diffraction of sound waves in the stratum corneum

The present study does not allow a final interpretation of the acoustic properties of tissue. Ultrasound echo signals detected by SAM (due to for example reflection, attenuation, scattering) are partly influenced by the mechanical properties of the tissue (e. g. stiffness, viscosity, elasticity). In the future the SAM method could help us to understand some of the physical properties of normal and altered biological tissues.

References

1. Bereiter-Hahn J, Buhles N (1987) Basic principles of interpretation of scanning acoustic images obtained from cell cultures and histological sections. In: Wanstecker K, et al. (eds) Imaging and visual documentation in medicine. Elsevier, Amsterdam, pp 537–543
2. Breitbart EW, Hicks R, Rehpennig W (1986) Möglichkeiten der Ultraschalldiagnostik in der Dermatologie. Z Hautkr 61 (4): 522–526
3. Buhles N, Altmeyer P (1988) Ultraschallmikroskopie an Hautschnitten. Z Hautkr 63 (11): 926–934

Acoustic Microscopy in Dermatology: Normal Skin Structures and Tumours

U. Matthes, S. Höxtermann, K. Hoffmann,
S. el-Gammal, E. Bruschke, and P. Altmeyer

Introduction

Ultrasound scanners for use in dermatology should have a high resolution. The currently used in vivo scanners operating at frequencies of up to 50 MHz are suitable to examine tissue compartments [1, 3, 6, 8, 9, 14, 19]. It is hoped that the use of very high frequency ultrasound scanners will provide important new information on the acoustic properties of individual cells and cell complexes. It is almost exactly 50 years since the Russian Sokolow [17, 18] first conceived the idea of using sound waves in the gigahertz range for microscopy but the generation of such high-frequency acoustic waves did not become possible until the 1960s. The first microscope based on ultrasound waves was built in 1974 [10, 12, 13, 18] and since then the principle has undergone further technical improvement and expansion. In 1984, the Ernst Leitz GmbH, together with Hoppe and Bereiter-Hahn [8, 20], developed such a microscope with the name ELSAM (Ernst Leitz Scanning Acoustic Microscope, Fig. 1).

ELSAM

Two different principles can be used in acoustic microscopy: either the waves transmitted through the specimen are recorded (transmission, acoustic microscopy), or the reflected waves (reflection acoustic microscopy). The latter method is employed in our acoustic microscope and, incidentally, in those generally used in medicine today. Reflection microscopy has the advantage that the transmitter and receiver are located in a single transducer lens system, while in transmission microscopy a confocal arrangement of two symmetrical lens elements is required between which the specimens are positioned. In the reflection microscope the sound waves pass as transverse wave packets through the concave sapphire lens, where they are focused. The diameter of the focus lies in the region of one wave length. After traversing the acoustic coupling medium, water, the focused beam strikes the object to be examined. The focal plane (z-axis) can be adjusted very precisely in 0.1 μm steps. In order to record the complete image, the ultrasound transducer integrated in the core piece (shown at the centre of Fig. 1) scans a field selected using a light microscope (Fig. 1) in a raster fashion, the lens being moved rapidly horizontally and transversely by a pair of moving coils.

The acoustic magnification factor ranges between 125 for an area of the specimen measuring about 900 x 700 µm and 2000 for an area of about 60 x 40 µm. The magnification can be set as required in six increments. A light microscope is used to select the area to be examined, and can then be moved aside by a pivot mechanism. In the same step, the acoustic transducer with the concave sapphire lens is positioned above the selected portion of the specimen and is thus ready for operation.

A luminescent control screen depicts the images generated in real time, and there is also a high-resolution television monitor, and a 35-mm camera for photographic documentation (see Fig. 1). The following software-driven functions can also be carried out from a control desk using the keyboard or a joystick: adjustment of frequency, choice of magnification, adjustment of z-axes (i.e. of focal plane), adjustment of brightness and contrast, setting to A-mode or DM-mode (i.e. pseudo-three-dimensional graphics).

Physical Principles

Sound waves, in contrast to electromagnetic waves, are elastic waves. In liquid and gaseous media they are propagated only as longitudinal waves, but in solids also as transverse waves.

The relationship between the input-output medium wavelength and resolution known to us from light and electron microscopy also holds here.

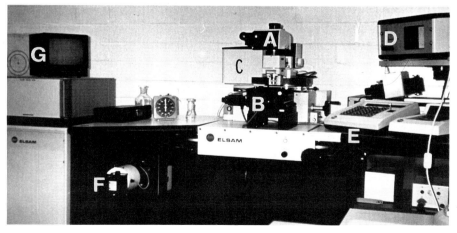

Fig. 1. Ernst Leitz Scanning Acoustic Microscope. *A* light microscope; *B* specimen stage; *C* scanner; *D* luminescent control screen; *E* control desk; *F* photographic equipment; *G* high-resolution control screen

The wavelength must be of the same order of magnitude as the size of the structure which is to be resolved. From the relationship between wavelength and frequency (see Fig. 2), it is apparent that ultrasound frequencies of at least 1–2 GHz must be generated if we are to obtain a resolution approximately equal to the resolving power of light microscopy. If high-frequency electromagnetic waves can be converted into sound waves with the same frequency, acoustic microscopy with wavelengths below 1.12M, i.e., in the range of light microscopic resolution, is possible. Modern transducer technology has created the prerequisites for this [4].

The principle of the acoustic microscope, like that of the optical microscope, is based on the fact that a wave alters its velocity when it passes from one medium to another. While, in the case of light waves, the ratio of the velocities in two different media (the refractive index) rarely exceeds 1.9 and is normally less than 1.5, the velocity of a sound wave can fall to 1/10 when passing from a solid to a liquid [21, 22]; in other words considerably higher refractive indices can be achieved with sound waves. It follows from this that, the image distortion of acoustic lenses will be much lower than that of optic lenses (Fig. 3).

Material

We examined material from human tissue biopsies. Half of the tissue was processed for normal routine diagnosis and half was frozen in liquid nitrogen and then stored at –80 °C. Unstained sections 5 µm thick were prepared on a cryostat shortly before examination and examined under the acoustic microscope. However, this preparation technique led to considerable

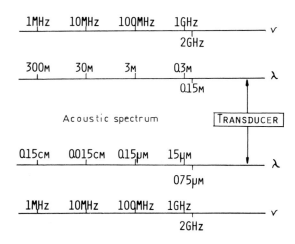

Fig. 2. The relationship between wavelength and frequency in acoustic and electromagnetic radiation (from [20])

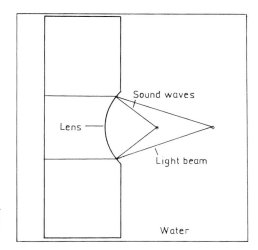

Fig. 3. The different focal lengths of sound and light on passage from a solid to a liquid at a concave surface.

preparation artefacts, particularly at higher magnifications. Partly for this reason and partly for greater convenience, we decided to use deparaffinized, likewise unstained sections 5–7 µm thick for the majority of the examinations. For the routine histological examinations, haematoxylin and eosin (HE), and van Gieson's elastin stains were used. The material examined was as follows: normal skin, 5; verruca seborrhoica, 5; basal cell carcinoma, 5; naevus cell naevus, 10; malignant melanoma, 25.

Method

Acoustic microscopy involves a completely different type of interaction with the object being examined and thus shows fundamentally different aspects than light and electron microscopy. Ultrasound waves are able to penetrate optically opaque material and thus tell us something about the interior of the object being examined. The acoustic images provide information on the elastic properties of the object (density, stiffness, acoustic attenuation). In materials science and electrical engineering acoustic microscopy is used to detect defects (e.g. microcracks, peeling, flaws), which was the purpose for which the microscope was originally developed. A further advantage lies in the possibility of non-destructive examination of living organisms [2, 8, 11, 13, 15, 16, 20].

First, the part of the object to be examined was selected using the light microscope (Fig. 1). The actual examination began after the ultrasound head had been moved into position. The sapphire lens was carefully advanced towards the object, first mechanically and then by joystick, to a distance of a few micrometers. The acoustic beam was then focused on the glass surface ($z = 0$). In this manner we were able to obtain largely standardized examination conditions.

Results

The acoustic image of the normal epidermis displays various phenomena. Figures 4 and 5 show the acoustic and optical micrographs of normal skin. At the top of Fig. 4 we see the total reflection of the glass slide, which appears white. The stratum corneum, like the regional connective tissue of the corium, is distinctly echo-poor, i.e. dark. In the epithelial band we can distinguish the stratum spinosum, stratum granulosum and stratum lucidum, the stratum spinosum being considerably more echogenic than the stratum granulosum. As expected, the keratin of the hair shaft, like the stratum corneum, is echo-poor, i.e. appears dark (Fig. 6).

Figure 7 shows a cryostat section containing sebaceous glands and a hair follicle. The sebaceous glands are highly echogenic whereas the distal region of the hair follicle is more echolucent, its echogenicity corresponding to that of the stratum corneum. The proximal region of the hair follicle contains echo-rich areas which probably represent tricholemmal cornification.

Figure 8 is an acoustic micrograph of an arteriole embedded in its surrounding tissue. The endothelium, the muscularis media and the echo-poor adventitia can be readily distinguished, the echogenicity of the adventitia corresponding to that of the surrounding collagenous connective tissue. The fatty tissue appears highly echogenic, resembling the total reflection of the glass slide. This is explained by the fact that the fat initially present was completely removed by the paraffin technique.

Figure 9 shows the corresponding light micrograph with HE staining.

In verruca seborrhoeica (Fig. 10) we again find the echo-poor stratum corneum which is retained here in the follicle. The keratin material in the pseudocysts, however, displays different acoustic characteristics. The tumour parenchyma of the verruca seborrhoeica is of similar echogenicity to normal epithelium.

Figures 11 and 12 show a naevus cell naevus of the compound type acoustic micrograph and in an HE-stained section, respectively. We see here the acanthotically thickened epithelium with the familiar reflectivity and, sharply demarcated, the highly echogenic nests of naevus cells. This pattern is seen throughout. It is interesting to note that the connective tissue stroma of the naevus cell naevus is considerably more echogenic than the underlying regional collagen. Light microscopy (Fig. 12) showed that the roundish echo-poor structure next to the naevus cell nest was an epithelial rosette.

Figure 13 shows a basal cell carcinoma nest underlying the epithelium and a hair follicle, which is shown at higher magnification in Fig. 6. This is a cryostat preparation. The cells of the basal cell carcinoma appear echo-poor. As in the naevus cell naevus, the stroma of the tumour is considerably more echogenic than the regional collagen.

Figures 14 and 15 show a highly pigmented malignant melanoma. The melanoma cell, like the naevus cell, is relatively echogenic. The pigment-laden melanoma cells are distinct from the unpigmented melanoma cells and are, surprisingly, echo-poor.

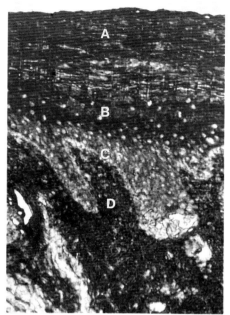
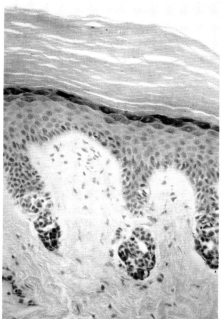

Fig. 4. Ultrasound image of the sole of foot, deparaffinized paraffin section, x 250. *A* stratum corneum; *B* stratum granulosum; *C* stratum spinosum; *D* connective tissue

Fig. 5. Histological reference section corresponding to Fig. 4. HE, x 250

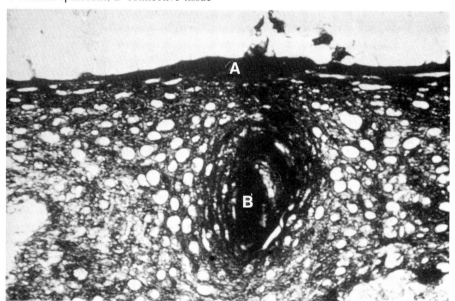

Fig. 6. Cryostat preparation of normal epithelial band, x 400. *A*, stratum corneum; *B*, hair shaft

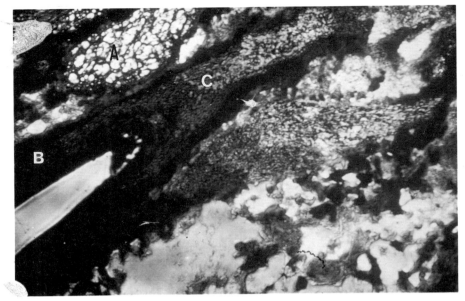

Fig. 7. Cryostat preparation of normal skin, x 600. *A*, sebaceous gland; *B*, proximal hair follicle; *C*, distal hair follicle

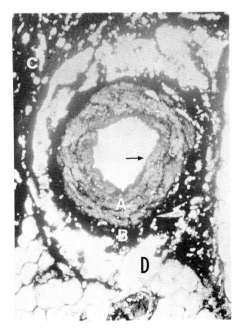

Fig. 8. Ultrasound image of an arteriole with surrounding tissue, paraffinized paraffin section, x 600. *arrow*, intima; *A*, muscularis media; *B*, advantitia; *C*, corial connective tissue; *D*, fatty tissue

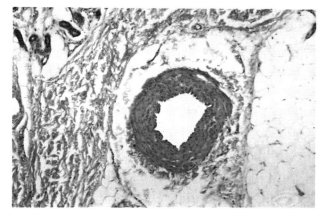

Fig. 9. Routine histological section corresponding to Fig. 8. HE, x 500

This detail image shows particularly clearly the different acoustic characteristics of stratum corneum, epithelial layer and melanoma nest.

Figure 16 shows a dense, inflammatory, mainly lymphocytic infiltrate at a magnification of about 400. In contrast to the melanoma cells, the lymphocytes appear echo-poor.

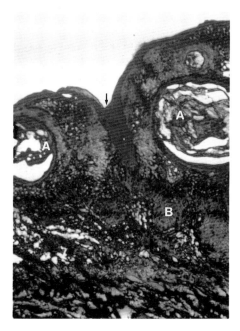

Fig. 10. Ultrasound image of a verruca seborrhoeica, deparaffinized paraffin section, x 400. *arrow*, retention of stratum corneum in follicle; *A*, pseudocysts; *B*, tumour parenchyma

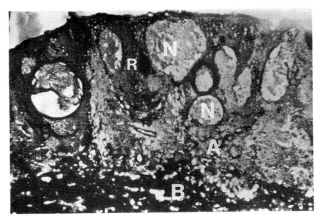

Fig. 11. Ultrasound image of a naevus cell naevus of the compound type, cryostat preparation, x 250. *N*, naevus cell nests; *A*, connective tissue stroma; *R*, epithelial rosette; *B*, connective tissue

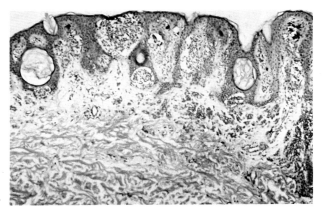

Fig. 12. Routine histological section corresponding to Fig. 11. HE, x 300

Discussion

In acoustic microscopy it is usually possible to relate the ultrasound image to the familiar light microscopic structures; staining is not necessary. During propagation through biological tissues ultrasound waves are subjected to various physical influences, the most important of which are reflection, refraction, scattering and absorption. As mentioned at the beginning, different refractive indices and thus different velocities of sound in the tissue structures contribute to the creation of the image. It is not possible to say at present precisely which physical phenomena are responsible for the differences in contrast.

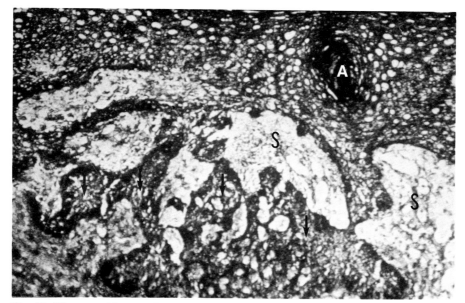

Fig. 13. Ultrasound image of a basal cell carcinoma, cryostat preparation, x 250. *arrows*, basal cell carcinoma cells; *A*, hair follicle; *S*, tumour stroma

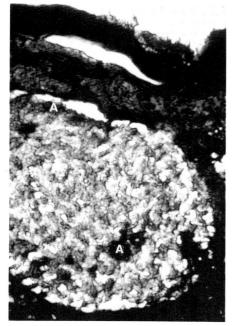

Fig. 14. Ultrasound image of a pigmented malignant melanoma, x 600. *A*, pigmented portions

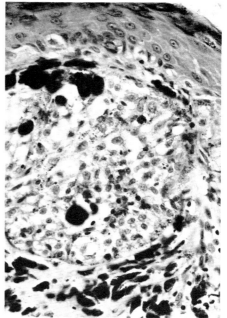

Fig. 15. Routine histological section corresponding to Fig. 14

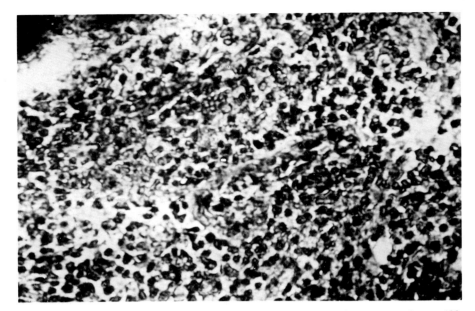

Fig. 16. Ultrasound image of a dense lymphocytic infiltrate, cryostat preparation, x 400

The markedly echo-poor pattern of the stratum corneum and of the keratinocytes was a consistent finding, as was the weak echogenicity of the regional collagenous connective tissue, although we cannot say with certainty whether this is due to marked absorption or diffuse scattering. Results comparable to those described here have also been obtained by acoustic transmission microscopy. The relatively marked echogenicity found in both the naevus cell naevus and the malignant melanoma is open to various interpretations. The most likely is that the ultrasound beam passes through the melanoma or the naevus tissue unhindered and that the highly reflective zones represent the strong reflection by the underlying glass slide. This interpretation would also correspond most closely to the ultrasound phenomena found in in vivo sonography. Our results conform largely to those of Buhles and Altmeyer 1987 [2]. A particularly interesting finding is that in both the naevus cell naevus and the basal cell carcinoma the fine fibrillary connective tissue of the stroma is considerably more echogenic than the regional collagen.

A particular difficulty in *in-vivo* ultrasound imaging is the distinction between tumour parenchyma and inflammatory infiltrate. Figure 16 shows impressively that a lymphocytic infiltrate can be identified clearly by acoustic microscopy. The lymphocytes appear echo-poor. There is thus a clear discrepancy compared with in vivo ultrasound procedures, which have not so far been able to distinguish between tumour and inflammatory reaction. It can be assumed that the reason for these discrepant findings is at least partially related to the method, i.e. to frequency and wavelength. If we assume that the ultrasound waves are able to pass through melanoma and naevus cells more or less unchanged, the results obtained in these two types of tumour are concordant with those of in vivo ultrasound, whereas both basal cell carcinoma and inflammatory cells interact with the sound waves in acoustic microscopy.

The high resolution of acoustic microscopy enables us to study the ultrasound properties of individual cells and cell complexes. Acoustic microscopy is thus able to provide important data on tissues which can supplement or even correct the findings obtained by *in-vivo* ultrasound methods.

References

1. Altmeyer P (1989) Dermatologische Ultraschalldiagnostik – gegenwärtiger Stand und Perspektiven. Z Hautkr 64: 727–728
2. Buhles N, Altmeyer P (1988) Ultraschallmikroskopie an Hautschnitten. Z Hautkr 63 (9):
3. Fornage DW, Deshaynes JL (1986) Ultrasound of normal skin. J Clin Ultrasound 14: 619–622
4. Hildebrand J A, Rugar D (1984) Measurement of cellular elastic properties by acoustic microscopy. J Micros 134 (3): 245–260
5. Hildebrand JA, Rugar D, Johnston RN, Quate CF (1981) Acoustic microscopy of living cells. Proc Natl Acad Sci USA 78 (3): 1656–1660
6. Hoffmann K, el-Gammal S, Altmeyer P (1989) 20 MHz B-scan Sonographie an Händen und Füßen. in: Altmeyer P, Schultz-Ehrenberg U, Luther H (eds) Handsymposium: Dermatologische Erkrankungen der Hände und Füße. Editiones Roche, Basel, pp 285–300
7. Hoffmann K, el-Gammal S, Matthes U, Altmeyer P (1989) 20 MHz Sonographie der Haut in der präoperativen Diagnostik. Z Hautkr 64: 851–858
8. Hoppe M, Bereiter-Hahn J (1985) Applications of scanning acoustic microscopy – survey and new aspects. IEEE Trans Sonics Ultrason 32: 289–301
9. Kessler LW (1974) Review of progress and applications in acoustic microscopy. J Acoust Soc Am 55 (5): 909–918
10. Kessler LW, Yuhas DE (1978) Principles and analytical capabilities of the scanning laser acoustic microscope (SLAM). Scanning Electron Microsc I: 555–559
11. Kolosov OV, Levin VM, Mayev RG, Senjushkina TA (1987) The use of acoustic microscopy for biological tissue characterisation. Ultrasound Med Biol 13 (8): 477–483
12. Lemons RA, Quate CF (1974) Acoustic microscope – scanning version. Appl Phys Lett 24: 163–165
13. Lemons RA, Qaute CF (1979) Acoustic microscopy. In: Mason WP, Thurston RN (eds) Physical acoustics. Principles and methods, vol 14. Academic Press, New York, pp 1–92
14. Payne PA (1983) Non-invasive skin measurement by ultrasound. RNM Images 13: 577–580
15. Quate CF (1979) The acoustic microscope. Sci Am 10: 58–66
16. Quate CF (1980) Microwaves, acoustics and scanning microscopy. In: Ash EA (ed) Scanned image microsocpy. Academic Press, London, pp 23–55

17. Sokolov S (1936) USSR patent
18. Sokolov S (1949) Acoustic microscopy. Dokl. Akad. Nouk SSSR 64: 333
19. Serup J, Northheved A (1985) Skin elasticity in localized skleroderma (Morphea). J Dermatol 12: 52–62
20. Thaer A, Hoppe M, Patzelt WJ (1982) Akustomikroskop ELSAM. Leitz Mitt Wiss Tech 8: 61-67
21. Weglein RD (1983) Integrated circuit inspection via acoustic microscopy. IEEE Trans Sonics Ultrason 30: 40–42
22. Weglein RD, Wilson RG (1978) Characteristic materials signatures by acoustic microscopy. Electron Lett 14: 352–354
23. Yamanaka K, Enomoto Y (1982) Observation of surface cracks with scanning acoustic microscope. J Appl Physiol 53: 846–850
24. Yin QR, Ilatt C, Briggs GAD (1982) Acoustic microscopy of ferroelectric ceramics. J Mater Sci 17: 2449–2452

From Ultrasound to Ultrastructure

K. Schmidt, M. Bacharach-Buhles, N. Buhles,
K. Hoffmann, and P. Altmeyer

Introduction

The principle of ultrasound diagnosis is the transformation of sound waves into visible light waves. The sound waves transverse different skin layers and become diffracted, reflected, scattered, and dampened at their surface borders due to different stiffness. The kind of modulation of the sound waves depends on the chemical composition, density, elasticity, form, and arrangement of the tissue structures [4].

After interaction of the sound waves with the tissue, several echo impulses are reflected and partly reach the sound generator where they are digitalized, e. g. by an IBM compatible computer, and reproduced as a "picture" made up of false colours. From this picture we clinicians try to perceive the different anatomical and pathological structures of the examined skin. However, it is unclear whether we are justified in assigning morphology to ultrasound patterns. Therefore, we tried to find a correlation between histological structures and their physical qualities, as expressed in ultrasound images.

Materials and Methods

In our study we examined various skin tumors – acral-lentiginous melanoma, superficial spreading melanoma, dysplastic melanocytic nevus, basal cell carcinoma, verrucous carcinoma, Bowen disease, verruca seborrheoica, and Kaposi's sarcoma – and a cryolesion by clinical inspection using light, ultrasound, and electron microscopy.

In this article we concentrate on presentation of the findings from superficial spreading melanoma, dysplastic melanocytic nevus, and basal cell carcinoma.

For our ultrasound examinations we employed two instruments, differing in their spatial resolution capacities and applicability: A 20 MHz device was used for in vivo measurements and the ELSAM, an ultrasound microscope, for the study of frozen sections.

The in vivo measurements were done using the DUB 20. It consists of a computer keyboard for electronic control and an applicator, which has incorporated a transducer which works at an average frequency of 20 MHz and is coupled to the region of examination using a water bath. The large axial resolution of 70 μm and the penetration depth of 7.5 mm result from the high frequency of 20 MHz.

In contrast to the axial resolution, the lateral resolution depends on the focus size of the "acoustic rays", i.e., on the quality of the acoustic lenses [5].

In our equipment it is about 200 μm. Futhermore, the spatial resolution depends on the recorded ultrasound information and on the quality of the screen.

After penetration of the tissue, the reflected part of the sound waves is received by the transducer. The analog signal is then digitalized, stored line by line in the computer and demodulated into the patterns of an image.

The equipment described here is able to provide representations in A-, B-, M- and HF-modes. In our study, we preferred the B-mode images of the color screen, in which gradations of colors from white to black are associated with 256 gradations of gray. White and blue correspond to high-echo signals, green to low-echo and black to the absence of echo signals.

After in vivo examination of the tumors, the patients were assigned to surgery. Subsequently, one part of the specimen was sent for routine histology. Another sample was frozen immediately in liquid nitrogen and stored at −70 °C to be cut into 7-μm-thick frozen sections with a freezing microtome for GHz examinations. For acoustic examinations we used the ELSAM (Ernst Leitz scanning acoustic microscope) which works at a frequency of 1.0 GHz, providing a lateral resolution of 1.2 μm and a magnification of 2000 [2, 6].

To correlate the ELSAM images with those of light microscopy, we embedded an adjacent part of the tissue in paraffin wax and prepared hematoxylin and eosin stained sections.

In the "acoustic pictures" we compared the areas appearing in white to black gradations with the reflection quality of glass as a reference value. Areas which reflect both the sound waves and glass appear as a bright pattern.

Another part of the tumor was fixed in glutaraldehyde (3%) over at least 4 h, rinsed, and then cured with a OsO4 solution (1%) for 1.5 h; the samples were embedded in Epon 812. Contrasting of the gold to silver ultrathin sections on the grid was done with uranyl acetate and lead nitrate. We then selected several of the tumor cells and photographed them with the EM9 (Zeiss) electron microscope. At a magnification of 12 400 we evaluated the electron microscopy pictures morphometrically with a scanner; the lowest surface area unit was 1 mm^2 (Fig. 1).

The whole cell surface was defined as 100%; the single organelles were subdivided into dense and translucent units and expressed as a percentage of the whole cell [12].

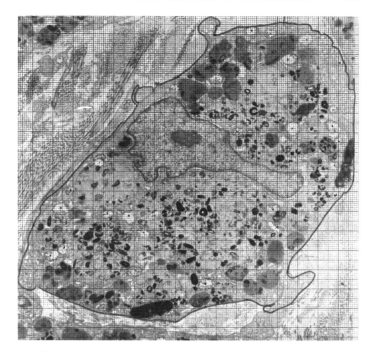

Fig. 1. Melanoma cell with an overlying scan of morphometric measurements. (x 4290)

Results

We found a correlation between the percentage of electron dense areas inside a cell and the reflection of sound waves. Histologically, the superficial spreading melanoma contains cells with a fine granular and vacuolized cytoplasm around a large irregularly shaped nucleus. These cells are found in the lower epidermis and upper dermis, embedded in an edematous connective tissue with many round infiltrate cells and pigment loaded melanophages [1, 18, 19].

The ultrastructure of the melanoma cell consists of ballooned mitochondriae and an enlarged and well-developed endoplasmic reticulum. Beside these translucent structures, the cell contains pigment granules, differing in degree of maturation and density (Fig. 2a) [8, 10, 14, 15].

In Fig. 3a we show the results of the morphometrical evaluation; the translucent cell area was 17.4 % and the dense area 39.1 %.

The acoustical picture of a melanoma nest is a homogeneous, transparent, echo-rich area clearly distinguishable from the adjacent tissue its lower echo intensity (Fig. 4). These supposed numerous signals are obtained from the reflection of the microscope slide [6]. The sound waves pass the bright tumor cells without hindrace, strike the glassy microscope slide, and are reflected.

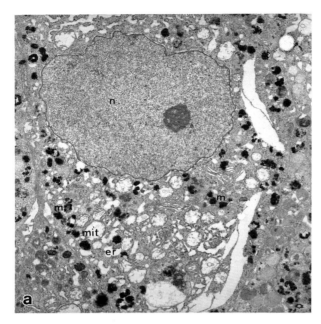
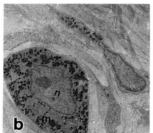
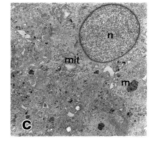

Fig. 2. *a* Ultrastructure of the melanoma cell with ballooned mitochondriae *(mit)*, enlarged endoplasmic reticulum *(er)*, and melanosomes *(m)* in different stages of maturation and density; *n*, nucleus (x 5590); *b* Oval type I nevus cell with many dense pigment granules; *n*, nucleus; *m*, melanosomes; *bl*, basal lamina (x 1992); *c* Dendritic type II nevus cell with few melanosomes; *n*, nucleus; *m*, melanosomes; *mit*, mitochondriae. (× 2790)

This means that the melanoma cell itself provides an echo-poor pattern in the GHz range.

In a dysplastic melanocytic nevus the nevus cells are arranged in well-circumscribed nests with large bright, irregularly shaped nuclei with prominent nucleoli, as demonstrated by toluidine blue staining. The surrounding connective tissue fibers are swollen edematously.

In comparison to melanoma cells, the cytoplasm of nevus cells is brighter and contains fewer pigment granules. Further on, we find fewer round cells and melanophages in the infiltrate of the nevus.

Ultrastructurally, the morphology of the single nevus cells is different. Therefore, we can distinguish between two types of nevus cells: The round to oval type I nevus cell (Fig. 2b) is poor in organelles and rich in pigment granules of different volume and density. The cytoplasm often shows intracytoplasmic luminae [8]. The nucleus is folded inward with one or more prominent nucleoli [7, 8, 15–17].

In the dendritic type II nevus cell (Fig. 2c), there are fewer melanosomes [14–16]. In contrast to the relatively few dense substructures, there are many translucent mitochondriae and an abundant endoplasmic reticulum. In dermal nevus cell nests, the close connections of pseudopodial processes appear as a mosaic-like picture [8].

Both types of nevus cells are delineated by a basal lamina [8]. The evaluations of the cell composition of the various nevus cells are shown in Figs. 3b and 3c. Here the different morphologies become obvious: a small translucent cell area of 5.8% cells, and 11.3% in type II and a dense area of 37.4% in type I and 25.5% in type II.

In the ELSAM image the nevus cell nest can also easily be distinguished from the adjacent tissue. Nevus cells yield a higher echo intensity than melanoma cells, which appear as an inhomogeneous cloudy area (Fig. 4) [2, 6].

We also analyzed a basal cell carcinoma taken from a female patient's back. Histologically, tumor cell lobes are seen in the dermal stroma surrounded by

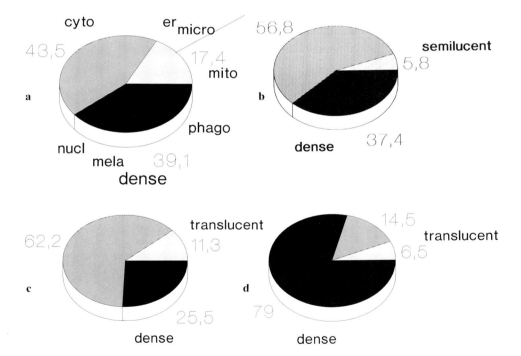

Fig. 3. a–d Cell composition (in %) of the *a* melanoma cell; *b* type I nevus cell (semi lucent and large dense areas); *c* type II nevus cell (with a smaller dense area than that of the type I cell); and *d* basal cell carcinoma (wherein the dense area clearly prevails). *cyto*, cytoplasm; *nucl*, nucleus; *mela*, melanosome; *phago*, phagosome; *mito*, mitochondriae; *er*, endoplasmatic reticulum

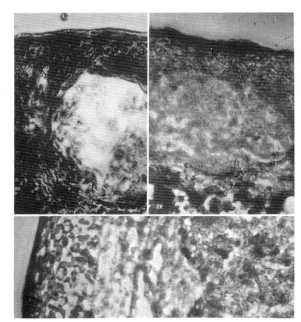

Fig. 4. ELSAM images of melanoma tumor nest *(left)*, nevus cell tumor nest *(right)*, 2nd basal cell carcinoma *(bottom, right)*

a huge infiltrate and ectatic blood vessels [8]. The typical palisade-like arrangement of the peripheral cell layer can, more or less, clearly be observed. Inside the tumor cell nest we find compact areas intermixed with loose areas, where the intercellular spaces are remarkably wide.

Ultrastructurally, a large irregular folded nucleus with two or more nucleoli is prominent. The surrounding cytoplasm is poor in organelles and there are few tonofilaments and desmosome-tonofilament complexes. The intercellulare spaces are widened and intercellular connections are provided by elongated cytoplasmic protrusions [7, 8]. The correlating morphometry values are shown in Fig. 3b. The translucent cell area is only 6.5%, compared to a dense area of 79%. The ELSAM image of the basal cell carcinoma shows a high-echo intensity, similar to that of the epidermis (Fig. 4) [6].

In summary the ELSAM images of the discussed tumors can be distinguished from one another by their echo reflections (Fig. 4). The lowest echo intensity was found in malignant melanoma, in which the highly visible echo intensity arises from the reflection of the glass slide. In comparison to malignant melanoma, the nevus cell nest yields a larger echo reflection and the islands of the basal cell carcinoma the largest [6].

Ultrastructurally, the melanoma cells have the largest translucent cell area (17.4%) followed by the nevus II cells (11.3%).

The basal cell carcinoma has the smallest translucent cell area (6.5%), but a clearly prevailing dense one.

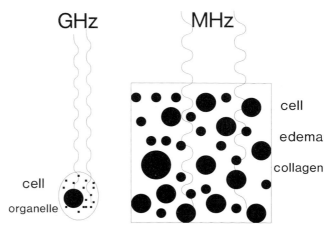

Fig. 5. Spatial resolution of ultrasound in GHz or MHz range, single cells and accumulation of cells

Regarding the correlation of ultrasound with the ultrastructure of the cell, this model cannot be applied for the 20 MHz range because both instruments differ in their spatial resolution capacity [2, 6, 8, 9].

Whereas the ELSAM is able to resolve single cells, the 20 MHz instrument recognizes an accumulation of cells only (Fig. 5). Therefore, we increased our counting area and evaluated an infiltrate area with abundant cells, connective tissue fibers, and edema.

Considering the various tumors analyzed by 20 MHz imaging, we always found an area poor in reflection in the region of the tumor, whereas the various tumors themselves partly produced internal echos [3, 5, 11, 13].

Light microscopically, all tumors are embedded in an infiltrate with differing numbers of various cells, dilated blood vessels, and edema. This infiltrate cannot be clearly distinguished from the tumorous tissue in the 20 MHz ultrasound images. Both structures appear as an area poor in reflection [3, 4].

Comparing the translucent area in malignant melanoma (17.4%) and in the infiltrate (19.1%) we see that both structures are roughly similar. If we consider the dense areas, we find of 43.5% in malignant melanoma and 31.1% in the infiltrate (Fig. 6).

Discussions

General Physical Observations

Transversing the skin, sound waves strike structures of different density and sound transmission properties. At the border surfaces of two adjacent

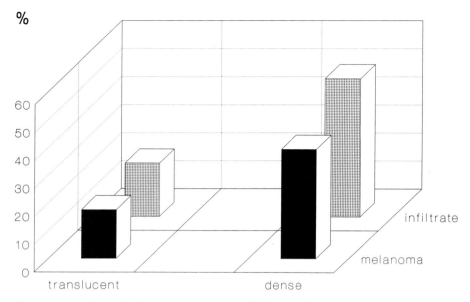

Fig. 6. Comparison of malignant melanoma and infiltrate with respect to the composition of dense or translucent substructures

substructures, e.g., water/stratum corneum, tumor/infiltrate, and infiltrate/dermis the sound waves are reflected [3].

Depending on the density, the spreading speed of sound waves changes when passing the various tissues and structures. The greater the difference in density between two closely lying substructures, the greater the amount of reflection [9].

Only that portion of reflection which is reflected vertically hits the transducer and can be measured, thereby determining the ultrasound image. Consequently, the largest number of echoes come from a tissue's border surfaces, which lie horizontal to the sound waves' transmission path. Influence which reduce the amount of direct reflection are a large number of membranous substructures of different densities and arrangement and changes of elasticity and fluidity inside a tissue. The greater the fluidity and the more border surfaces the fewer the vertical sound reflections, resulting in an image with fewer patterns. The reflection due to water filled organelles is less than that of dense structures. Numerous membranous organelles cause a high degree of scattering.

Change in Density and Sound Reflection

Inside tumorous and inflammatory tissue we find a variation of all aforesaid physical properties.

The morphometric measurements show that a different composition of dense, translucent, and semilucent areals exist inside cells of various tumors. In melanoma cells, we find a dense cell area of 43.5 %, while nevus cells have a larger dense area with (56.8 % in type I and 62.2 % in type II). The largest dense area percentage (79 %) can be found in basal cell carcinoma cells (Fig. 3 a–d). With respect to the GHz images of the various tumors (Fig. 4), we can easily recognize a direct correlation between the percent density of a cell and the reflection of sound waves. Malignant melanoma, with the smallest dense area of the three tumors has the least echoes. The nevus has a higher density and more echoes. In the basal cell carcinoma we find the highest echo intensity, resulting in an image full of contrasts. The obvious conclusion is: the larger the dense area of the cell in electron microscopy, the greater the sound reflection in ultrasound microscopy.

In the MHz range, the dense substructures of cells cannot be seen because of the lower resolution of 200 μm. Tumor nests, with many dense cells, are embedded in an infiltrate, which also consists of closely lying dense cells. Since the borders of the single cells cannot be distinguished, the 20 MHz equipment recognizes both structures, the tumor and the infiltrate, as areas of similar density. In our evaluation we found a density of 43.5 % in the melanoma itself and 31.3 % in the infiltrate area (Fig. 6). Without a significant gradation of density between both structures, we do not really have a border surface and hence no reflection of sound waves. These ideas are corroberated in the 20 MHz images in which the nests of malignant melanoma as well as the infiltrate appear absent of echo patterns.

Number of border Surfaces and Sound Reflection

In the tumors discussed here the dense or translucent portion belongs to a number of different organelles. The distribution can be seen in the ultrastructural image of the tumor cells; it is not evaluated numerically (Fig. 2 a–c).

In the melanoma cell (Fig. 2 a) the dense area consists of a large nucleus and a few pigment granules. The translucent area consists of many membranous liquid filled organelles. In nevus cells we find many pigment granules beside the nucleus in the dense region of type I cells (Fig. 2 b), in contrast to the few melanosomes found in type II cells (Fig. 2 c). The number of translucent liquid filled organelles is less in both types of nevus cells compared melanoma cells.

We found the fewest organelles in basal cell carcinoma cells. Here, the large dense area consists of a large nucleus.

Regarding the ELSAM images of the various tumors (Fig. 1), it is obvious that melanoma cells, with the most organelles that appear as translucent vesicles, yield the fewest echo reflections. While the number of substructures decreases from nevus to basal cell carcinoma, the echo reflection increases inversely. The more membranous organelles inside a cell the higher the scattering and the fewer vertical sound reflections.

We do not want to enter into the particulars of the 20 MHz range here. Due to the lower resolution capacity, the consideration of border surfaces in single cells or a cell's organelles cannot explain the sound phenomena in this region.

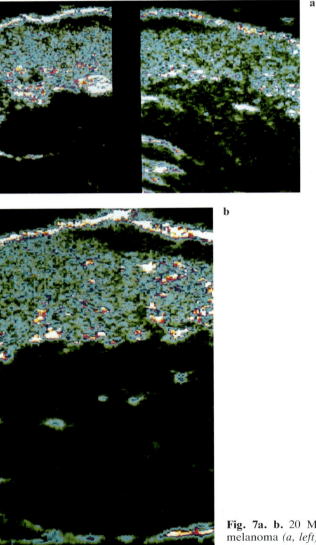

Fig. 7a. b. 20 MHz image of malignant melanoma *(a, left)*, and dysplastic melanocytic nevus *(a, right)*, and basal cell carcinoma *(b)*

Change in Fluidity, Elasticity, and Sound Reflection

Ultrastructurally, melanoma cells mainly contain ballooned mitochondriae and a dilated endoplasmic reticulum which means an increased of amount liquid inside the cell (Fig. 2a).

The echo reflection of liquid structures is lower than that of dense ones. Here we find another correlation with the low-echo intensity of melanoma cells analyzed in the GHz range. The cytoplasm of melanoma cells contains many membranous liquid filled organelles; the ELSAM image thus represents an echo-poor pattern (Fig. 4).

Histologically, the tumor cell nests are surrounded by an edematous infiltrate. This means that the sound waves pass from the liquid-rich tumor cell nests into the infiltrate which is also liquid-rich. Due to the same physical qualities of both structures we see no reflection by scanning the affected tissue. Here we find an explanation for the loss of signals inside the area of tumor and infiltrate and for the insufficient discrimination between tumor and infiltrate in MHz measurements.

The increased amount of liquid produces a loosening inside the cell and tissue, resulting in destruction of membranous border surfaces. The destructions cause a decrease in elasticity, which produces a diminished echo reflection.

In conclusion, we find a low-echo reflection in the GHz range if the cells contain many membranous substructures and if the translucent area prevails over the dense one. An increase of fluidity, resulting in a loosening of the structure and a change in elasticity, promotes the loss of echo signals.

In the 20 MHz range we have to consider an accumulation of cells, the physical qualities inside the area, and the change in density between two adjacent areas. The final result is that 20 MHz equipment cannot distinguish between benign and malignant tumors nor between tumor and adjacent infiltrate because the physical quality of both tissues is similar.

Even if the electron density alone cannot explain all ultrasound phenomena, it surely provides one key for the decoding of our ultrasound images. In addition, it demonstrates that we need high frequency equipment to resolve the small structures of the skin.

References

1. Balch CM, Milton GW (1985) Cutaneous melanoma. Lippincott, Philadelphia
2. Bereiter-Hahn J, Buhles N (1987) Basic principles of interpretation of scanning acoustic images obtained from cell cultures and histological sections. In: Wamsteker K et al. (eds) Imaging and visual documentation in medicine. Elsevier, Amsterdam, pp 537–543
3. Breitbart EW, Rehpenning W (1983) Möglichkeiten und Grenzen der Ultraschalldiagnostik zur in vivo Bestimmung der Invasionstiefe des malignen Melanoms. Z Hautkr 58 (13): 975–987
4. Breitbart EW, Hicks R, Rehpenning W (1986) Möglichkeiten der Ultraschalldiagnostik in der Dermatologie. Z Hautkr 61 (8): 522–526

5. Breitbart EW, Müller CE, Hicks R, Vieluf D (1989) Neue Entwicklungen der Ultraschalldiagnostik in der Dermatologie. Aktuel Dermatol 15: 57–61
6. Buhles N, Altmeyer P (1988) Ultraschallmikroskopie an Hautschnitten. Z Hautkr 63 (11): 926–934
7. Daroczy J, Racz I (1987) Diagnostic electron microscopy in practical Dermatology. Akademiaikiado, Budapest
8. Fornage BD, Deshayes JL (1986) Ultrasound of normal skin. J Clin Ultrasound 14: 619–622
9. Hoffmann K, el-Gammal S, Altmeyer P (1989) 20 MHz-Sonographie an Händen und Füßen. In: Altmeyer P et al. (eds) Dermatologische Erkrankungen der Hände und Füße, Handsymposion. Editiones "Roche", Basel, pp 285–300
10. Hunter JAA, Zaynoun S, Paterson WD, Bleehen SS, Mackie R, Cochran AJ (1978) Cellular fine structure in the invasive nodules of different histogenetic types of amlignant melananoma. Br J Dermatol 98: 255–272
11. Kraus W, Nake-Elias A, Schramm P (1985) Diagnostische Fortschritte bei malignen Melanomen durch die hochauflösende Real-Time-Sonographie. Hautarzt 36: 386–392
12. Reith A, Mayhew PM (1988) Steriology and norphometry in electron microscopy. Problems and solution. Hemisphere, New York
13. Sander C, Tschochohei H, Hagedorn M (1989) Zur Epidemiologie des dysplastischen Nävus. Hautarzt 40: 758–760
14. Schwaighofer B, Pohl-Mark H, Frühwald F, Stiglbauer R (1987) Der diagnostische Stellenwert des Ultraschalls beim malignen Melanom. Fortschr Rothgenstr 146 (4): 409–411
15. Seki T, Rhodes AR, Fitzpatrick TB (1986) Electron microscopic observation of intraepidermal melanocytes in dysplastic melanocytic nevi, superficial spreading melanoma, typical acquired nevomelanocytic nevi, and normal skin. Jpn J Dermatol 96: 410
16. Strasser W, Wokalek H, Vanscheidt W, Schöpf E (1987) B-Scan-Ultraschall in der Dermatologie. Hautarzt 38: 660–663
17. Takahashi H, Horikoshi T, Jimbow K (1985) Fine structural characterization of melanosomes in dysplastic nevi. Cancer 56: 111–123
18. Takahashi H, Yamana K, Maeda K, Akutsu Y, Horikoshi T, Jimbow K (1987) Dysplastic melanocytic nevus. Electron-microscopic observation as a diagnostic tool. Am J Dermatopathol (3): 189–196
19. Wolff H, Schmeller W (1985) Cutaneous melanoma. Lippincott, Philadelphia.

Three-Dimensional Computer Reconstructions

Principles of Three-Dimensional Reconstructions from High-Resolution Ultrasound in Dermatology*

S. EL-GAMMAL, K. HOFFMANN, J. KENKMANN, P. ALTMEYER, A. HÖSS, and H. ERMERT

Introduction

When the first high frequency A-scan ultrasound imaging systems became available in dermatology [1], interpretation of the voltage oscillation curve was reduced to thickness measurements of the cutis, subcutaneous fatty tissue and muscle fascia. In those years especially images of the corium-subcutis interface were likely to be misinterpreted due to fatty tissue inlets or hair follicle structures. With the advent of two-dimensional high-resolution ultrasound imaging systems, the interpretation has become much easier. However, apart from gross pathological structures (e.g. tumours, inflammatory conditions), little progress in image interpretation was made because the ultrasound images greatly differ from traditional dermatohistology. But by correlating *in vivo* ultrasound images with histological sections taken from the very same skin region, different smaller anatomical or pathological structures can also be discerned using ultrasound. Presently, this correlation is still necessary to prove and understand the way different structures are represented in the ultrasound image and also for discarding artefacts which are due to structure image interference (e.g. speckle) combined with a limited resolution. It is to be expected in future that with further experience, histological methods will become increasingly obsolete for image interpretation. High-resolution ultrasound will only then become a truly non-invasive method.

During this period of knowledge aquisition, we have become increasingly aware that different skin structures have a specific shape in space and are oriented in a particular way. The loss of skin tension and elasticity modifies structure shape and appearance in histology compared with *in vivo* methods. Our knowledge of the skin architecture is therefore based upon "histological artefacts" to date.

Thus, it is important to study the existing, living three-dimensional architecture of different anatomical skin structures and pathological conditions to understand structure shape and orientation *in vivo*.

---

* Essential parts of this publication are part of the dissertation of Mrs. Kenkmann (hair follicle reconstructions).

Axis Definitions

Today, single transducers (and not transducer arrays) are commonly used in dermatology. These transducers work in pulse-echo mode as transmitter/receiver (Fig. 1a). Accordingly, the in-depth (axial) image information is gained by transforming the time elapsed between the acoustic pulse and the returning echo into spacial distances (z-axis) by assuming a *constant sound speed* in different tissues. Note that this assumption is among other reasons responsible for the inaccuracies of skin measurements compared with caliper or post-mortem measurements. In fact, sound speed actually varies by about 10 % in different biological tissues of the skin [25]. Note that in other structures, like bone, sound velocity is about twice that in soft tissues.

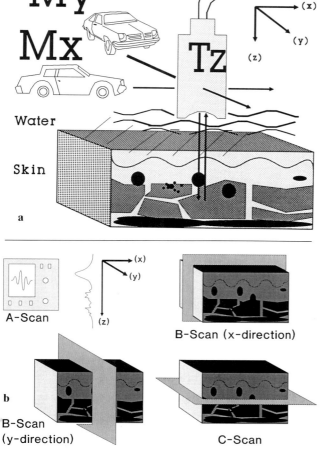

Fig. 1 a, b. The applicator and different scanning modes. **a** Axis definitions of the applicator. Two stepper motors *(M)* move the transducer *(T)* laterally over the skin surface. The z-axis is calculated by transforming the time lapse of the returning echo signal into a distance representation. While the z-axis is oriented vertically, the x- and y-axes are oriented horizontally in relation to the skin surface. All axes are orthogonal to each other.
b A-, B- and C-scan. The A-scan is a solitary amplitude modulated echo signal which has been transformed into a distance representation. B-scans use many A-scans which are aligned to one another forming a two-dimensional image. Every A-scan is reduced to a single line by transforming the echo signal amplitude into a brightness modulation of the points along the line. The C-scan is defined as horizontal section through the skin. The two B-scan planes and the C-scan plane are orthogonal to each other

By moving this transducer laterally in one direction (e.g. x-axis) grossly parallel to the skin surface, multiple A-scans (*a*mplitude) can be obtained. Every scan is then demodulated and its signal amplitude is transformed into a brightness modulation. By placing many such lines side by side, we finally obtain a two-dimensional B-scan (*b*rightness) image (Fig. 1b).

If two motors are used to move the transducer over a surface area (Fig. 1a), a tissue block can be sectioned in a variety of ways. Different scanning strategies are now conceivable for moving the transducer over a plane pitched by the x- and y-axis (Fig. 1a). Firstly, however, we should discuss some specifications of signal processing and resolution to enable judgement of these different scanning strategies.

Signal Processing

When an image is to be processed by computers, it is often described as a matrix, or some other discrete data structure. The first problem is therefore the conversion of a continuous signal (e.g. the received echo signal) into a discrete form. This involves two processes: *sampling*, which is the selection of a discrete grid of points in continuous time or space to represent a signal, and *quantization*, which is the mapping of the signal amplitude into integer values.

Only values of the signal at those selected points are then used for further processing. The following question arises: which sampling frequency/distance is adequate for a particular signal? Shannon demonstrated that the sampling frequency must be at least twice the maximum frequency of the analog signal. In the English-language-literature this theorem is also known as Nyquist sampling rate [2].

Note that this theorem does not suggest a way of reconstructing a continuous signal from its discrete samples. It only states that this is possible. In fact, fairly sophisticated techniques are needed to reconstruct a signal when it is sampled at the minimum frequency. If restricted to a particular form of reconstruction, the sampling frequency may have to be well above the minimum which is suggested by Shannon's sampling theorem.

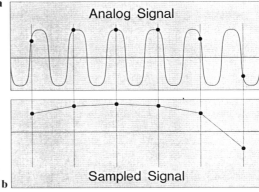

Fig. 2 a, b. Aliasing phenomena. The original analog signal (**a**) and the sampled signal (**b**). Due to a sampling frequency that was only a little different from the frequency of the original signal, the interconnecting curve between sampled points *(b)* gives the illusion of a low-frequency signal

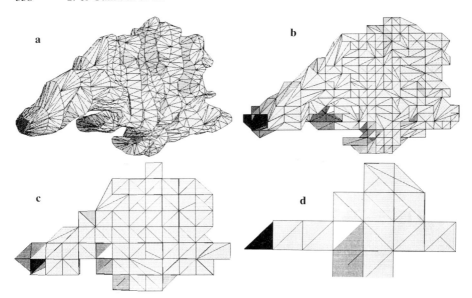

Fig. 3 a–d. Scaling phenomena. When structures have to be transformed from an analog drawing onto a discrete integer grid, inadequate scaling can alter the shape of those structures. **a** hair follicle in telogen state with its sebaceous gland scaled at optimum. In the other figure parts the scaling was reduced by 10 (**b**) by 20 (**c**) by 40 (**d**). Zooming after transformation could only enlarge the already faulty shape (**b–d**)

If the sampling interval does not satisfy these conditions, then a distortion of the spectrum occurs. High frequencies are folded onto lower frequencies, producing a phenomenon known as *aliasing*. Figure 2 illustrates this effect in the one-dimensional case: a high-frequency signal appears as a low-frequency signal after sampling at too low rate. The aliasing phenomenon can simulate nonexisting structures.

A different effect occurs when a coarse discrete grid is used during the sampling process. This grid is well above the minimum sampling frequency discussed earlier. Figure 3 displays a similar effect for a three-dimensional object. Here an object with floating-point coordinates was scaled and converted into the integer space. During this mathematical transformation truncating takes place, thereby producing rounding off errors. These errors become critical when, due to an inadequate scaling factor, small structures are transformed to an integer grid[2]. Figure 3 demonstrates that structures can even change their shape when transformed into the integer space. Zooming after sampling may then enlarge the faulty shape further.

Figure 4 compares two commercially sold high-frequency ultrasound systems with the 50-MHz experimental system used in our laboratory. It becomes apparent that images can only be partially compared. This

---

[2] An integer grid is a multidimensional array of discrete values as elements, such as 0, 1, 2, ...

	DUB 20	Dermascan	50 MHz
Transducer			
centre-frequency	20 MHz*	20 MHz*	40 MHz*
bandwidth (−6 dB)	10 MHz*	15 MHz*	30 MHz*
material	ceramic	ceramic	PVDF
Signal processing			
sampling rate	100 MHz	60 MHz	200 MHz
quantization	8 bits	6 bits	10 bits
sampling points	1024	1024	1024
Demodulation	digital	analog	digital
Interpolation	no	no	yes
graphics	raster display	raster display	raster display
false colour coding	yes	yes	yes
Applicator			
water path	yes	yes	yes
membrane	no	yes	no
contact gel	no	yes	no
B-probe			
sampling interval	100 um	50 um	
sampling length	12.8 mm	12.1 mm	
sampling positions	128	224	
real-time B-scan	no	yes	
C-probe			
sampling inverval		100 um	10 um..500 um
sampling area x*y		2.24*2.24 cm²	1.5*1.7 cm²
sampling points x		224	16..4096
sampling points y		max. 224	16..4096

Fig. 4. Comparison of two commercially available high-frequency ultrasound systems (DUB20; Dermascan C) with the 50-MHz equipment. (*) these measurements were made using a glass plate located in the focal plane of the transducer. Attenuation effects in biological tissues cause a significant shifting of the centre frequency to lower frequencies

particularly holds for the resolution of the ultrasound system. In general, resolution describes the minimum distance between two point sources which can be discerned as being distinct. To present, no general biological phantom has been accepted in dermatology; the resolution of different ultrasound equipment cannot be compared. Furthermore, experimental data suggest that the centre frequency is lower in biological tissue than in the testing objects used in materials science to define the transducer characteristics (refer to Höß et al., in this volume).

Resolution and Volume/Surface Calculations

Resolution also has a direct impact on volume and surface calculations; a situation which, at first glance, is not obvious. To study these effects, we will reduce a three-dimensional object (volume, surface area) into a two-dimensional section (section area, structure contour). Figure 5 depicts different sectioned structures which all have the same section area but a different structure contour length. In Fig. 5b, the contour length is more than twice as long as that in Fig. 5a. Both Figures differ in their pointgrid resolution. It becomes apparent that with higher resolution, the section area asymptotically reaches a fixed value, whereas the structure contour appears to augment ad infinitum. Going back to the three-dimensional space, the same characteristics hold for the volume and surface area. A good example is the gut of an animal, where the luminal surface area multiplies exponentially in moving from the macroscopical to the electron-microscopical level, since every epithelial cell has densely packed microvilli on its luminal surface. This finding also has consequences for biology and molecular biology. Since different particles (cells, macromolecules, small molecules) differ in size, they also "see" a different surface area of the same biological structure with which they interfere.

It can therefore be concluded that surface area calculations in the three-dimensional space are strongly resolution dependent and thus can only be compared in reconstructions of same resolution. Volume calculations are, on the other hand, less resolution dependent.

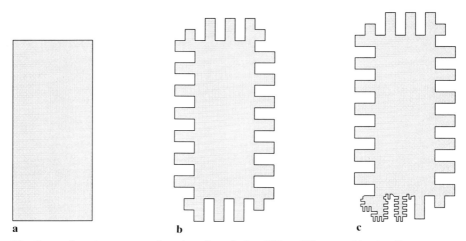

Fig. 5 a–c. Structure contour length and resolution. When different grid point distances are used *(b, c)*, the structure contour length can increase significantly in the two-dimensional space although the structure area has remained constant. The contour length in **b** is more than double the length of that in **a**. When an even finer grid is used, the contour length can increase even further (**c**). The same effect occurs in the three-dimensional space, where the object surface area measured is influenced by the resolution, although its volume remains nearly constant

Scanning Strategies

To study an object three dimensionally, the object must be sectioned from different sides. For a reliable reconstruction it is necessary to know the exact orientation of these sections in space. Different strategies of sectioning are conceivable. To compare them, a rectangular point grid with a minimum distance between two points of one unit length (uL) is defined.

The exact orientation of every section poses special mechanical problems for the ultrasound applicator. One of the most simple methods consists of rotating a B-scan applicator (e.g. sector scanner) around an axially oriented vector. Figure 6 illustrates a simple, symmetical rotation body from several perspectives. Each section is thus defined by its rotation angle and the rotation axis (Fig. 7 a, c). This method was recently used in gynaecology [23]. One of the main disadvantages of this reconstruction technique is, however, that the resolution diminishes proportionally to the distance from the rotation axis. Furthermore, in coming closer to the rotation centre structures are oversampled. To reconstruct a tissue block with a resolution of 1 uL (in x, y and z direction), a total of $(x+y-2)$ rotation sections are needed. For reconstructions using parallel sections, a minimum of (x) or (y) sections are necessary (Fig. 7 b, d).

This confirms that reconstructions from parallel sections are superior to reconstructions from rotational sections because clear statements are available about the resolution and also unnecessary oversampling around the rotational axis can be prevented.

The mechanics, however, have to be built much more precisely so as to position the transducer exactly. Problems arise from the different free-moving mechanical parts. With further reduction of the distance between neighbouring points, these factors become increasingly disturbing. It may then be advantageous to use uni-directional scans (Fig. 8 a). Indeed, this

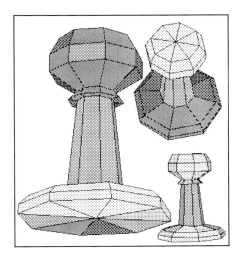

Fig. 6. Simple symmetrical rotation bodies. Three perspectives of the same object. The surfaces are shaded using patterns of different point density to give an illusion of depth

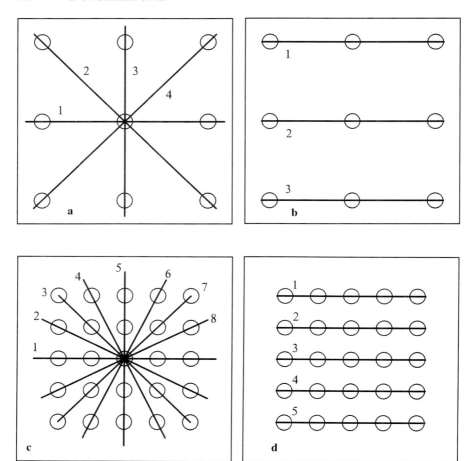

Figs. 7 a–d. Comparison between rotation and parallel sectioning methods. To resolve "n" points in the x-axis and "m" points in the y-axis, a total of (n+m−2) sections are needed for reconstructions from rotational sections (**a, c**), whereas only (n) or (m) sections are needed to reconstruct from parallel sections (**b, d**). *Numbers* represent sections

principle was used in the past by matrix printers when they were printing in near-letter quality. When the mechanical parts are exact enough, the skin can be scanned bidirectionally (Fig. 8b), which reduces scanning time.

In conclusion, we need applicators which perform parallel B-scan ultrasound sections of the skin in sequence. Presented below are several solutions for different high-resolution B-scan equipment available:

1. DUB 20 (Taberna Pro Medicum, Lüneburg, FRG). At present, only a B-scan applicator is available for this machine. By mounting this applicator into a holder consisting of a screw to move the applicator

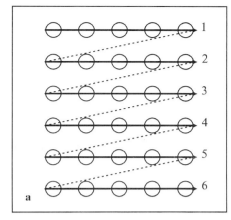
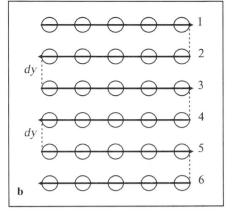
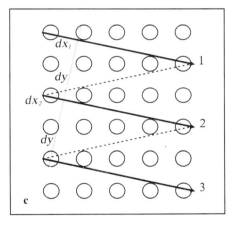

Fig. 8 a–c. Scanning methods for serial sections. **a** Uni-directional scanning neglects the mechanical game. **b** Bi-directional scanning is faster but requires precise mechanics. **c** The zig-zag movement of the Dermascan C. Only every second B-scan image is parallel. Furthermore, neighbouring sections are translated by dx in the x-axis. *Numbers* represent sections

laterally, parallel serial B-scan sections (section distance 250 μm –1 mm) are made available manually. This reconstruction method was used by Pawlak et al. (this volume).

Recently, Taberna pro Medicum has advertised a new applicator which is supposed to move the transducer 12.8 mm in the x-direction (used for B scans) and 10 mm in the y-direction, thereby making a few parallel sections available. It has been claimed that this new applicator is quite small.

2. Dermascan C (Cortex Technology, Denmark). This ultrasound imaging system uses a rather large applicator, which scans over an area of 2.24 × 2.24 cm in real-time using two linear motors. The rotational movement of the motors is transformed into a oscillation movement. To correct for this inconstant movement speed, the fast-moving axis has been equipped with a distance measuring system which is based on a light diode to synchronize the equidistant digitizing between neighbouring transducer positions. The total area is scanned in a zig-zag fashion (Fig. 8c). This gives rise to

special geometrical problems for reconstructions: 1. only even numbered (or odd numbered) sections are parallel between them; 2. the sections have to be shifted by a varying value dx which depends on the speed of the second linear motor. Since this motor also produces an oscillation movement, only a certain number of sections can be considered parallel to another. Alternatively, the second linear motor is used in a start/stop mode. The sections are then sampled after every full stop. This, however, only works adequately if a similar electronic measuring system is also used for the second linear motor. As this start/stop procedure has to be done manually, it has to be questioned whether it would have been more advantageous to use a linear motor in one direction (fast component) and a stepper motor in the other (slow component). It is to be expected that Cortex Technology will offer such an applicator for the Dermascan C soon.
3. 50-MHz Ultrasound Imaging System. The electronic setup has been described elsewhere (Höß et al., this volume). To obtain B-scan images with high resolution, the 50-MHz ultrasound imaging system is equipped with two perpendicularly oriented stepper motors which move the transducer over an area of 1.5 × 1.7 cm using two helices (position accuracy 10 μm). Compared with linear motors, the acceleration/deceler-

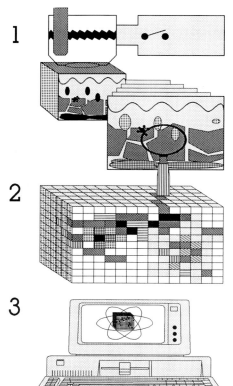

Fig. 9. Voxel reconstruction procedure. After demodulating all sections within the data cube from RF-B-scan images into a LF-images *(1)* a smaller segment within the primary data cube can be selected for further analysis and data processing using image analytical methods *(2)* This cube segment can then be rotated over any arbitrary axis while being perspectively projected onto the monitor screen *(3)*

Fig. 10. Structure boundary reconstruction procedure using parallel B-Scan ultrasound sections in sequence. In a first step, many parallel sections of the skin were obtained using an applicator with two stepper motors *(1)*. All sections were photographed one by one from the monitor and projected onto a drawing tablet using a slide projector *(2)*. Now, all structures of interest within each section were copied onto paper, named by a system of indices and entered into the Atari Mega ST4 computer using a digitizing tablet *(3)*. The program ANAT3D finally reconstructs a three-dimensional surface model which can be studied from any arbitrary view point *(4)*

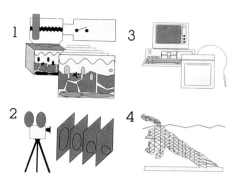

ation procedure of stepper motors is time consuming. On the other hand it becomes possible to average 16 A-scans per position, thereby correcting for the bad signal-to-noise-ratio of the polyvenylidenedifluoride (PVDF) transducer as compared to ceramic transducers.

Having agreed on parallel sections in sequence, two different reconstruction methods are principally available today. They are characterized by the order in which the data processing and image analysis takes place.

Voxel reconstruction methods (Fig. 9) apply image analytical methods and filtering on the complete dataset prior to image viewing. As a consequence, a fast computer with a large memory is needed for this type of three-dimensional image processing.

The second procedure (Fig. 10) reduces the data prior to reconstruction. In the simplest case, contours and point clouds are extracted manually. Image analytical methods extracting contour approximations using polygons (e.g. point and connectivity list) may be helpful during this phase (refer to "New Concepts and Developments", this volume). This data condensation brings about an enormous data reduction, allowing also microcomputers to reconstruct realistic object sceneries in an acceptable time period. Note that in both methods the coordinate system which is used to describe the spacial orientation of different structures has changed using the program VOXEL3D/ANAT3D (Fig. 11). Both methods shall now be discussed in detail.

Voxel Reconstruction Methods

The basic element of this reconstruction method is the voxel, an unity-quader or cube (Fig. 9). Many of these bricks are piled to form a tissue block. Every voxel has an associated grey scale which represents the mean grey-scale level of its tissue volume. In general, integer grey scales between 0 (black) and 255 (white) are used. From physiology it is known that the human eye can

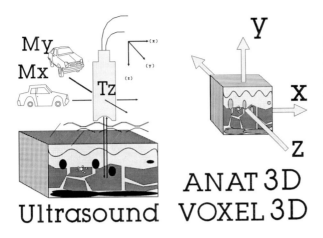

Fig. 11. The programs VOXEL3D / ANAT3D. Note the coordinate axes change which occurs when passing from the applicator axis definition *(left)* to the program axis definition *(right)*. Note that the applicator uses a right-handed coordinate system, whereas both programs use a left-handed coordinate system. In addition, the axis notation (x, y, z) has been altered

differentiate only about 32 black-and-white grey levels within a single visual field [17], 255 grey-levels are therefore considered sufficient. One voxel therefore uses one byte (equals eight bits[3]) of memory.

When the voxel side length is halved in order to double the resolution, the computer memory necessary to represent the tissue quader multiplies by eight. On the other hand computer processing time also increases significantly using larger cube grids. It is therefore necessary to fill the grid quader with the tissue structures to be analyzed as much as possible in order to receive a detailed reconstruction and reduce the needed resources. The amount of memory necessary for a tissue cube with side length 100 units (i.e. $100 \times 100 \times 100$ points in x,y,z-axis) is 1 Mbyte.

One of the simplest ways to study a data cube is to section it in various planes (Fig. 1 b) and compare them. Apart from a series of two orthogonally oriented B-scan sections, a section plane grossly parallel to the skin surface, called C-scan (*c*omputed) is available. Sophisticated programs can even evaluate different obliquely oriented sections.

Materials and Methods

To demonstate the potential of voxel reconstructions, the program VOXEL3D was developed under Windows 3.0 on a 80386 IBM-compatible computer. A skin tissue cube of $2 \times 2 \times 4.8$ mm (80×80 A-scans, digitized with 1024 points) was registered using the 50-MHz ultrasound imaging system. The A-scans were then demodulated. In this primary data cube, the distance between neighbouring points in lateral direction comprises 25 µm, and in axial direction 5 µm. To correct for the unequal spacing in the x,- y- and z-axes, the primary 6.4 Mbyte data (1024 (axially; z) * 80 (laterally; x) * 80

---

[3] Abbreviation for binary digit.

(laterally; y) points) was further reduced by averaging points along the z-axis. Although random access memory is still quite expensive, huge external media for computers are affordable. It is essential to optimize data access on the external device in larger voxel models, since most external media (e.g. hard disk, floppy disk, magnetic tape) store the information in blocks, which are sequentially processed. In most cases, it is advantageous to extract a small cube segment (Fig. 9) or use a coarse grid displaying the structures of interest for further processing. This reduces computer processing time significantly during object rotation/manipulation.

Different approaches to visualize the complete three-dimensional data array on a two-dimensional monitor screen are conceivable. To study the principles of voxel reconstruction we shall concentrate on a simple way to make the data grid visible. Every point of the three-dimensional voxel array shall be represented as hexagonal. Since our monitor is a raster display, a simple painter algorithm[4] can be used to represent the array. This algorithm requires that the grid points are sorted in such an order that those further away from the viewer are drawn first. Therefore, a method must be developed which determines which points of the data cube are the furthest away. Figure 12a illustrates a fairly simple method. Imagine a cube placed into the coordinate system in such a way that its sides are parallel with the orthogonal axes of the coordinate system and so that its diagonals intersect at the origin of the coordinate system. All eight corners of the rectangular tissue block can now be numbered by a system of indices (Fig. 12a). The first index represents the x-axis (positive, negative), and the second and third index the y- and z-axis, respectively. When this cube is rotated over a user defined axis, at least one of the eight corners will lie furthest away from the viewer. This edge defines for every axis the direction of data processing along the sides of the data block (i.e. incrementation or decrementation). By comparing the second and third furthest corner with the furthest edge of the rectangle, it is possible to detect which one of the axes has changed its sign from positive to negative or vice versa (Fig. 12b). This procedure determines the chronological order in which the side axes of the three-dimensional grid array are incremented/decremented.

As has been stated earlier, voxel reconstructions also involve image processing methods for further data reduction. This program VOXEL3D has implemented two different aspects for the point data representation. Both the radius and the grey scale of the hexagon representing the grid point can be varied. In Fig. 13 the hexagonal diameter was modulated by the white intensity of the grey-scale level of the particular voxel element to be represented within the cube array. Its shade was evaluated as the mean value of the grey-coded distance of this particular voxel from the screen plane (giving an illusion of depth) and the hexagonal radius (to focus the image on strong reflexes).

---

4 An algorithm is an instruction sequence which solves a task, like a recipe to cook a meal.

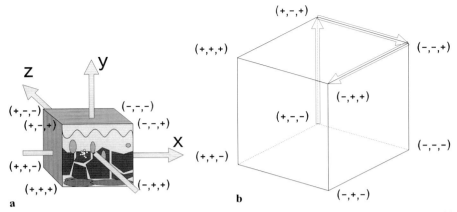

Fig. 12 a, b. Voxel reconstruction procedure. *(a)* The corners of the three-dimensional grid array are numbered by a set of indices, describing the direction (positive, negative) to proceed along the x, y, z sides of the cube when, due to user defined grid rotation this corner is the one which is furthest away. *(b)* Comparing the change of indices from the furthest corner to the second furthest, and from the second furthest to the third furthest corner, the correct order of axis processing (x, y, z-axis) can be detected *(arrows)*

To increase the transparency of the model, it is advantageous to apply on the cube array a trigger grey level and a filter to reduce noise. The trigger level serves to either reject a point (e.g. grey level below trigger value) during the painting process, or to draw the point (e.g. equals to or above trigger value). In principle, different image analytical concepts have been expanded from the discrete plane (refer to "New Concepts and Developments", this volume) to the three-dimensional space.

As the user spends some time looking at different views and structural combinations, a special effort is necessary for maximum comfort and speed during this period. To speed up this object orientation, the point grid is reduced to a quader with yellow sides except for three sides orthogonally to each other: these sides are red (x-axis), green (y-axis) and blue (z-axis) and join in a common origin. Once the optimal perspective is found, the computer is told to draw the cube. When large cubes are used, the drawing process may take several minutes for a single perspective.

Results

Figure 14 shows different orthogonal sections through the tissue cube of normal skin registered using the 50-MHz equipment. Figure 14a delineates their approximal location along the borders of the tissue cube. Note the apparently randomly scattered undulating echo lines within the corium in the B-scan sections (Fig. 14b–g). In the C-scan sections, however, globular

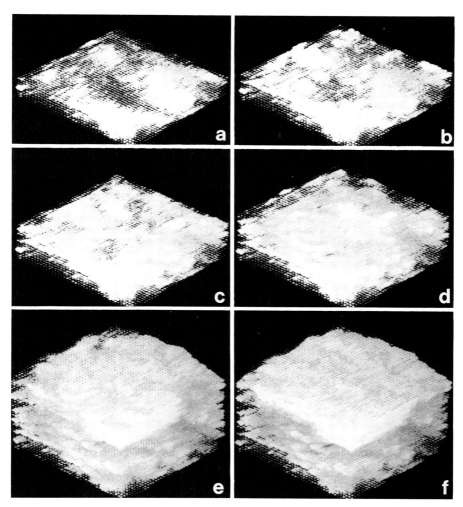

Fig. 13 a–f. Perspective voxel reconstruction of a normal skin tissue block. The tissue cube has been rotated and tilted; it therefore appears somehow compressed. When the drawing process is interrupted, the shape of the echo reflexes in different regions of the corium becomes apparent. In the lower portion of the corium, discus-shaped reflexes are present *(a, b)*. The middle position exhibits fewer reflexes *(c, d)*. In the upper portion of the corium, oblique, discus-shaped, partly irregular reflexes are apparent which merge into the skin entry echo. In *(e)* the painting process has been interrupted in the upper region of the skin entry echo. *(f)* The complete cube. The cube was rotated by 4° in *(f)*. *e, f* A stereo pair which can be observed by crossing the eyes

structures become apparent (Fig. 14 h–s). Both findings suggest that the echo reflexes form discus-shaped undulating, partly irregular-shaped ovaloids within the corium.

Using voxel reconstruction methods, we shall now visualize a 40×40×40-elements data cube taken mainly from the corium. Figure 13 shows the voxel cube drawing interrupted at different stages during the painting process. Large, partly irregular, discus-shaped ovaloids are observed at the lower corium (Fig. 13 a, b). Above, regions with fewer reflexes are apparent. The upper corium exhibits multiple smaller irregularly shaped echo-ovaloids (Fig. 13 c). Some of them connect obliquely to the skin entry echo layer. In Fig. 13 e the drawing process was interrupted in the "upper skin entry echo layer". Figure 13f finally shows the entire voxel cube. The cube was rotated by 4° between Figs. 13 e (right eye) and f (left eye). The images form a stereo pair. By crossing the eyes, the borders of the cube can be appreciated three-dimensionally, exhibiting the lower density of strong echo reflexes in the middle of the corium.

Discussion

Voxel reconstruction methods have found wide application in computer tomography (CT) [10] to study mainly bone anatomy [11, 12, 24], and magnetic resonance imaging (MRI) to study in particular brain anatomy [3, 13]. Whereas CT and MRI sections exhibit structures which have a specific texture with rather sharp boundaries, the received ultrasound signal is strongly influenced by angular reflection properties at tissue boundaries and absorption phenomena due to tissue layers above the structure of interest. In ultrasound, tissue boundaries produce different artefacts (e.g. a structure border may vanish when it is obliquely oriented in relation to the ultrasound

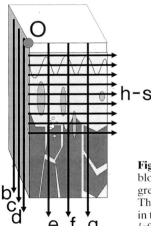

Fig. 14. Different sections through a 2×2×4.8-mm tissue block of normal skin. A false color grey-scale coding (black-green-blue-red-yellow) was used.
The letters **a–s** denote the approximate position of the sections in the tissue block. All distances were measured from the *upper left corner O* of the cube.

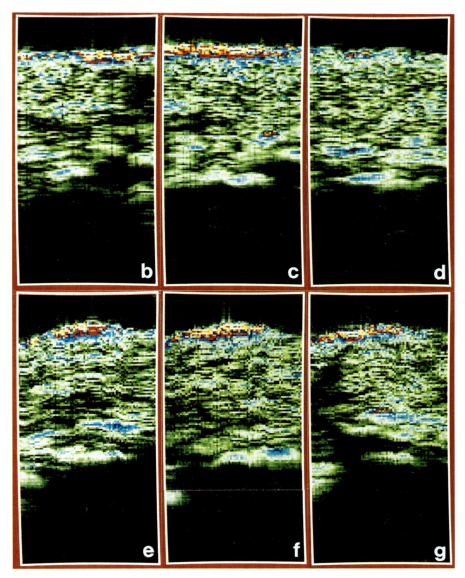

Fig. 14 b–g. Two groups of orthogonally oriented B-scan sections, with their section plane at 0.5 (**b**), 1.0 (**c**), 1.5 (**d**) and 0.5 (**e**), 1.0 (**f**), 1.5 (**g**) mm from the origin. Skin entry echo (upper white-blue border), corium (black-green-blue layer), subcutaneous fatty tissue (black region at bottom of image). Note the undulating echo lines in the corium which become larger at greater distance from the skin entry echo.

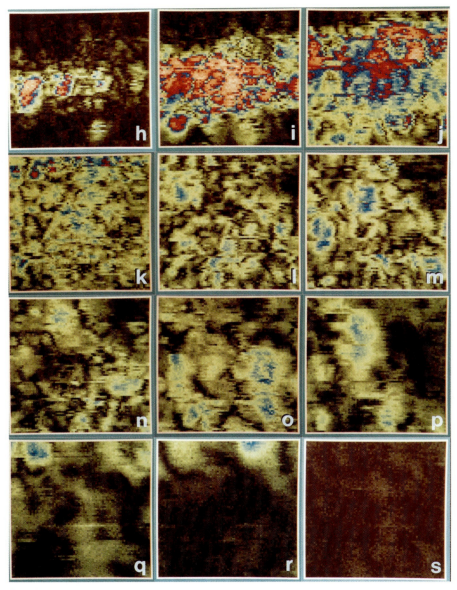

Fig. 14 h-s. C-scan sections at different levels. Every section is 5 μm thick according to the time window used. The distance of the sections from the upper corner is 0.4 (**h**), 0.5 (**i**), 0.6 (**j**), 0.8 (**k**), 1.0 (**l**), 1.25 (**m**), 1.5 (**n**), 1.75 (**o**), 2.25 (**p**), 2.5 (**q**), 2.75 (**r**), 3.25 (**s**) mm. Note the globular aspect of the skin entry echo (**h–j**). Small globular and irregular shaped echoes predominate in the upper corium (**k–m**). The middle of the corium shows fewer echo globules (**n, o**). In fact, this finding is not as obvious in the B-scan sections (**b–g**) due to the slightly oblique orientation of the corium/subcutis border. The subcutaneous fatty tissue (**s**) exhibits nearly no echo signal

beam), which make voxel reconstructions difficult to interpret, since all these artefacts are included in the ultrasound B-scan image and may give a more prominent contrast than the structure of interest.

For small structures such as echo reflexes within the corium, sections along the three orthogonal axes can help in the interpretation of the orientation of these reflexes. Figures 13 and 14 reveal that these reflexes are oriented as undulating discus-shaped ovaloids grossly parallel to the skin surface. This finding is in accordance to the scanning electron microscopic studies of human dermis under normal and uni-axial strain by Finlay [8]. He observed that collagen fibre bundles in the corium run almost parallel to the epidermal surface. With further loading in the direction of the initial bundle orientation, more and more randomly oriented bundles fully align themselves in the direction of the load. Skin biopsies on the other hand showed apparently randomly oriented undulating collagen bundles in their unstressed state.

In addition, Finlay [8] observed a closer collagen bundle packing at the junction of the corium and underlying fat. This finding could explain why, using ultrasound, stronger corial reflexes were observed in the lower part of the corium.

Structure Boundary Reconstruction Methods

A quite different approach is followed in structure boundary reconstructions. Often the interaction between only a few biological structures is of interest. The image information can then be reduced to the essential: a few contours and maybe several point clouds. This condensation to the main image elements affords quite sophisticated image analytical methods. One of the best image analytical systems available is our own visual perception system.

Using this concept, Katschenko [15] proposed a simple method to build realistic models in 1886: the tissue containing the structure is sectioned parallel in sequence, and every structure of interest in each cross-section is scaled and copied onto a transparant sheet of glass, wood or plastic, eventually trimming the material to the shape of the structure. The layers are then stacked one onto another, thereby forming a three-dimensional replica. Indeed, many anatomical studies were performed using this technique. This manual reconstruction method has, however, three major disadvantages:
1. a skilled artistic talent is required;
2. when many sections are required, the transparency of plastic becomes a limiting factor;
3. quantitative information (e.g. surface or volume) is not easily available.

These disadvantages can be overcome by combining parallel sections and computer reconstruction techniques. Consequently many different three-dimensional modelling program packages [review: 14], mostly for mainframes, have been proposed. The vast majority of the programs however used simple hidden-line algorithms. Note that the contours of a structure are greatly influenced by the orientation of the section plane. Our mind can therefore be easily mislead about the true shape of a structure when simple line reconstructions are used. We suggest, therefore, that computer modelling should include surface reconstruction procedures, since biological structures are delimited by surfaces [5]. Although the program ANAT3D was primarily developed on an Atari Mega ST4 computer, a version running under Microsoft Windows 3.0 is now available [6]. Presently all ultrasound images are entered into the computer using a digitizing tablet (Fig. 10). The new version uses a frame grabber to instantaneously digitize the video image, thereby making the intermediate paper copy obsolete. In combination with image preprocessing and filtering to extract the structure contours (refer to "New Concepts and Developments", this volume), the time necessary for the reconstruction can be significantly reduced, making this method more suitable for routine diagnostic examinations.

The present paper presents three-dimensional surface models from hair follicle studies using a 50-MHz experimental ultrasound system.

Materials and Methods

For the following reconstructions mainly hair follicles of the lower limb were studied. We chose this skin region because the corium is quite thick and well delimited towards the subcutaneous fatty tissue, making it easy to follow the hair canal in the corium.

For B-scan image recording, we used a 50-MHz ultrasound imaging system. The penetration depth at centre frequency (40 MHz) is about 4 mm, the axial resolution 37.5 μm and the lateral resolution 125 μm in biological tissue. Two computer-controlled stepper motors were used to move the focused active 50-MHz PVDF transducer parallel to the skin surface in bidirectional mode (Fig. 1 a). The minimum step width is 15 μm and the maximum scanning area 1.5 × 1.7 cm. For hair follicle reconstructions, equidistant 50-μm B-scan sections were processed. Although this oversampling is redundant, it helps in defining precisely the borders of the hair appendages. The B-scan sections were then photographed from the monitor.

The contours of all structures of interest within each section were then copied on paper using a slide projector (Paximat, FRG). The corners of the picture were marked as fiducial points. Finally, all structures were named by a system of indices. The digitizing tablet (1st CRP Koruk, FRG) was calibrated using the fiducial points to correct for the different axial and lateral scaling. This calibration was necessary for the computer to be able to convert all point coordinates into SI units, ranging from 10^{-37} to 10^{37} m. Finally, the contours of different structures were entered into an Atari MegaST4 computer (Atari Corp, Sunnyvale, Calif., USA) as single points (x/y-coordinates) interconnected by lines (polygons) using a cross-hair button cursor. For further data reduction, equidistant sampling has been abandoned. Note the coordinate system transformation occurring from the transducer axis definition to the ANAT3D axis definition (Fig. 11). The program ANAT3D orders all sections by their z-coordinate and adapts single sections within the section pile. The further processing steps have been described elsewere [7].

For the final reconstruction, all structures of interest within the structure list and all sections necessary within the section pile are selected. For every single structure, the user decides whether it is reconstructed either as a surface model (Fig. 15 d–f), a wire-frame model (Fig. 15 c), a line-contour model (Fig. 15 a) or a point cloud. Combining these different presentation modes, structures within structures may easily be studied. Analogous to any viewing instrument (e.g. TEM, LM, SEM), scaling is essential to study all structures of interest at a reasonable magnification. For the following calculations, all structures chosen are treated as a single object. In the first step the program therefore evaluates the smallest and largest x,y,z-

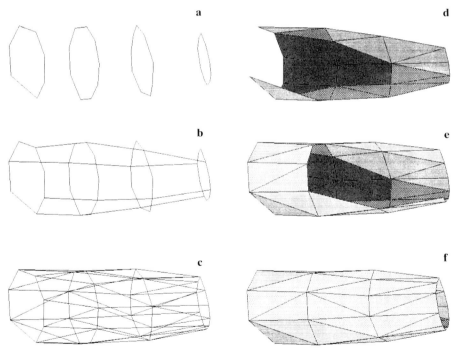

Fig. 15 a–f. The surface triangulation procedure. **a** Contour lines of a single structure in adjacent sections. **b** In this example, all contours have been broken into four line segments using segmentation points. To make these points visible, they have been interconnected by lines between the contours. **c** Corresponding line segments in neighbouring sections have been completed by a wire-frame which delimits triangular patches. **d–f** Painting sequence. After sorting all triangles according to their depth, they are drawn using a painter algorithm. Different surface patterns were used for the triangles to improve in-depth perception

coordinates of the object. Secondly, a translation is calculated which moves the object into the coordinate origin. Finally, a scaling factor is evaluated which enlarges the object so that it fits into an imaginary cube of predefined diameter.

Note that for optimal object scaling, the object dimensions have to be known *a priori*. To avoid object shape deformation (Fig. 3), the object data must therefore be processed by the computer twice. On the other hand, automatic object centring has been implemented by adding a matrix translation prior to the user defined object rotation. This translation can correct for minor variations of the objects dimensions by selecting and deselecting structures in the structure list. Now the object can be rotated over any user defined axis without danger of moving out of the viewport of the screen (Fig. 16). Moving the screen along the z-axis enlarges or diminishes the perspective projection of the object.

To speed up graphics, all real coordinates are then transformed into integer coordinates (−32000...32000), using the previously defined translation and scaling constants and are then placed into a point buffer. Points connected by lines (e.g. structure contour polygons) are placed into the line buffer as a sequence of point numbers. According to the chosen presentation mode, every structure contour is broken into surface patches of triangles (surface mode; Fig. 15f) or line segments (wire-frame or contour-line). Different point cloud presentation modes are also available [6]. This data is stored as a sequence of connected point numbers in a surface buffer. A maximum of 16000 points, 30000 lines and 32000 surfaces can be involved in a single image. A sophisticated machine language program embedded in a graphics environment (GEM, Digital Research, USA) implements high-speed rotation and scaling of the reconstructed object. As the user spends most of the time looking at different views and structural combinations, a special effort is

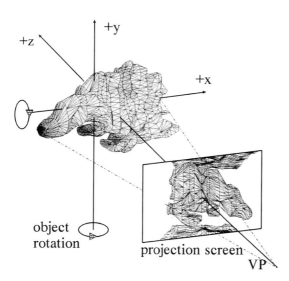

Fig. 16. The mathematical model implemented in the program ANAT3D. The object is translated into the coordinate origin and scaled to fill an imaginary cube. After user defined rotation, the object is projected onto a screen. By moving the screen along the z-axis in positive direction, the object projection is enlarged. *VP*, vanishing point used for perspective

necessary for maximum comfort and speed during this period. We implemented perspective three-dimensional-red-green stereo images for real-time object manipulation. Once the optimal view has been found by the user, the computer is told to redraw all structures using the surface buffer. As a first step all lines and surfaces are sorted according to their mean z-coordinate and drawn using a painter algorithm. The lines are now shaded in-depth to enhance the perspective impression while the surfaces are shaded according to a user defined virtual point light source. Volume and surface calculations are available.

Results

Figure 17 b–e shows four cross-sections of a vellus hair follicle on the lower limb of a young woman, whereas Fig. 17 a exhibits a longitudinal section. The arrows mark the positions of the cross-sections 17 b–e. In the ultrasound B-scans the thickness of the skin entry echo is about 50–70 μm. Respiration artefacts are seen because the enregistration of a tissue block is time consuming. The corium is about 1.5 mm thick. At this body location the border between corium and subcutis is sharp. The hair follicle canal in the

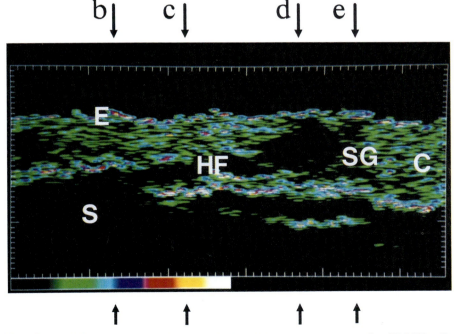

Fig. 17 a–e. Different cross-sections of a hair follicle in anagen state using 50 MHz. *E*, epidermis; *C*, corium; *S*, subcutaneous fatty tissue; *H*, hair; *HF*, hair follicle; *SG*, sebaceous gland. The *arrows* mark the different positions of the transversal sections (**b–e**) within the longitudinal section (**a**) of the hair follicle and sebaceous gland

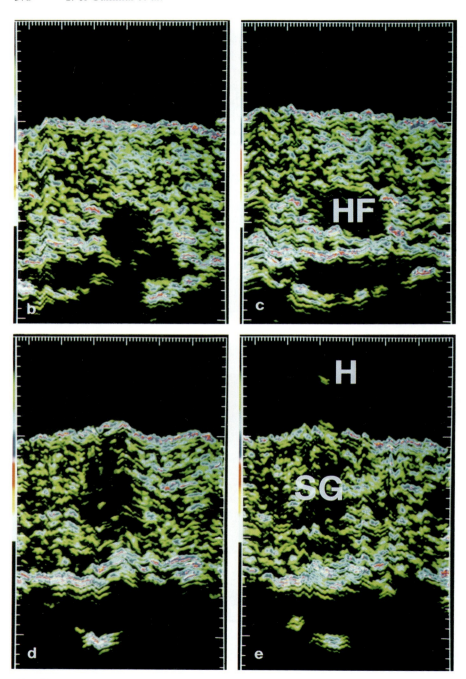

Fig. 17 b–e

corium can be easily followed. Figure 17b shows a sharply delimited trifoliate echo-poor structure at the corium-subcutis interface. The middle part can be followed as a hair follicle canal in successive sections (Fig. 17c–e). Figure 1c exhibits the hair canal half-way through the corium. In the upper subcutis connective tissue septa are present. Figure 17d shows the greatest diameter of the hair follicle canal. The cross-sectional ovaloid contour diameter varied between 1.7×0.6 mm and 2×1 mm.

Figure 17e finally exhibits a cross-section of a sebaceous gland. The sebaceous gland is more echo rich and less well delineated to the surrounding corium in comparison to the hair canal. Note the echo-rich ovaloid structure in the water path, which is discontinuously visualised within the obliquely oriented hair follicle canal (Fig. 17 b–d). The follicle canal is oriented at an angle of about 30° within the corium (Fig. 17a). This value was measured after correcting the unequal scaling in the lateral and axial directions. A connective tissue septum is seen in the upper part of the subcutis. The hair above the skin surface has not been sectioned in this plane (Fig. 17a) and therefore cannot be observed.

Figure 18 a–c illustrates a hair follicle (violet) in anagen state with its sebaceous gland (yellow) in the wire-frame mode. The lower violet wire-frame corresponds to the corium-subcutis interface (Fig. 18 b+c). The upper green and blue lines represent the borders of the skin entry echo. The hair follicle canal is oriented obliquely and reveals a hair (red-yellow, surface mode) in its upper part, which can only be followed partly in the hair canal and above the skin. This phenomenon was found in all hair follicles. In

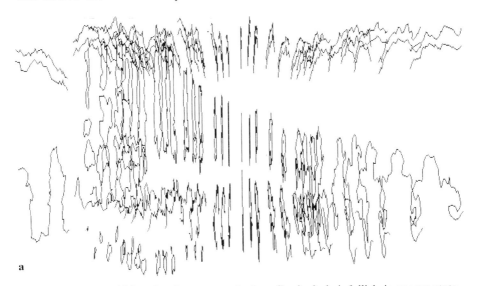

Fig. 18. Line-model (**a**) and surface reconstructions (**b, c**) of a hair follicle in anagen state, *E*, epidermis; *C*, corium; *S*, subcutaneous fatty tissue; *H*, hair, *HF*, hair follicle; *SG*, sebaceous gland. The in-depth shaded, wire-frame presentation mode makes is easy to follow structures within structures (**b, c**).

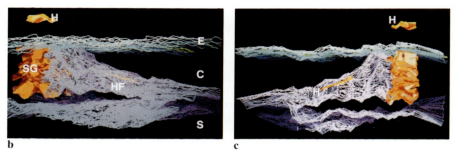

Fig. 18 b–c. b) Note the obliquely oriented hair follicle *(HF)* passing through the corium *(C)*. In **c** the front plane of the hair follicle was omitted, thereby exhibiting the interior of the hair follicle. The hair *(H)* can only be followed discontinuously. Note the lobular structure of the sebaceous gland *(SG)*

Fig. 18c only the back plane of the hair canal was reconstructed so that the visible hair segment can easily be followed in the hair canal. Figure 19a shows another hair follicle in anagen state obliquely from above (lower limb of a young man). Figure 19b–d show closeups of the sebaceous gland. Note its lobular structure.

Note that it is often insufficient to use line models, even when combined with hidden-line algorithms. If, for example, the section pile is oriented perpendicular to the viewer, no information can be gathered from the line

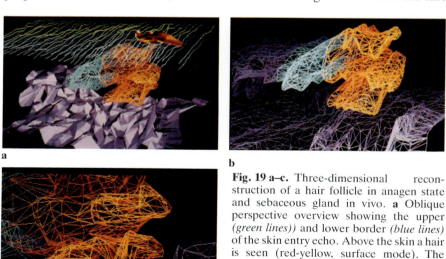

Fig. 19 a–c. Three-dimensional reconstruction of a hair follicle in anagen state and sebaceous gland in vivo. **a** Oblique perspective overview showing the upper *(green lines))* and lower border *(blue lines)* of the skin entry echo. Above the skin a hair is seen (red-yellow, surface mode). The corium-subcutis interface is shown as a *violet surface*. In the corium a hair follicle *(blue wire-frame)* and sebaceous gland *(red-yellow wire-frame)* are observed. Note the lobular shape of the sebaceous gland *(red-brown wire-frame)* at higher magnification **(b, c).** By adding the hair follicle *(blue wire-frame)* and the corium-subcutis interface *(violet wire-frame)*, the grouping of these different structures can be analysed

model (Fig. 18a). Using surface triangulation algorithms and hidden-surface removal it is possible to study the same computer model from any arbitrary point of view (Fig. 18b).

Figure 20 exhibits a hair follicle in telogen state. The hair follicle bulb is lying in the middle of the corium and the sebaceous gland is oriented to the left. Note the large sebaceous gland in comparison to the small hair canal. Due to the change of the presentation mode into shaded surface mode (Fig. 20b), its lobular shape is easily visualised. The echolucent hair canal ends in the corium. Here, the hair canal is represented in blue, the large sebaceous gland in yellow. The M. arrector pili has not yet been identified.

Discussion

Using ultrasound, structure boundary three-dimensional models are superior to voxel reconstruction models because ultrasound artefacts due to reflection, absorption and attenuation can be eliminated. High-resolution ultra-

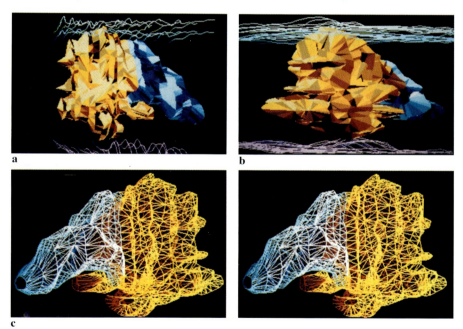

Fig. 20 a–c. Three-dimensional reconstruction of a hair follicle state in telogen in vivo. Lateral view **(a)**; front view **(b)**. The skin entry echo is represented by the *upper green and blue lines*, the corium-subcutis interface by the *lower violet lines*. The hair follicle bulb *(blue surface mode)* is retracted from the subcutaneous fatty tissue into the corium. Note the disproportionally large sebaceous gland *(red-brown-yellow surfaces)* in comparison to the hair follicle. **c** Stereo image pair (0/4° of the hair follicle bulb in telogen state *(blue wire-frame)* and the sebaceous gland *(brown-yellow wire-frame)*. When looking through the holes of the wire-frame in the front plane, the back wall of both structures can be observed, thereby giving a hint about their true spatial proportions

sound (e.g. skin tumours; Pawlak et al., this volume) and ultrasound imaging at frequencies below 20 MHz profit from this method (e.g. inner organs and vessel structures; Hammentgen et al., this volume).

We suggest that a structure boundary reconstruction program should include different possible presentation modes for every individual structure, since transparency algorithms are elegant but very time consuming [20]. The approximation of structure boundaries with polygons brings about an enormous data reduction. Vectorized three-dimensional surface area reconstructions can be accomplished today by microcomputers in an acceptable time period. It must be pointed out, however, that although volume calculations are quite precise on these models, surface area calculations can be rather inexact, especially when the sections of the section pile are far away from each other in relation to the distance between neighbouring points of the polygon contour of the structure [9].

By combining different presentation modes for different structures in an object, structures within structures are easily analysed. Figures 19, 20 show that the combination of different modes improves structure interpretation considerably. Furthermore, by selectively omitting structures, the region of interest can easily be studied from any perspective.

Hair follicles have already been identified as echo-poor structures in the dermis [1, 4]. However, the sebaceous gland could not be clearly delimited and differentiated from the hair canal [19, 21]. By combining high-resolution 50-MHz ultrasound B-scan sections and three-dimensional reconstruction techniques, it is possible to study the spacial interrelationship of different structures of the hair complex [16]. This additional information makes it possible to differentiate between the hair canal (Figs. 17 b–d; 18 b, c) and the sebaceous gland (Figs. 177 e; 19 b, c) due to their location and echogenicity. The hair canal is a sharply demarcated structure passing through the corium. The sebaceous gland is unsharply bordered and shows diffuse inner reflexes. Three-dimensional structure boundary reconstructions reveal the lobular structure of the sebaceous gland in vivo. Due to the skin tension and elasticity, the sebaceous gland has a flatter shape in vivo than observed in histology. The hair itself cannot be followed continuously as echo-intence structure from the skin surface into the hair canal – where it is oriented obliquely to the ultrasound beam, it cannot be detected. We think that the echo-rich structures within the hair canal represent parts of the hair.

The three-dimensional structure boundary computer models therefore provide further hints about the shape and functional state of the hair follicle (Figs. 18–20). Due to the differing length of the hair canal, hairs in anagen and telogen state can be differentiated. We expect that high-resolution ultrasound will have an impact on diagnostics and therapeutic control of hair follicle diseases. This non-invasive method could supplement trichograms. Furthermore ultrasound examinations are less tedious for the patient than punch biopsies and can easily be repeated. Thus the extent, regression and and progression of a pathological process can be analysed easily non-invasively.

Conclusion

By combining ultrasound B-scan sections with computer techniques, it is possible to develop three-dimensional computer replicas from skin structures and tumours in vivo. After reviewing different sectioning strategies, it becomes apparent that parallel sectioning in sequence is best suited for an accurate modelling with a minimum of sections necessary. A section pile of parallel 50-MHz B-scan images of the human skin *in-vivo* was used to study voxel and structure boundary reconstruction methods.

The ultrasound texture of the corium was studied using voxel reconstruction program VOXEL3D. The echo reflexes were more pronounced in the lower and upper region of the corium. Within the corium, they are oriented parallel to the skin surface and form undulating layers. Correspondingly, C-scan sections through the corium reveal ovaloid structures in the corium.

Computer modelling with structure boundary reconstructions was accomplished using the program ANAT3D. Hair follicles in telogen and anagen state could be distinguished. Furthermore, the lobular structure of the sebaceous gland was easily identified. Volume and surface calculations were also available.

Using ultrasound, structure boundary reconstructions are superior to voxel reconstructions because different ultrasound artefacts can be eliminated. We expect that with further automation using image analytical tools three-dimensional reconstructions from high-resolution ultrasound sections can become a powerful tool in the study of normal and pathological skin appendages, skin tumours and inflammatory diseases non-invasively.

Acknowledgements. The program ANAT3D was written by Dr. med. S. el-Gammal. It runs either on an Atari MegaST4 under GEM or on IBM-compatible computers under Windows 3.0 (SIS3D™). For further information please contact: Soft-Imaging-Software GmbH, Breul 1–3, W-4400 Münster, FRG.
The program VOXEL3D was recently written by Dr. med. S. el-Gammal and is still under further development (Beta-Version).

References

1. Alexander H, Miller DL (1979) Determining skin thickness with pulsed ultrasound. J Invest Dermatol 72: 17–19
2. Birgham OE (1974) The fast Fourier tranform. Prentice-Hall, Englewood Cliffs, p 85
3. Cline HE, Dumoulin CL, Hart HR, Lorensen WE, Ludke S (1987) 3D reconstruction of the brain from magnetic resonance images using a connectivity algorithm. Magn Res on Imaging 5: 345–352
4. Dines KA, Sheets PW, Brink JA, Hanke CW, Condra KA, Clendenon JL, Gross A, Smith DJ, Franklin TD (1984) High frequency ultrasonic imaging of skin: experimental results. Ultrason Imaging 6: 408–434
5. El-Gammal S (1987) ANAT3D: a computer programm. In: Elsner N, Creutzfeld O (eds) New frontiers in brain research. Thieme, Stuttgart, p 46

6. El-Gammal S (1990) ANAT3D: on-line computer demonstrations of shaded three-dimensional models under Microsoft Windows. In: Elsner N, Roth G (eds) Brain – perception – Cognition. Thieme, Stuttgart, p 530
7. El-Gammal S, Altmeyer P, Hinrichsen K (1989) ANAT3D: shaded three-dimensional surface reconstructions from serial sections. Applications in morphology and histopathology. Acta Stereol 8: 543–550
8. Finlay B (1969) Scanning electron microscopy of the human dermis under uni-axial strain. BioMed Eng 4 322–327
9. Funnell WRJ (1984) On the calculation of surface areas of objects reconstructed from serial sections. J Neurosci Methods 11: 205–210
10. Herman GT, Liu HK (1979) Three-dimensional display of human organs from computed tomograms. Comput Graph Image Proc 9: 1–21
11. Hirschfelder H (1989) Dreidimensionale (3D) Oberflächenrekonstruktion aus computertomographischen Schnittbildern. Orthopädie 18: 18–23
12. Hoehne KH, Delapaz RL, Bernstein R, Taylor RC (1987) Combined surface display and reformatting for the three-dimensional analysis of tomogrpahic data. Invest Radiol 22: 658–664
13. Hu X, Tan KK, Levin DN, Galhotra S, Mullan JF, Hekmatpanah J, Spire JP (1990) Three-dimensional magnetic resonance images of the brain: application in neurosurgical planning. J Neurosurg 72: 433–440
14. Huijsmans DP, Lamers WH, Los JA, Strackee J (1986) Toward computerized morphometric facilities. A review of 58 software packages for computer-aided three-dimensional reconstruction, quantification, and picture generation from parallel serial sections. Anat Rec 216: 449–470
15. Kastschenko N (1886) Methode zur genauen Rekonstruktion kleinerer makroskopischer Gegenstände. Arch Anat [Physiol Abt] 388–394
16. Kenkmann J, el-Gammal S, Hoffmann K, Altmeyer P (1990) A 50 MHz ultrasonic imaging system for dermatology – 3D reconstructions of the hair-complex. Zentralbl Haut Geschlechtskr 157: 330
17. Lullies H, Trincker D (1977) Taschenbuch der Physiologie, vol 3/2. Fischer, Stuttgart
18. Miyauchi S, Miki Y (1983) Normal human skin echogram. Arch Dermatol Res 275: 345–349
19. Murakami S, Miki Y (1989) Human skin histology using high-resolution echography. JCU 17: 77–82
20. Newman WM, Sproull RF (1984) Principles of interactive computer graphics. McGraw-Hill, London, pp 389–410
21. Quereleux B, Léveque JL, de Rigal J (1988) In vivo cross-sectional ultrasonic imaging of human skin. Dermatologica 177: 332–337.
22. Sohn C, Grotepaß J, Schneider W, Sohn G, Funk A, Jensch P, Fendel H, Ameling W, Jung H (1988) Dreidimensionale Darstellung in der Ultraschalldiagnostik. Erste Ergebnisse. Dtsch Med. Wochenschr 113: 1743–1747
23. Sohn S, Rudofsky G (1989) Die dreidimensionale Ultraschalldiagnostik – ein neues Verfahren für die klinische Routine? Ultraschall Klin Prax 4: 219–224
24. Vannier ME, Gado MH, Marsh JL (1984) Three-dimensional CT reconstruction images for craniofacial surgical planning. Radiology 150: 179–184
25. Wessels G, Weber P (1983) Physikalische Grundlagen. In: Braun B, Günther R, Schwenk B (eds) Ultraschalldiagnostik. Lehrbuch und Atlas. Ecomed, Landsberg

Three-Dimensional Reconstruction of Serial Ultrasound Images of the Skin*

F.M. PAWLAK, K. HOFFMANN, S. EL-GAMMAL, and P. ALTMEYER

Introduction

New high-resolution scanners for use in dermatology are now able to construct two-dimensional images. In this form of imaging the echo signal is converted to brightness values (B-scan) [2, 3]. The previously used A-mode scanners produced one-dimensional images which were suitable mainly for determining skin thickness [1, 14, 16]. However, as exact correlation of fine-structural and ultrasound sections is not possible, many questions regarding the evaluation of two-dimensional ultrasound scans remain open.

Medicine has always been very interested in three-dimensional representations of morphologically interesting structures. The shape, extent and degree of infiltration of a pathological process can be analysed better on the basis of a three-dimensional model than with a conventional two-dimensional image. In the past, models made of various materials such as plaster of Paris, cardboard and polystyrene have been used for three-dimensional representation in pathology and anatomy. Kastschenko used series of transparent films for three-dimensional reconstructions as far back as 1886[12].

Innovations in microelectronics have procured programs for computer reconstruction which enable three-dimensional representations to be used in diagnostic imaging. We applied such a reconstruction program to serial ultrasound images of the skin which we obtained with a high-resolution 20-MHz ultrasound scanner.

The aim of this investigation was to examine whether three-dimensional reconstruction of the 20-MHz ultrasound scans is actually possible and whether the reconstruction improves the morphological information provided by the two-dimensional scans.

Material and Methods

In total ten series of ultrasound sections were reconstructed. After reconstruction of normal skin and circumscribed scleroderma we focused our attention on skin tumours. The following tumours were examined: a nodular melanoma, a superficial spreading melanoma, a superficial basal cell

---

* This publication contains significant parts of the dissertation of Frank-Michael Pawlak.

carcinoma, a haemangioma, a Kaposi's sarcoma, a verruca seborrhoica and a naevus cell naevus. All the skin regions examined were on the trunk.

We performed the ultrasound examinations with a digital ultrasound scanner (DUB-20, Taberna pro Medicum, Lüneburg). The scanner consists of a 20-MHz ultrasound pulser/receiver unit (Panametrics), a digital oscilloscope with GPIB interface (2430 Tektronics) and an 80286 Tandon processor. The image storage was on diskette and hard disk. The pulse-motor-driven transducer is advanced through the 12.8 mm water path. In this water path it transmits and receives echo signals which it converts to a sectional image after digitization. The echo signals received correspond to reflection at interfaces between tissues of different impedance. The depth of penetration of the sound waves of the scanner is 7 mm, which covers epidermis, dermis, subcutis, and sometimes muscle fascia. The maximum axial resolution is 80 µm, the lateral resolution 200 µm. The scanner converts the echo amplitudes received into brightness values. The grey-scale generally used in ultrasound is replaced by a false colour code (black = echolucent, through green, blue, red, yellow to white = echo-rich). This coding permits evaluation of even slight differences in the echogenicity of tissues. The dimensions of a region of interest or a structure of interest can be measured directly using measuring lines which can be displayed on the screen. The image shown on the screen is compressed, with different magnification factors for width (approx. 8 x) and depth (approx. 24 x).

The three-dimensional reconstruction required known distances between the individual images in the series of sonographic sections. In order to guarantee such precise movement of the transducer over the area of skin to be examined we used a specially designed transducer holder (Fig. 1). This consists of an immobile anchoring plate for attachment to the skin and a

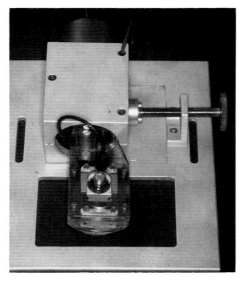

Fig. 1. The ultrasound transducer in the holder specially designed for the purpose of three-dimensional reconstruction

mobile unit which holds the transducer. The transducer is moved over the skin in an opening in the anchoring plate. The mobile portion is driven by a stainless steel spindle. One complete revolution of the spindle advances the transducer exactly 1000 μm. A scale permits preparation of a series of ultrasound sections with a minimum distance between scans of 250 μm.

In order to ensure secure positioning of the holder, all examinations were performed in the region of the trunk. The forward feed selected gave intervals of 250 and 500 μm between the individual images. When recording a series of ultrasound sections of a skin tumour, for example, attention was paid that the first and last images, were recorded in healthy skin. We obtained on average 15–30 sections per tumour.

The ultrasound sections on the screen of the scanner were photographed. Structures of interest were selected on the photographs and the outlines transferred to tracing paper. The outlines of the structures were named for later input into the computer. Particular attention must be paid here to branching and fusion of the structures. In the subsequent reconstruction, the computer combines structure outlines with the same names to form a three-dimensional model. After exact labelling of all individual sections, we entered the contours of the following structures into the computer using a digital graphics tablet:

1. Boundary structures serving orientation purposes, e.g. upper and lower limits of the entry echo, corium/subcutis interface, muscle fascia
2. Morphologically or pathomorphologically interesting structures, e.g. tumours, bands of fibrous septa in the subcutis.

After preliminary calibration of the digitizing graphics tablet, the different scaling used in the ultrasound image for width and depth was corrected so that the computer now processes the contours of the structures without compression. After this calibration, the contours of the selected structures were entered into the Atari-Mega ST4 computer section by section using the graticule of the graphics tablet. The computer input included entry of the name and specification of the colour and geometric type (point, open or closed line) of each structure.

The program ANAT3D then sorts all sections according to their distance from the previous section on the basis of their z-coordinates in the batch. Using translation and rotation the sections entered are fitted to each other and the contours of the structures better aligned. Segmentation-points are used to break the contours into segments. These segments of the same structure in adjacent sections are superimposed during the later reconstruction process.

By triangulation of the contours or contour segments of the same structure in adjacent sections, the computer reconstructs a surface/volume model. Surface area and volume of the structure can also be computed. Various modelling modes are available to visualize a structure: surface area reconstruction, lattice model, perimeter model or point cloud. The reconstructions can be moved in real time and projected on the monitor as three-dimensional

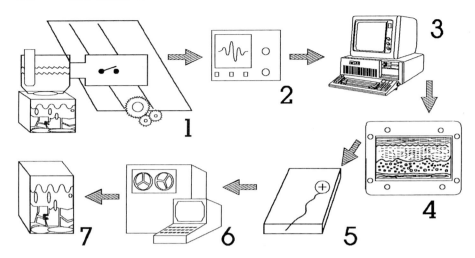

Fig. 2. Reconstruction procedure. Creation of a series of ultrasound sections of the area of skin to be examined *(1)*, digitization of the received frequencies to form a B-scan *(2, 3)*, photographic documentation *(4)*, input of the structures of interest via digitizer tablet *(5)* and construction of a three-dimensional computer model using the program ANAT3D *(6, 7)*

red-green stereo pictures. When an interesting vantage point is found, the object is redrawn as surface model illuminated by a virtual point light source. This leads to a distribution of colour on the object which gives the impression of depth. The complete reconstruction on the monitor is recorded photographically. Figure 2 summarizes the stages involved in reconstructing the three-dimensional images.

Results

Patient

In a healthy 28-year-old man, undiseased skin in the region of the upper epigastrium was examined by ultrasound. Figure 3 shows one image from the series of ultrasound sections. At the top of the scan we see as a homogeneous, black echolucent space the water path through which the ultrasound signal travels before it strikes the skin (W). Beneath this is an almost uniformly white, highly reflective entry echo (E) representing the transition between water path and skin. It is formed by summation of echoes arising on the one hand from the epidermis itself, on the other hand from the impedance jump at the interface between water and the stratum corneum.

Above this skin entry echo we see an elongated echo-rich structure (H). This structure appears to be superimposed on the entry echo without

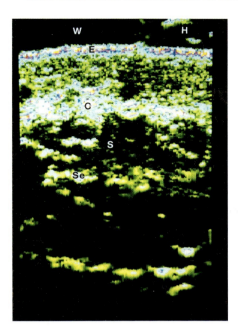

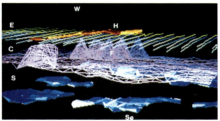

Fig. 3. Ultrasound scan of healthy abdominal skin. *W*, water path; *E*, entry echo; *C*, corium; *S*, subcutis; *Se*, bands of fibrous septa; *H*, hair

Fig. 4. Corresponding three-dimensional reconstruction. *W*, water path; *E* entry echo; *C*, corium; *S*, subcutis; *Se*, bands of fibrous septa; *H*, hair; *F*, projections of fatty tissue

being connected with it. Below the entry echo is an inhomogeneous layer corresponding to the corium (C). The predominant green colour is interspersed with individual white (echo-rich) and black (echo-poor) regions. There then follows a largely homogeneous black, i.e. echo-poor, zone which represents the subcutis. This region is interspersed with bizarre islet-like echo-rich (green/white) structures (Se).

Figure 4 shows the corresponding three-dimensional reconstruction of the healthy abdominal skin. The reconstruction was based on a series of 20 ultrasound sections made at intervals of 500 µm. Here, a lateral view was chosen. The upper and lower boundaries of the entry echo are shown in the form of two lines (E). On the basis of these double lines, the sonographic plane of section can be reconstructed. The elongated echo-rich structure superimposed on the entry echo can be followed through several individual sections. It is depicted on the double lines representing the entry echo as a red fibre-like structure shown in surface mode (H). After reconstruction, it was possible to classify this structure as a hair.

Double lines also indicate the upper limit of the corium. The lattice structure coloured white at the "front" and blue at the "back" represents the lower limit of the corium. The space actually corresponding to the corium thus lies between the double lines and the lattice structure (C). Below this lies the space corresponding to the subcutis (S). The tent-like elevations of the lattice structure represent projections of the subcutis into the corium. The structures in the subcutis described in the sonogram as highly reflective and islet-like appear in surface presentation mode as blue tubular formations (Se). We had already been able to follow the contours of these structures in detail from picture to picture in the series of ultrasound sections. The three-dimensional reconstruction showed their course in the subcutis more clearly: they traverse the subcutis in a tubelike fashion and are all oriented in the same direction. Some of the structures continue unbranched through several sections, some diverge to form thinner strands, and other converge and form thicker strands. On the basis of the three-dimensional reconstruction, these structures can be classified as fibrous septa.

Patient 2

Figure 5 shows a 3 × 3.5 mm senile haemangioma in the right upper abdomen of a 74-year-old patient. In the ultrasound scan of the haemangioma (Fig. 6), the corium is visible as an sonographical inhomogeneous zone (C) below the white band-like entry echo. Highly reflective (white) areas and less echogenic (green and black) areas alternate. Below this lies a homogeneous echo-poor layer corresponding to the subcutis (S). The tumour (T) is shown as a black echo-poor drop-shaped area. In this scan the tumour occupies two-thirds of the corium and projects above the level of the remaining entry echo in the form of a relatively pointed structure. Above the apex of the tumour the entry echo is attenuated or in parts completely interrupted.

Figure 7 shows the three-dimensional reconstruction of the haemangioma viewed from the side. The series of ultrasound sections comprised 15 images obtained at intervals of 500 μm. The upper and lower limits of the entry echo are shown as lines (E). On the basis of these lines, the individual sections can

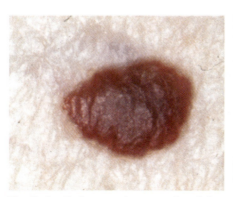

Fig. 5. Senile haemangioma on the abdomen of a 72-year-old patient

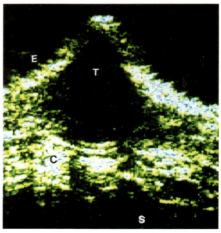

Fig. 6. Ultrasound scan of the haemangioma. *E*, entry echo; *C*, corium; *S*, subcutis; *T*, tumour

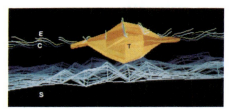

Fig. 7. Three-dimensional reconstruction of the senile haemangioma, lateral view (ultrasound plane of section at 90° to focal plane). Labels as in Fig. 6

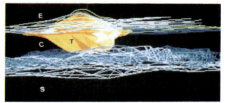

Fig. 8. Reconstruction of the haemangioma after lateral rotation through 30°. Labels as in Fig. 6

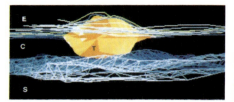

Fig. 9. Reconstruction of the haemangioma after lateral rotation through 60°. Labels as in Fig. 6

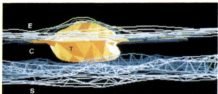

Fig. 10. Reconstruction of the haemangioma after lateral rotation through 90°. Labels as in Fig. 6

be identified. The lower boundary of the corium (C) is shown as a lattice structure. Below this lies the space corresponding to the subcutis (S). The tumour is shown as a yellow structure in the surface presentation mode (T). Its shape is reminiscent of a biconvex lens. The middle portion occupies practically the entire corium. At the edges, the tumour becomes thinner and appears drawn out like the brim of a hat. It occupies a third to a quarter of the corium. In Fig. 8, 9, and 10 the reconstruction has been rotated laterally through 30°, 60°, and 90°. The biconvex shape of the haemangioma and the hatbrim-like processes remain when the image is rotated. Further rotation of the computer model on the screen confirms this regular architecture of the haemangioma.

Patient 3

An ulcerated nodular malignant melanoma was found on the scapula of a 72-year-old patient. The tumour appeared as a roundish-oval nodule 15 mm long and 12 mm wide. It had homogeneous dark brown pigmentation and central ulceration (Fig. 11). Histology showed it to be an ulcerated, 2.4-mm-thick, nodular melanoma (Clark level 3–4, Fig. 12).

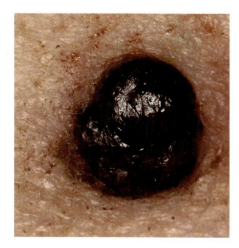

Fig. 11. Nodular melanoma on the back of a 72-year-old patient

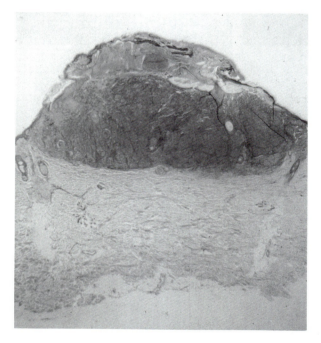

Fig. 12. Histology of the melanoma

In the ultrasound scan (Fig. 13) a bright, entry echo line (E) that is attenuated or effaced in the region of the tumour is visible below the water path (W). Below this is the corium (C). The upper corium is interspersed with fewer bright echo-rich spots. The lower corium thus appears more echolucent. Below the corium, the subcutis is shown as a echo-poor (black) homogeneous zone (S). The tumour appears as a circular echolucent area

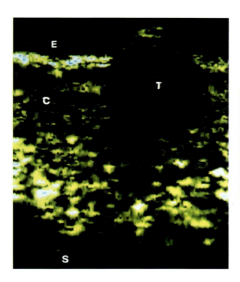

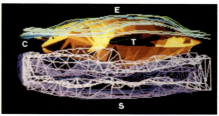

Fig. 13. Ultrasound scan of the melanoma. Labels as in Fig. 6

Fig. 14. Three-dimensional reconstruction of the melanoma. The selected view corresponds approximately to the perspective of the ultrasound scan and histological section. Labels as in Fig. 6

without internal echoes (T). In this section the tumour occupies about half of the corium.

The three-dimensional reconstruction of the tumour was based on a series of 20 ultrasound sections. On account of the size of the melanoma, an interval of 1000 μm between the individual images was chosen. The first and last sections of the ultrasound series were obtained in healthy skin. The tumour was studied in its entirety.

Figure 14 shows a three-dimensional reconstruction of the tumour as seen from the front, which corresponds to a perspective where the histological and ultrasound section plane lie parallel to the focal plane. The entry echo is shown in line mode. The lower echo-rich region of the corium is shown in lattice mode. The space below the lattice structure corresponds to the subcutis. The tumour (T) is depicted in shaded surface presentation mode. The shapes of the tumour in the reconstruction and in the histological section are comparable. The circular appearance of the tumour in the ultrasound scan compared with the spindle-like appearance in the histological section and the 3D computer reconstruction is due to the lateral compression of the ultrasound image. This compression was compensated by the reconstruction program.

Figures 15 and 16 show the same reconstruction of the tumour after lateral rotation 45° and 90°. In these views the tumour appears as an elongated structure. By rotating the tumour on the computer screen, the tumour region with the greatest width and depth could be determined and measured on the ultrasound screen and later in the corresponding ultrasound section. The maximum tumour thickness as measured sonometrically was 2.6 mm. For this particular malignant melanoma, the computer calculated a tumour surface area of 272 mm^2 and a tumour volume of 240 mm^3.

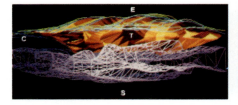 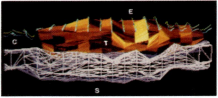

Fig. 15. Reconstruction of the melanoma after lateral rotation through 45 degrees. Labels as in Fig. 6

Fig. 16. Reconstruction of the melanoma after lateral rotation through 90 degrees. Labels as in Fig. 6

Discussion

In their search for information to supplement macroscopic and histological findings, dermatologists have turned their attention to high-resolution B-scan ultrasound of the skin. This reproducible noninvasive method gives a new insight into the structures of both healthy and diseased skin. The first results obtained with this new method have already been published [2–4, 9–11].

In order to determine whether the information obtained in 20-MHz ultrasound images can be supplemented by third-dimensional topography, we combined series of ultrasound sections of the skin with reconstruction methods for 3D modelling. The computer program ANAT3D which we used has already demonstrated its efficiency in other areas [6–8].

The ultrasound sections obtained with our mechanical transducer holder were suitable for reconstruction. The form and mutual relationships of structures of both healthy and diseased skin can be evaluated in a three-dimensional computer model. Distances of 250–1000 µm between the individual sections proved sufficient to follow structures measuring 5–25 mm on the ultrasound sections and to depict them as three-dimensional computer models. Distances of 250 µm between images proved to be most suitable (the ultrasound scanner having a lateral resolution of 200 µm). Here, even the details of tumour contours and fibrous septa could be followed from ultrasound image to ultrasound image.

Some structures in the sonograms could not initially be related to a definite morphological structure. The three-dimensional reconstruction of these structures, particularly the possibility of observing the reconstructed structure during rotation on the computer screen, is of assistance in interpreting the ultrasound B-scans.

Other working groups had previously described echo-rich oblique islet-like structures in the subcutis [3]. On the basis of the three-dimensional reconstruction, we were able to classify these formations in the subcutis with certainty as bands of fibrous septa. The 3D model also permitted us to study the behaviour of these fibrous bands, their convergence and divergence and their particular orientation. Round echo-rich structures above the entry echo were found in the reconstruction to be long cylindric structures distinct from the entry echo. The three-dimensional reconstruction confirmed the assumption from ultrasound images that they represent hairs. Hence, in certain respects, three-dimensional reconstruction can supplement the information obtained by ultrasound B-scan images of the skin.

The width and depth of pathological skin structures, e.g. skin tumours, can be determined with 20-MHz ultrasound. In the case of skin tumours, it is interesting to know the maximum length, width and depth of a tumour. Using a series of ultrasound B-scan sections for a three-dimensional reconstruction of the tumour, it is possible to identify and measure the maximum width and depth with greater certainty than by an unsystematic ultrasound examination of the tumour. The program ANAT3D is able to compute the shape, surface area and volume of the reconstructed structures. In our opinion, these measurements are of particular importance concerning skin tumours, particularly malignant melanomas.

Conventional prognostic staging of malignant melanomas is based on the depth of invasion of the tumour [5]. The Clark level and the tumour thickness according to Breslow are generally used as prognostic parameters for malignant melanomas and is likely that the computed surface area and volume of a tumour are also of prognostic significance. We therefore propose that for malignant melanoma these two computed values should be combined to form a new prognostic parameter which we term "invasive tumour mass". The number of cases we investigated to date is, however, too small to prove the actual prognostic value of this parameter. In particular, we have not yet been able to show whether tumour volume or tumour surface area has a greater influence on prognosis.

A current limitation of three-dimensional reconstruction of ultrasound images of the skin using our mechanical device is that, so far, only skin structures in the region of the trunk have been reconstructed. The head and extremities do not provide a sufficiently stable base for the designed transducer holder. Moreover, the reconstruction procedure is still very elaborate. In particular, the input of the contours of the structures of interest by means of the digital graphics tablet is very time consuming. Programs which permit tracing the outline directly from the ultrasound screen without intermediate drawing operations would considerably simplify the procedure (refer to "Principles of 3D reconstructions", in this volume).

Three-dimensional reconstruction from parallel sectioned B-scan ultrasound images of the skin is possible and, as such, of great promise. The computer models are able to give us information on the shape of a structure examined in vivo. The three-dimensional reconstruction facilitates the interpretation of structures sectioned on individual ultrasound scans. In future, the measurement of the invasive tumour mass in larger numbers of cases will show whether this new parameter is indeed of prognostic significance for malignant melanoma.

References

1. Alexander H, Miller DL (1979) Determining skin thichness by pulsed ultrasound. IJ Invest Dermatol 72: 17–19
2. Altmeyer P (1989) Dermatologische Ultraschalldiagnostik – gegenwärtiger Stand und Perspektiven. Z Hautkr 64: 727–728 (editorial)
3. Altmeyer P, Hoffmann K, el-Gammal S (1990) Sonographie der Haut. Münch Med Wochenschr 132 (18): 14–22
4. Breitbart EW, Müller CE, Hicks R, Vieluf D (1989) Neue Entwicklungen der Ultraschalldiagnostik in der Dermatologie. Aktuel Dermatol 15: 57–61
5. Breslow A (1970) Thickness, cross sectional areas and depth of invasion in the prognosis of cutanous melanoma. Ann Surg 172: 902–908
6. el-Gammal S (1987) ANAT3D: a computerprogram. In: Elsner N, Creutzfeld O (eds) New frontiers in brain research. Thieme, Stuttgart, p 46
7. el-Gammal S, Altmeyer P, Hinrichsen K (1989) ANAT3D: shaded three-dimensional surface reconstructions from serial sections. Applications in morphology and histopathology. Acta Stereol 8: 543–550
8. el-Gammal S, Bacharach-Buhles M, Altmeyer P (1989) 3D-Computerrekonstruktionen bei Pustulosis palmoplantaris. In: Altmeyer P, Schultz-Ehrenburg U, Luther H (eds) Handsymposion: Dermatologische Erkrankungen der Hände und der Füße. Editiones Roche, Basel, pp 285–300
9. Hoffmann K, el-Gammal S, Matthes U, Altmeyer P (1989) Digitale 20-MHz-Sonographie der Haut in der präoperativen Diagnostik. Z Hautkr 64: 851–858
10. Hoffmann K, el-Gammal S, Altmeyer P (1990) B-scan Sonographie in der Dermatologie. Hautarzt 41: W7–W16
11. Hoffmann K, Stücker M, el-Gammal S, Altmeyer P (1990) Digitale 20-MHz-Sonographie des Basalioms. Hautarzt 41: 334–339
12. Kastschenko N (1886) Methode zur genauen Rekonstruktion kleinerer makroskopischer Gegenstände. Arch Anat Physiol Abt 1886: 388–394
13. Miyauchi S, Tada M, Miki Y (1983) Echographic evaluation of nodular lesions of the skin. J Dermatol 10: 221–227
14. Payne PA (1985) Medical and industrial applications of high resolution ultrasound. J Phys E: Sci Instrum 18: 465–473
15. Quereleux B, Léveque JL, de Rigal J (1988) In vivo cross sectional ultrasonic images of human skin. Dermatologica 177: 332–337
16. Tan CY, Statham B, Marks R, Payne PA (1982) Skin thickness measurement by pulsed ultrasound: its reproducibility, validation and variability. Br J Dermatol 106: 657–667

New Developments

New Concepts and Developments in High-Resolution Ultrasound

S. el-Gammal, K. Hoffmann, A. Höss, R. Hammentgen, P. Altmeyer, and H. Ermert

Introduction

Contrary to internal medicine and surgical subjects, in whom ultrasound imaging methods have found wide application fields in the past decades, sonography has received only little attention in dermatology.

As a matter of fact, dermatologists used ultrasound imaging systems only to examine lymph nodes at 5–7.5 MHz in the follow-up of patients who had skin tumours [26] or to examine different conditions of the testes in andrology [29, 41]. Because image interpretation was often quite difficult, most dermatologists ignored ultrasound imaging methods completely and preferred to delegate this examination to the radiology and internal medicine department.

For a few years now high-resolution ultrasound equipment has been available to examine the skin architecture *in vivo*. The interest in this new technique has increased trying to reach to the limits of this method in tumour diagnosis and inflammatory diseases [e.g. 2, 5, 14, 42].

Multifrequent Ultrasound Equipment for Dermatology

At the beginning only a small group of engineering departments and laboratories were able to design, construct, and use high-resolution ultrasound imaging systems. Recently, however, commercial 20 MHz B-scan imaging systems have become available. They are now used in different dermatological clinics, thereby improving our clinical-sonographic knowledge in dermatology considerably. To study connective tissue diseases and pathological changes in the corium the resolution of 20-MHz systems is suffucent. The progression and regression of scleroderma plaques, for example, can be followed during therapy [14, 33, 42]. Especially in patients, where the connective tissue layers involved lie deeper (e.g. sclerofascia), simple methods like the observation of a lilac ring are insufficient. Until recently, the doctor had to rely upon deep punch biopsies and indirect methods such as biochemical blood examination (antibodies etc.) in these cases. Using high-frequency ultrasound the lesions can now be studied directly [42].

Great attention has been devoted to the sonographic appearance of malignant melanoma [5, 6, 25, 43]. Although the malignant melanoma is a rare malignant tumour, its incidence rate has increased as no other tumour has, except for lung cancer in female smokers [44]. Therefore the early detection of this tumour is of primordial importance for the survival of the patient. After diagnosis, the maximal tumour thickness is used to determine the minimal operative security distance. The tumour thickness is also one of the main factors used to distingnish between high-risk and low-risk tumours concerning their metastatic potential [7]. In fact, 20-MHz ultrasound is well suited for measurements of in-depth tumour penetration. However, 20-MHz ultrasound cannot differentiate between tumour and infiltrate. It therefore tends to measure "too thick" tumours. On the other hand very thin tumours (melanoma in situ) may also be missed due to the insufficient resolution.

Concerning the semi-malignant basal cell carcinoma, the axial and lateral expansion of the echo-poor area (corresponding to the tumour parenchyma, stroma and infiltrate) can be delimited easily [23]. It is therefore no longer necessary to make circular biopsies to determine the lateral borders of the tumour. Here, again, 20-MHz ultrasound cannot differentiate between tumour parenchyma and infiltrate.

Also other tumours (naevocellular naevi, angioma) can be studied as long as they are limited to the corium [22]. All these tumours show a more or less echolucent area in a region of multiple, apparently randomly scattered corial echo reflexes. However, with a few exceptions, it would be rather hazardous to use the tumour texture for differential diagnosis or to lineate the tumour parenchyma and infiltrate at the present state of technology. We have to accept that 20-MHz ultrasound is presently mainly suited to define the location of a large tumorous process within the corium and to judge certain ultrasound phenomena such as in-depth signal attenuation or enhancement along the borders of the tumour's process.

On the other hand, by increasing the frequency to 50-MHz and improving the electronical and mechanical setup, epidermal structures can also be studied [16]. There are even differences among the texture of the corium, infiltrate and tumour in selected cases. Now, epidermal atrophy can be characterized and measured, and the degree, distribution and extension of acanthosis can be followed in vivo.

We therefore need multifrequency ultrasound equipment in dermatology to study the different parts of the skin adequately (Fig. 1). For lymph nodes 5- to 7.5-MHz could be used (Fig. 2a), 20-MHz for corial and subcutaneous structures and 50- to 100-MHz for epidermal and upper corial processes. Finally, epiluminescent microscopy can close the gap between ultrasound and macroscopy by exhibiting the skin surface architecture and supporting the analysis of pigment anormalities (Fig. 2b).

5..10 MHz:	fatty tissue arteries, veins lymphnodes musculature
10..30 MHz:	subcutaneous fatty tissue corium arterioles, venules
50..80 MHz:	epidermal structures mucosa upper corium
Epiluminescent-microscopy:	skin surface mucous surface pigmentation

Fig. 1. Application fields and frequency spectra of ultrasound in dermatology. Epiluminescent microscopy closes the gap between macroscopy and ultrasound

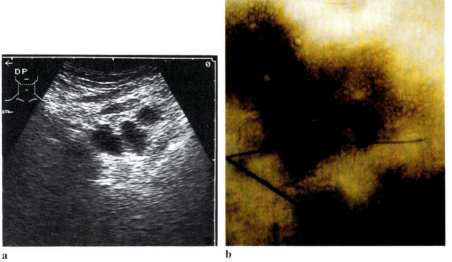

a b

Fig. 2a, b. Different aspects of the skin. Whereas ultrasound above 20 MHz is well suited to study epidermal and corial structures of the skin, lower-frequency ultrasound (7.5–15 MHz) is used to study deeper subcutaneous structures. On the other hand, epiluminescent microscopy closes the gap between macroscopy and high-resolution ultrasound (50-80 MHz). (**a**) Lymph nodes of a patient with an infraclavicular malignant melanoma; (**b**) malignant melanoma visualized with a Scopeman fibreoptic microscope using immersion oil and a glass plate

Ecto-Sonography
  Dermatology
  Ophthalmology
  Internal medicine

Endo-Sonography
  Cardiology
  Gastroenterology
  Gynaecology
  Otolaryngology
  Pneumology
  Proctology
  Urology

Fig. 3. New high-frequency ($> = 7.5$ MHz) ultrasound B-scan application fields in medicine

High-Resolution Endosonography

High-resolution ultrasound is also very helpful in other medical disciplines (Fig. 3). In gastroenterology, for example, the first endosonographic fibreoptic flexible endoscopes (7.5 MHz) were presented in 1980 by three independent research groups [15, 21, 45]. These instruments can provide

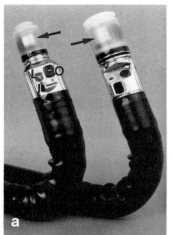
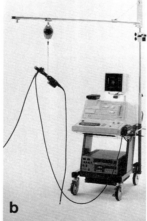
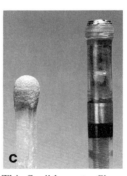

Fig. 4a–c. Gastroenterological endosonographic equipment. (**a**) This flexible gastrofibrescope for ultrasound examination (GF_{Type} UM3) allows endoscopic imaging (L, light source; O, optical system), 7.5/12-MHz ultrasound imaging (S) and has a 2-mm instrument channel (I). A ballon, fixed like a car tyre around the rotating ultrasound transducer (*arrow*), can be filled with water to study the architecture of the mucous wall of the gastrointestinal tract using ultrasound. The ultrasound transducer is rotated over 360°, making radial scanning images available. (**b**) The endoscopic ultrasound system EU-M3 is used for image processing and visualization. (**c**) This tiny endosonographic catheter can be advanced into the choledochus duct. It consists of an ultrasound transducer with a 45° mirror which rotates over 360° like a radar system. (Courtesy of Olympus Optical Co. Europe GmbH)

information as to whether a stomach cancer has invaded the muscularis propria or the serosa [11]. Figure 4 a–c shows gastroenterological endoscopes working at 7.5 and 12 MHz with sector scanners mounted on the lateral border of the tip. This flexible tube allows classical endoscopic imaging, has a working channel to take punch biopsies, and enables ultrasound analysis of the inner organ wall. A balloon at the tip of the endoscope can be filled with water to study the mucous wall. Figure 4c shows a miniature endosonographic catheter which can be introduced into the ductus choledochus.

In comparison to transthoracal echocardiography, which is done using 2.5–3.75 (up to 5) MHz; "higher frequency" 5- to 7.5-MHz transducer arrays are used in transesophageal echocardiography. Figures 5 and 6 show

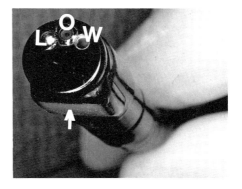

Fig. 5. Monoplanar transesophageal echocardiography. The flexible tube allows simultaneous endoscopic imaging (*L*, light source, *O*, optical system) and has a water channel to clean the optics (*W*). Note the linear transducer array (*arrow*) mounted at the lateral border of the tip. Since correct intubation of the esophagus is facilitated under visual control, this method is quite safe

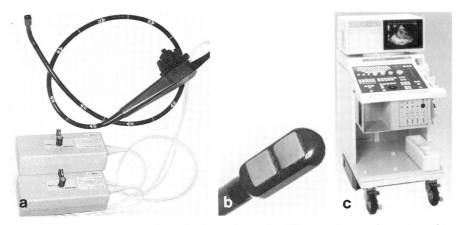

Fig. 6a–c. Biplanar transesophageal echocardiography. The complete equipment consists of the flexible tube and two connectors (**a**) which are mounted to a Hellige/Aloka cardiovascular phased array sector scanner colour Doppler SSD-870 (**b**). The flexible tube has two transducer arrays mounted perpendicular to each other lateral on its tip (**c**). The intubation of the esophagus is done without visual control. (Courtesy of Hellige/Aloka)

different cardiographic endoscopes with 3.5- and 5-MHz sector scanners mounted at their tip. Using this flexible tube, the cardiovascular system can be studied transesophageally without having the air-filled lungs obstructing the view. The equipment in Fig. 6 uses two 5-MHz sector scanners oriented perpendicularly to each other. By rotating, retracting and advancing the "endoapplicator" different views of, for example, the heart are available. The simultaneous ECG registration enables a comparison of similar phases in the repeating cardiac cycle. Different heart positions during systole and diastole can be studied easily. Please refer to "Biplanar Transesophageal Echocardiography" (TEE; this volume) for further details. Reichert et al. [38] used 7.5-MHz sector scanners to study the coronary arteries transesophageally.

High-Resolution Angiosonography

Recently, it has become possible to study the vessels morphologically and haemodynamically. The morphology is studied using B-scan techniques and the flow is analysed using Doppler techniques. With higher frequency the morphology is better resolved due to the improved axial resolution. Using Doppler techniques it is just the opposite: low frequencies enable a more precise quantification. New transducer crystals are now available which emit low frequencies for flow measurements and high frequencies for B-scan imaging sequentially (Figs. 7a, b; 8a–d). Doppler techniques include the

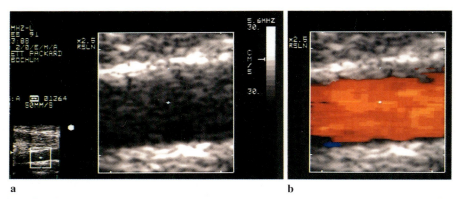

Fig. 7a–d. Angiosonographic equipment, ecto-sonography. (**a**) Linear B-scan section (7.5 MHz) taken from the internal carotid artery in longitudinal direction (young man). (**b**) A nearly laminar blood flow is observed in the internal carotid artery using a linear scanning mode (5.6 MHz). Towards the center of the vessel, the blood flow is slightly faster (more yellowish colours). **c + d** Sector B-scan of the aorta registered transesophageally (5 MHz). Although the flow is in principle quite laminar in the transverse section of the aorta (**c**), the angular changes during transducer rotation produce a Doppler colour shifting artefact in the longitudinal section (**d**). Note this flow colour change from light blue to dark blue to black to dark red and to red within the aorta. The images were registered with a Hewlett Packard 77030A colour Doppler ultrasound system (linear scanner, *a b*) and a Hellige/Aloka SSD-870 colour Doppler ultrasound system (sector scanner, *c d*)

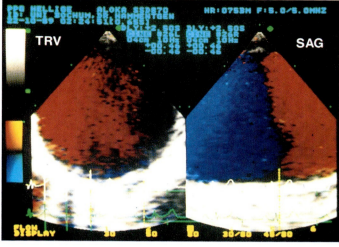

Fig. 7c, d

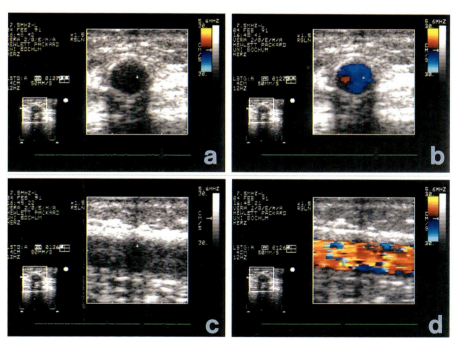

Fig. 8a–d. Angiosonographic equipment, ecto-sonography. Extra-anatomical axillobifemoral bypass studied by linear scanning (Hewlett Packard 77030A ultrasound system). 7.5-MHz transverse (**a**) and longitudinal (**c**) B-scan section. Turbulent flow in transverse (**b**) and longitudinal (**d**) colour-coded flow images (5.6 MHz). The turbulence is especially apparent in *d*, where the colour suddenly changes from red to blue

conventional Doppler pulsed wave (PW) and continuous wave (CW) or the colour flow imaging. When many transducers lying close together are used (e.g. transducer array), they can be activated in such a way that the resulting pulse corresponds to a sector scan or to a linear scan (Kreitz, this volume). In a sector scanning mode, all A-scan lines are oriented radially originating from a centre point, whereas in linear scanning techniques the A-scan lines are parallel to each other.

Figures 7a, b show a colour-coded duplex scan in longitudinal direction of the common carotid artery using a linear scanning mode. Note the homogeneous colour flow display in Fig. 7b, since the blood flow shows nearly no turbulence and the angle of the Doppler signal in relation to the vessel remains constant. Figure 7c depicts the thoracic aorta analysed with a sector scanning technique transesophageally (see also [20]). Note the colour change from red to blue resulting from the flow direction change due to the changing angle of the sector line in relation to the homogeneous blood flow.

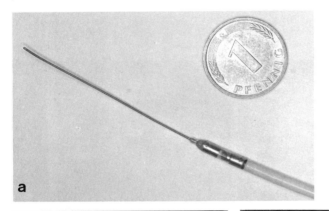

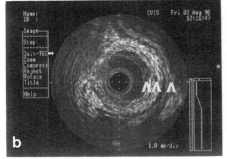 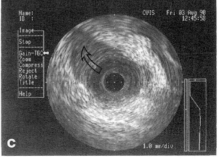

Fig. 9a–c. Angiosonographic equipment, intravascular ultrasound. **a** The transducer is oriented perpendicular to the longitudinal axis of the catheter. A motor rotates the transducer over 360° like a radar system. The fine wire at the tip of the catheter stabilizes the applicator during scanning. The catheter has a diameter of about 2.5 mm. **b** A 20-MHz 360° sector scan image of an artery in vitro. Note the three layers of the vessel wall: intima, media, adventitia (*arrows*). **c** Bifurcation of an artery (*arrow*)

In contrast to this ecto-sonography of vessels (c.f. Fig. 3), recently also "intravascular ultrasonography" (IVUS) of the blood vessels has become possible. Figure 7a shows a miniaturized catheter with a 20-MHz ultrasound transducer used for this techique (Hammentgen et al., this volume). A motor rotates an ultrasound transducer over 360° like a radar system. The vessel wall lamination can be visualized (Fig. 9b). Arteriosclerotic plaques and other pathological conditions can be examined directly. Note the artery bifurcation in Fig. 9c. To study the walls' architecture of the heart intravascularly, low-frequency (5 MHz) catheters have also been used [27].

New perspectives become apparent when several ultrasound images (using the sector scanning method) are combined. For example, the geometrical processing of the same region of interest analysed from different scanning directions within the same plane provides new ultrasound images which have fewer artefacts. Furthermore, when several colour-coded duplex images within the same plane are combined, the true direction of the flow can be calculated in the overlapping image region [17, 39, 40].

Apart from such image-improving methods which require several different B-scan ultrasound perspectives of the same region of interest, a sequence of B-scan images registered by translating the applicator can be used to reconstruct the three-dimensional shape of the structures of interest (el-Gammal et al., Hammentgen et al., Pawlak et al., this volume).

Promoting High-Resolution Ultrasound in Dermatology

We have to become aware that high-resolution ultrasound in dermatology has many unique advantages over other disciplines such as endosonography or angiosonography. Because the skin is directly accessible, it is possible to make an precisely oriented excision biopsy from the skin region registered with ultrasound thus enabling a direct comparison between the ultrasound image and histological section. We expect that ultrasound tissue differentiation in dermatology will promote other fields of high-frequency ultrasound where image interpretation has posed problems up to now. In the following chapters we shall therefore discuss the principal concepts of image formation and then introduce the reader to the different image processing methods as an aid to understanding the difficulties of pattern recognition in ultrasound images.

Concepts for Acoustic Image Interpretation

In clinical practice the differentiation of normal and pathological tissue is essential. It was hoped in the past that tissue characteristics would correlate directly with ultrasound parameters. However, ultrasound energy interacts in many different ways with the tissue. Two major parameters influence the

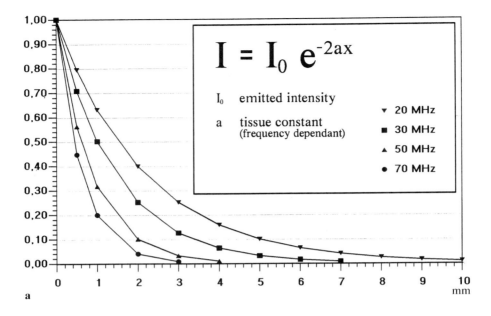

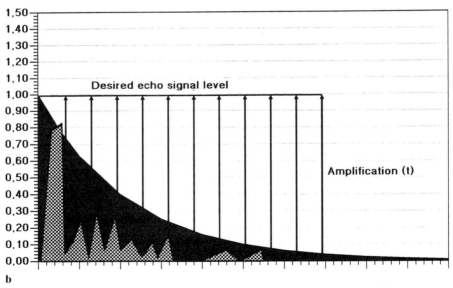

Fig. 10a, b. a Absorption in relation to in-depth signal penetration (in millimeters) in a homogeneous tissue. The *curves* have been drawn until 0.01 (= 1%; -40 dB) of the initial energy I_0 (1.00 = 100%) is left. Note the *steep curve* at high frequencies and the low signal in-depth penetration. **b** The time-gain compensation (*arrows*) is used to correct for the signal attenuation of the signals emanating from greater depth prior to sampling and quantization. If different tissue layers are present (*schematic signal* in the foreground), the amplification curve may have to be corrected adequately

received ultrasound signal: signal attenuation due to absorption and/or scattering and reflection. While reflection takes place mainly at the boundaries of tissue compartments with different impedance, signal attenuation is related primarily to tissue "stiffness" or homogeneity to ultrasound. For homogeneous tissue the absorption can be described by an e-function (Fig. 10a). This chart shows furthermore that the frequency of the acoustic signal influences in-depth signal penetration. Image interpretation is further complicated by the fact that the acoustic parameters of tissue are not constant under different experimental conditions. They depend upon frequency and other physical variables such as tissue temperature (Fig. 11), epidermis humidity (Fig. 12), skin elasticity and tension [16]. In order for these acoustic parameters to provide a unique signature of a specific tissue type, they must also be determined or kept constant to obtain comparable results.

Figure 11 shows that the in-depth signal attenuation at first approximation is proportional to the temperature of the water, which is used as coupling medium. An increase of the water bath temperature in the applicator seems to be a method to improve the amplitude of the received echo signal. Figure 11a–c were recorded at a water bath temperature of 5°C, 20°C and 35°C, respectively. To eliminate artefacts which are due to a time- or temperature-dependent soaking of the upper skin layers, the measuring window of the applicator was sealed with a membrane before filling it with water. This membrane is observed as white interrupted line above the skin entry echo (Fig. 11). It can easily be seen, that with increasing water temperature the intensity of the skin entry echo and the corial reflexes augment. Even echo reflexes from the connective tissue (routes) in the subcutaneous fatty tissue have become prominent. This visual impression is confirmed by Fig. 11d. It exhibits representative A-scans within the images Figs. 11a–c. It can be seen that echoes received with a time lapse of 2.8 ms are amplified with increasing temperature. It is difficult to choose exactly corresponding A-scans in the three images. Nevertheless, this effect was reproducible in all A-scan triplets and therefore is not a coincidence.

Figure 12 exhibits exactly the same skin region from the forearm after applying a creamy ointment (Fig. 12a) and after 24 h application under occlusive bandage (Fig. 12b). Note that the echo reflexes of the corium have become more intense. The skin entry echo line, on the other hand, exhibits many interruptions and has become less intense.

A survey of the consequences and deduction of similar experiments is discussed in the dissertation of Auer [3].

Measuring Acoustic Properties

At this time, little progress has been made in establishing a theoretical description of the interactions of ultrasound with biological tissues [12, 13, 37].

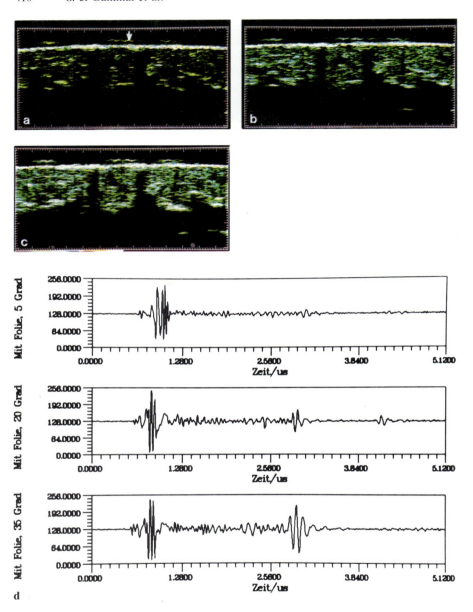

Fig. 11a–d. Water temperature and 50-MHz ultrasound of normal skin. The same skin region was studied using a (a) 5 °C, (b) 20 °C and (c) 35 °C water bath. The *longer bars* at the picture *borders* correspond to 1 mm, the *smaller bars* to 100 μm. To exclude artefacts due to skin humidity (i.e. variable water penetration into upper skin layers related to water temperature), the skin scanning window of the applicator was sealed with a membrane (*arrow*) inhibiting any direct contact of the water bath with the skin. (d) Single A-scans of approximately the same image region taken from *a–c*. Note that with higher water temperature stronger reflexes from deeper skin regins are observed

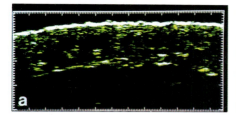 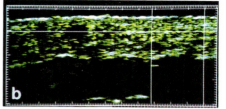

Fig. 12a, b. Sonographic texture and skin humidity. Normal skin a few minutes after applying a creamy ointment (**a**). Same skin region 24 h after application of the same ointment under occlusion (**b**). Note that the echo reflexes of the corium have become more intense. On the other hand, the skin entry echo line now exhibits interruptions and has become less intense (see *enlarged insert* at the *lower right corner* of *b*)

Most descriptions of acoustic interactions assume an ideal, linear, homogeneous liquid medium which does not really apply to the inhomogeneous biological tissue. Values for attenuation, velocity and impedance as a function of frequency have been measured for many body organs and tissues (Kuttruff, this volume). Generally, the attenuation and velocity increases in proportion to the relative content of protein and collagen and decreases in proportion to the water content.

The influence of the frequency on various acoustic parameters has also been used to characterize biological tissue. One of the most popular methods uses an echo system which emits broad-band acoustic pulses. Either the transmission or the backscattered ultrasound signal is processed further.

Acoustic microscopy (e.g. 1.1 GHz) can provide information about the absorption and reflection of acoustic waves by different micromorphological structures, including cells [10]. Although the biological tissue shows a different texture at different frequencies, this method gives a hint about the echogenicity of different tissue components. This information can help us to interpret 20- and 50-MHz ultrasound images. Figure 13 shows the acoustic image of a basal cell carcinoma. A histological, deparaffinized section was

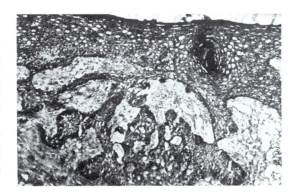

Fig. 13. Acoustic microscopy at 1.1 GHz of a basal cell carcinoma. Note the finger-like (*dark*) epithelial tumour buds which have grown into the upper and middle corium. The parenchyma of the basal cell carcinoma exhibits ultrasound characteristics identical to those of the epidermis. The stroma of the basal cell carcinoma is observed as *white area*

placed on a reflecting glass surface. Light image regions therefore correspond to areas with no tissue or echolucent tissue and dark regions to tissue areas which have either absorbed all energy or scattered the energy diffusely. The tumour nests of the basal cell carcinoma have a sonographic behaviour similar to that of the stratum spinosum. Since the histological sections are 6–8 μm thick, the topography of the sectioned area strongly overlaps the acoustic signal emanating from the biological tissue due to the angular reflection.

Alternatively the frequency spectrum of the beam is analysed before and after the passage through the specimen [24]. The entire frequency/attenuation characteristic may then be obtained with a single measurement.

Texture of Sonicated Tissue

Collagen seems to be the main source for the echo reflexes in soft tissue. Fields and Dunn [18] could demonstate that the supporting tissue has a thousand times higher bulk modulus or "stiffness" than the surrounding parenchyma. Since collagen and other proteins form the connective tissue skeleton in soft tissue, one would expect that different organs show a different backscattered texture. In cancer the tumour tissue can replace normal collagen tissue, thereby forming regions of reduced echogenicity. In a skin scar, which is accompanied by a increase of collagen fibres, one should expect more echo reflexes. We observed, however, that a skin scar is echo-poor. This finding illustrates that the orientation of the collagenous fibres in space strongly influences the sonographic texture of the corium. In a scar or wound, the new collagenous fibres are unordered; the region therefore remains echo-poor.

Scanning electron microscopic studies [9] show that the orientation of the collagen fibres in the corium of the skin changes under different tension forces. Brown [9] observed that the dermal fibres reorientate, straighten, become aligned and compacted in response to the increasing strain. This effect could explain the higher echogenicity of the skin during tension observed in ultrasound [16].

Because the wavelength of the ultrasound signal is in the dimensions of the studied structures, reflection, absorption and scattering phenomena produce interference patterns in the grey-level picture. These effects change the spacial distribution of the grey-levels, especially when movement (heart contraction, respiration) occurs. We therefore can conclude that the *concentration, spatial orientation* and *packing of the collagen fibres* strongly influence the backscattered texture in soft tissue.

A-Scan Sampling and Quantization

As has been stated earlier, the relation between the in-depth signal penetration and the absorption or "stiffness" of homogeneous tissue can be described by an e-function (Fig. 10a). Note that the tissue specific constant "a" increases with raising frequency linearly to quadratically. It can be seen from the curve that for the first millimeters the curve's gradient angle is very steep (Fig. 10a). Consequently a time-gain compensation (TGC) is needed to amplify the echo signal to an acceptable level (Fig. 10b). Most ultrasound imaging systems use microprocessors for image viewing. It is therefore necessary to transform at a certain point the analog signal into a discrete form. This involves two processes: *sampling*, which is the selection of a discrete grid of points in continuous time and *quantization*, which is the mapping of the signal amplitude into discrete values. Most high-frequent analog-to-digital converters have only a reduced set of quantization levels. To keep the signal well above the noise level, it is therefore advantageous to use a TGC prior to the mentioned conversion.

From the two commercial ultrasound imaging systems, only the Dermascan C has a TGC amplifier (Fig. 14).

Radio-Frequency Image Preprocessing

Prior to viewing the ultrasound image, a certain amount of data processing has to be done on the primary radio-frequency image.

Many commercial systems, especially those working in real-time, reduce this preprocessing to a simple rectification (e.g. using four diodes) and low-pass filtering (e.g. using a condensator) of the A-scan signal prior to the analog-to-digital sampling. This procedure is quite fast and inexpensive since the radio-frequency signal peaks are averaged out. Furthermore the sampling frequency can be reduced in comparison to the radio-frequency A-scans because of the low-pass filtering. Inexpensive analog-to-digital converters with a reduced set of quantization levels (e.g. 64 grey levels) can be used. A typical example in high frequency ultrasound is the Dermascan C Sonoscanner (Cortex Technology, Denmark) working in real-time (Fig. 14). However, fast analog image processing can only be done at the cost of image quality. In particular more sophisticated image processing can be accomplished when the full dynamic range of the radio-frequency picture is available. In these cases the A-scan signal is digitized and sampled using high sampling rates and many quantization levels. After preprocessing the radio-frequency signal, the envelope detection is done as last step to transform the radio-frequency image into the low-frequency image.

Filtering

To choose the appropriate filter, a spectrum analysis of the ultrasound image is necessary (see Appendix, Image transformation).

On the DUB20 different demodulation modes can be chosen. Figure 15b, c demonstrates the effect on the radio-frequency image (Fig. 15a). Correct

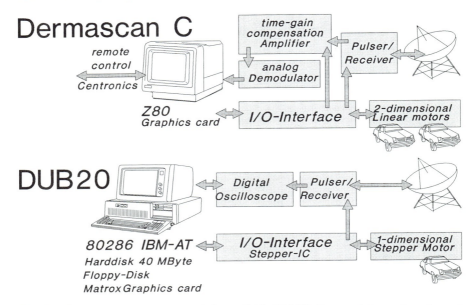

Fig. 14. Technical setup of commercially available 20-MHz B-scan ultrasound equipment for dermatology. Dermascan C (Cortex Technology, Denmark) and DUB20 (Taberna pro medicum, FRG)

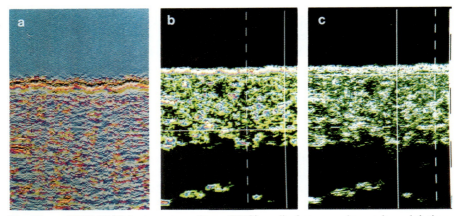

Fig. 15a–c. DUB 20 (Taberna pro medicum, FRG), radio-frequency image demodulation. **a** Radio-frequency image of the skin in the gluteal region of a 56-year-old man. The baseline corresponds to blue colours, green-black corresponds to a deflection of the high-frequency echo signal to negative values, red and white, to positive values. Two different demodulation modes were applied on the same radio-frequency image. They differ mainly in the algorithm for low-pass filtering and envelope detection used. The mean grey level was measured in the rectangle delimited by two *dotted* and two *continuous lines*. In demodulation mode 0 (**b**) the mean grey level measured was 67, in demodulation mode 1 (**c**) it was 40.5 (total range: 255 grey levels). The envelope detection (demodulation) is superior in *b* (demodulation mode 0)

low-pass filtering is done in Fig. 15b. Figure 15c exhibits plenty of horizontal stripes in the different ovaloid echoes, especially apparent in the connective tissue (routes) of the subcutaneous fatty tissue.

Although the radio-frequency images are available on the DUB20 (Taberna pro Medicum, FRG; Fig. 14b), its present computer program is rather limited. The following steps therefore only apply to our 50-MHz experimental system.

Frequency-dependent signal enhancement. This method could even correct for a frequency dependent echo signal attenuation in the biological tissue. It should be noted, however, that this kind of signal processing also increases the high frequency noise in the images. We therefore propose to develop a mathematical model for *in-depth dependent frequency amplification*.

Radio-Frequency Image Reconstruction. Because spherically focused transducers are mainly used in high frequency ultrasound imaging systems, the images tend to become unsharp outside the focal range. This effect makes texture analysis quite difficult, because the texture contrast and brightness in influenced by the distance of the focal plane (refer to Fig. 17a). To correct for this artefact, time-consuming holographic reconstruction methods are necessary. When the shape of the ultrasound beam is known, fine sampling in lateral direction (x, y-axis) makes it possible to determine the cummulative influence of line segments in adjacent A-scans of the original picture for every point in the new synthetic picture.

Pictorial Data Processing

To understand basic concepts of pictorial data processing it is useful to classify this field into two main areas: structure descriptions and images. Figure 16 shows the basic different transformation processes applicable in these two

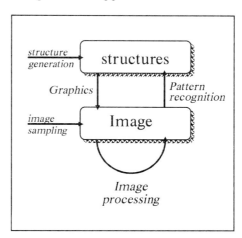

Fig. 16. Interactions between structures and images

areas. Note that complex[1] programs use often different elements at the same time.

We shall define *image input* as the process of sampling and quantization of an image. Accordingly, new nonpictorial structure descriptions are created by *structure generation* (Fig. 16).

Graphics deal with the generation of images from nonpictorial data. A few examples are, in order of increasing complexity: plots and functions of experimental data, computer animation and computer sceneries. Note while plots are static with time, computer animation displays moving image patches, while computer sceneries create the illusion of depth and shading.

Image processing deals with algorithms[2] where both input and output are pictures. For example over- or underexposed ultrasound pictures can be improved with contrast enhancement techniques. We may for example take an image with a wide range of illumination and reduce it in a first step into an image with only two levels of illumination for further shape analysis. In other situations we may even create a new image from another set, such as reconstructing cross-section images of the human body from projected X-ray pictures (e.g. computed tomography).

Pictorial pattern recognition finally deals with methods which produce either a description of the image and/or an assignment of picture elements to a particular class. To a certain extent, pattern recognition can be considered to be the inverse problem of computer graphics; a picture is transformed into an abstract description, e.g. a set of numbers, a group of symbols, or a graph. Further processing of this data finally results in assigning the original picture element to one of several classes.

Presently, only little experience on analytical methods suitable for high-resolution ultrasound images is available. The last chapters can therefore only develop general concepts for pattern description and expert systems using high-resolution ultrasound in dermatology. We shall see in future whether these or analogous techniques will be of any use in dermatology. For the different image analytical techniques mentioned please refer to the appendix.

Ultrasound Texture Description

The skin is an inhomogenous structure composed of different tissue layers and skin appendages. These different parts produce different echo phenomena, which interfere between them. Furthermore angular reflection phenomena can strongly influence the received echo signal in high-resolution

---

1 The reader should not confuse the complexity of the program with what is often called computational complexity – the computational effort (in time) required for its execution.
2 An algorithm is a instruction sequence which solves a task, such as a recipe to cook a meal.

ultrasound. The distribution, orientation and relative change in intensity are probably the main factors which can vary in a region of interest and can enable some kind of tissue differentiation. In the past years, different research groups have focused on image processing tools to reach these goals using ultrasound in medicine [28, 46, 47].

By extrapolating on high-frequency ultrasound in dermatology, the following concept can be formulated:
1. Regions of interest have to be compared with histology to differentiate between, for example, tumour masses and infiltrate. Here the histologically seen areas have to be projected onto the ultrasound pictures to define the regions of interest.
2. Different regions of interest in different images have to be compared. These areas can be rather irregular in shape and have a variable surface area. It is therefore advisable to keep amplification and different physical factors constant.
3. The texture of the irregularly shaped areas has to be described by a set of parameters. Different statistical methods such as the histogram of grey-level distribution, frequency analysis or co-occurrence matrices can be useful at this stage.

Image Normalization

Since the texture information is coded in the grey-level changes of the picture, it is influenced by the sound energy reaching the organ under study. The patient specific layers of the skin as well as the varying characteristics of the coupling medium do influence the image strongly (refer to Figs. 10, 11). It is therefore necessary to normalize the ultrasound images. For the texture analysis of the thyroid gland, for example, Zielke et al. [47] used the mean skin grey level to normalize the ultrasound images.

In dermatology the water path, fatty tissue and to a lesser extent the corial texture can be used to normalize the ultrasound image. Whereas those methods use extrinsic (external) parameters to render pictures comparable, intrinsic methods which use some statistical data extracted from the pictures are sometimes useful. Histogram equalization, which is presented in the appendix, should be used cautiously, however, because it introduces nonlinear contrast enhancement to improve the images qualitatively.

Elaborate texture analysis algorithms use multipart[3] techniques, which extract statistical data on the texture in different regions to evaluate an estimate about the variability of normal tissue in different individuals. These parameters can then be used either to immediately correct every image using image transformation methods or alternatively are considered as classification correction factors.

---
3 It is better to speak of "two part" than of "two-pass" image processing methods because two different algorithms are used in sequence.

Texture Extraction

Because of the stratified inhomogeneous nature of the skin, regions of interest are commonly defined interactively by the user. The extracted features within the region of interest can now be classified into four different groups, according to similar mathematical characteristics (refer to Fig. 18):

1. Statistics of first order are represented by features which describe the shape of the grey-level histogram in the region of interest. They describe the mean grey-level as well as other values (standard deviation etc.) and allow a differentiation of texture with different grey-level distributions.
2. Features of second order describe the local interdependence of grey levels between them (e.g. co-occurrence matrix) and therefore judge the inner characteristics of the sonographic texture.
3. Regularity, shape and distribution of the echo signal can be analysed using segmentation procedures to extract a binary (class 2) picture. This picture can then be reduced to a class 3 image and analysed using shape descriptors (see Appendix).
4. It is often useful do define a fourth class of classifiers which can be used by the physician to describe his expertise [47].

Figure 17 shows an example of such image processing. In Fig. 17a a region of interest was defined (red line) interactively within a malignant melanoma. By setting a grey-level threshold (Fig. 17b) within the region of interest, a bilevel image occurs. Using connectivity algorithms, different echopoor regions were extracted within the tumour region. These areas were sorted by their size in decreasing order (Fig. 17c). The larger areas could correspond to a certain extent to the tumour cell conglomerates seen in histology.

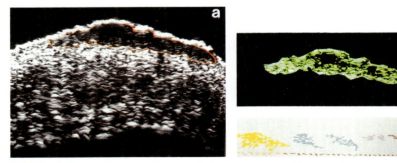

Fig. 17a–c. Image segmentation by thresholding on a 50-MHz ultrasound image of a malignant melanoma. **a** After defining the boundaries of a region of interactively manually (*red line*), a binary (class 2) image is calculated by grey-level thresholding (**b**). Using connectivity analysis, different *dark region* patches can be extracted, which have been sorted here in decreasing order into six colour coded classes according to their surface area (**c**)

Expert Systems

Most decision systems are based on multiplication factors which describe the influence of the different parameters for tissue differentiation. When the parameters show a high selectivity, their influence on a certain diagnosis is strong. The multiplication factors are evaluated by comparing the different parameters, with the diagnosis validated by dermato-histopathology.

In comparison to binary decision systems, which make a choice between two alternatives in a predefined region of interest, the differentiation of different structures within a region of interest seems to be much more difficult. For this purpose the region of interest has to be subdivided into (overlapping) smaller regions. Note, however, that for statistical analysis these regions cannot be too small either. This poses special problems at the present state of technology, since the regions of interest in dermatological high-resolution ultrasound are already quite small.

Nevertheless, the potential of expert systems can be judged in internal medicine: inflammatory liver tissue could be differentiated from normal liver tissue in vivo using a 3.5-MHz ultrasound scanner with 87% sensitivity [28]. In thyroid lesions the overall accuracy of differentiation between malignant and benign nodules was over 80% [32].

Conclusion

High-resolution ultrasound in vivo has opened new perspectives in dermatology. While corial structures and subcutaneous connective tissue septa with their blood vessel routes can be studied easily using 20 MHz, a further differentiation of epidermal and upper corial structures is – due to the insufficient resolution – impossible. By increasing the frequency up to 50 or 80 MHz and improving the electronical and mechanical setup, these structures can also be studied. We will therefore need in future multifrequent ultrasound equipment in dermatology to study lymph nodes (e.g. 5–7.5 MHz), subcutaneous and corial structures (e.g. 15–30 MHz) and upper corial and epidermal structures (50–100 MHz). Epiluminescent microscopy finally closes the gap between high-resolution ultrasound of the upper epidermal layers and macroscopy.

On the other hand, due to the easy access of the skin we have the unique chance in dermatology to directly compare the ultrasound picture in vivo with dermatohistopathology. We therefore believe that the results of image analysis on high-resolution ultrasound images of the skin will promote other application fields like endosonography and angiosonography.

Presently different image pre- and postprocessing methods for texture analysis and classification of the "region of interest" in ultrasound images are needed and have to be developed. These software tools will hopefully allow pattern recognition and the development of expert systems which support the physician in making a correct diagnosis.

Appendix: Principles of Image Processing

This appendix describes a subset of different image processing procedures commonly used. Since this book is intended to introduce the reader to the state-of-the-art of technology of high-resolution ultrasound, we decided to include this appendix. Those readers familiar with image processing techniques will forgive the sometimes oversimplified description, which intends to give an overview in a nonmathematical manner for medical staff. The following text is an excerpt of different textbooks of image processing and computer graphics [19, 34–36]. For an exact mathematical definition of the algorithms the reader is therefore referred to the standard textbooks mentioned. Most examples presented in this chapter were developed on an SIS image analysis system executing under MS-DOS 3.3 on an 80386 IBM-compatible computer equipped with a MATROX PIP graphics card. In those cases where particular, more sophisticated image processing methods were needed, the images were processed by the program MANI(pulate)2D under WINDOWS 3.0. The program MANI2D was implemented by Dr. S. el-Gammal.

To classify the different basic algorithms (refer to footnote page 412) and study their influence on the pictures, it is useful to distinguish three classes of images (Fig. 18). This classification has less to do with the human visual perception of the images than with the way they are represented and processed by the computer. Pattern recognition often involves several classes. Moving from class 1 to class 3 by passing class 2, the level of abstraction concerning the picture information increases.

Class 1 (grey and color scale) images are, for example, normal photographs or video pictures. Such images are close copy of "reality". The pictures are stored as large matrices[1] with integer elements[2] for which the term picture element, *pixel*, is commonly used. Colour pictures can be represented either as three matrices (red, green, blue), or as one matrix where different bits[3] of each element correspond to different colours. Usually, the human eye cannot distinguish levels of illumination that differ by less than 1 % so that a byte[4] per colour per pixel is considered sufficient. As a matter of fact, most people can only differentiate about 32 grey levels within their visual field [30] without changing the iris opening. In high-resolution ultrasound false colour coding is therefore often used to make small grey-level variations visible.

---

1 Two-dimensional discrete number field.
2 An integer value is a discrete number without a fraction part, e.g. 1, 2, 3,....
3 *bi*nary digi*t* (bit); basic element of every computermemory. This element can only have one of two states: 0 or 1 (binary system).
4 One byte equals 8 bits. A total of 256 (2^8) grey/colour levels, ranging from 0 to 255, can be represented with one byte.

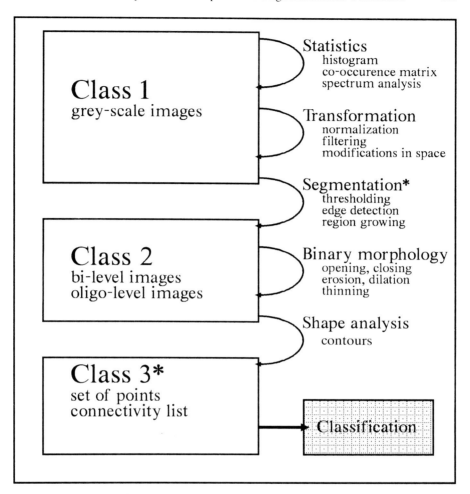

Fig. 18. Image classes and applicable transformations (*) Note that segmentation can be accomplished for different criteria (e.g. regions of same texture, same grey level, etc.). This step therefore defines what kind of data is available in the class 3 image. Using shape descriptor algorithms a data reduction becomes possible prior to classification.

Class 2 (oligo[5]- or bilevel) pictures can be represented as "maps", since they contain well-defined uniform regions such as a certain colour level. For example in geology such a bilevel map could differentiate between water and terrestrial surfaces. Bilevel pictures can be further simplified because the "0" map and "1" map exclude themselves mutually. Bilevel pictures can therefore be represented as matrices with one bit per element. We shall see

---

5 *Oligo (latin)*, which means a few (colour) levels.

later that to solve connectivity problems, bilevel pictures have to be treated as two separate maps.

Class 3 (charts, curves, polygons) pictures deal with point sequences (x, y-coordinates) and a connectivity list. The points may be joined by straight lines or simple curve approximations. This type of image is often used in graphics applications. For example the polygonal contour of a state (e.g. France) is a class 3 picture. Although the internal representation of the image data in the computer is class 3, it may be displayed as a class 1 or 2 image on the screen.

We shall now review the different kinds of image processing procedures which can be applied to each of the three image classes (Fig. 18).

1. Grey-Scale (Class 1) Images

Two major types of grey-scale image processing are available (Fig. 18): transformations within the same class (e.g. *filtering* or *image enhancement*) and transformations of a class 1 image to a class 2 image (e.g. *segmentation*). Most of these algorithms use, directly or indirectly, statistical data extracted from images. We shall therefore begin by presenting three of these statistical methods, the *histogram* or occurrence distribution graph of grey levels, the *co-occurrence matrix* of grey level pairs at pixel pairs and the spectrum analysis. Their application in image transformation and segmentation will then be studied.

The image analytical methods on class 1 images will be demonstrated on two different examples (Fig. 19). In many instances, these methods were not too convincing on ultrasound images. We therefore decided to include a video image with uniform areas (Fig. 19a).

1.1. Statistical Methods

1.1.1. Histograms

Algorithm. The histogram H(L) represents the occurrence distribution graph of the grey or brightness levels "L" in the current image or region of interest. For monochrome pictures we shall define that L can vary between 0 (very dark) and some value greater than zero (very bright).

When regions of different size have to be compared using histograms, a normalization becomes necessary. In those cases, the relative probability H(1) is used in the histogram. The number of points within every grey-level class is divided by the total numer of points within the studied region.

Simplified, every point is sorted according to its grey level into one of different grey level classes. The histogram is a curve which represents the number of points within every grey level class (grey level "densitometry" curve).

Examples. Figure 21b shows the histogram of Fig. 21a. Note the two peaks which show that dark and white pixels predominate. Figure 21 is, except

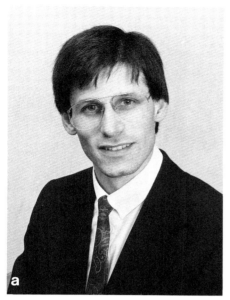
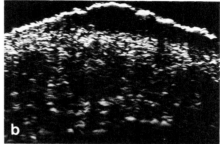

Fig. 19a, b. Image analytical methods. The two examples used in this appendix. **a** The Portrait was digitized using a CF8 Kappa video camera. Due to the geometrical characteristics of this camera, the image is compressed by a factor of 0.7 in the x-axis (the rectangles in Fig. 20a are in reality squares). **b** A 50-MHz grey-level ultrasound image of a malignant melanoma (low-frequency image). Note that the image becomes unsharp towards higher depth. At the same time the maximal intensity of the echo signal decreases at greater distance from the skin surface

for the lower left corner, homogeneously illuminated. False colour coding of the grey levels is a simple way to visualize the linear illumination gradient from left to right in Fig. 20. Note that unequal illumination (Fig. 20c) did deteriorate the two peaks seen in the grey-level histogram of the uniformly illuminated image (Fig. 21b).

Figure 22b (and Fig. 22c) shows the grey-level histogram of an ultrasound image of a malignant melanoma. Note the logarithmic distribution of grey levels. This effect seems to be the result of two synergistic influences:
1. Because the ultrasound transducer is focused, the images become increasingly unsharp when moving away from the perpendicularly oriented focus plane (lower image portion of Fig. 19b). This effect is accompanied by numerous, wide, ovoid echo reflexes which have a reduced maximum amplitude;
2. furthermore, the signal attenuation in homogeneous tissue (Fig. 10a) becomes increasingly nonlinear at higher frequencies (see Chap. "A-Scan Sampling and Quantization"). The ordinary time-gain compensation does not correct this frequency-dependent nonlinearity.

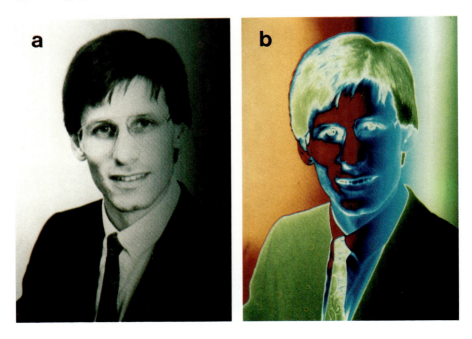

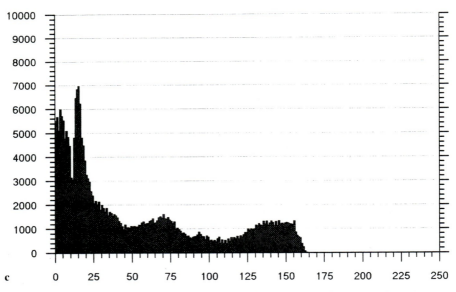

Fig. 20a–c. Statistical image analytical methods. **a** Unequally illuminated grey-level image. **b** False-colour grey-level codation makes the illumination gradient visible. **c** Histogram. Occurrence distribution graph of the grey levels of a. The x-axis denotes the grey levels (1–249), the y-axis the number of points with have a particular grey-level within the picture. **c** Histogram. In comparison to the histogram of Fig. 21, this histogram exhibits ill-defined peaks

1.1.2. Co-occurrence Matrices

Algorithm. This two-dimensional matrix is an estimation table about the co-occurence of a grey-level pair within a region of interest or image. We denote such a matrix by $Mr(L_A, L_B)$, where "r" stands for the relation between the points A and B. Such matrices can be quite large, depending on the number of quantization levels used. One may consider only the immediate neighbour(s) of a pixel or ignore the orientation completely and average the matrices obtained for various orientations.

When using co-occurrence matrices, their large dimension can cause problems. It is possible to overcome these difficulties by introducing a coarser grid using grey-level classes.

When regions of different size have to be compared, a normalization becomes necessary. The number of points of every element in the matrix is then divided by the total number of points within the region studied.

Simplified, the grey level class of both points describes an element in a matrix which is then incremented. The co-occurence matrix is a surface which represents the number of points within every matrix element.

Examples. Since the co-occurrence matrix for all grey-levels is rather large (250×250 elements), we shall restrict ourselves to 32×32 grey-level classes (eight grey levels per class). Figure 21c shows the co-occurrence matrix of the entire photograph (Fig. 19a). Peaks mainly along the diagonal (upper left to lower right) within the entire photograph give a hint about the uniformity of regions. Peaks which are spread far away from the diagonal are a hint for an inhomogeneous area. When the peaks become grouped around a single point along the diagonal, the region must have a quite uniform grey level.

In Figure 21a the photograph (Fig. 19a) was divided into small rectangles on which the co-occurrence matrix algorithm was applied. The photograph is

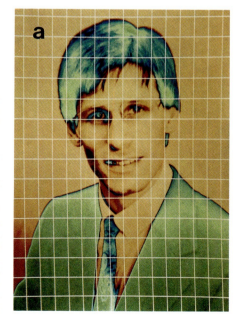

Fig. 21a–d. Statistical image analytical methods. **a** False colour grey-level coding of the video-digitized photo of Fig. 19a exhibits quite an homogeneous illumination. **b** Histogram. The occurrence distribution graph of grey levels of Fig. 19a/21a shows two peaks far apart, denoting two large uniform areas in the picture (*white background, black foreground*). **c** Co-occurrence matrix of grey-level pairs at neighbouring horizontal pixel pairs of the total image. Every element of this matrix represents a class of eight consequtive grey levels (of a total of 256 levels). Note the two peaks along the diagonal of the 32 ×32 matrix, denoting that there are mainly two uniform regions. **d** Co-occurrence matrix of grey-level pairs at neighbouring horizontal pixel pairs. The rectangles in *a* denote small picture regions which were analysed independantly. Points which lie close to the main

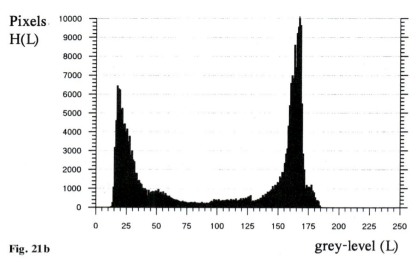

Fig. 21 b

grey-level (L)

Fig. 21 c

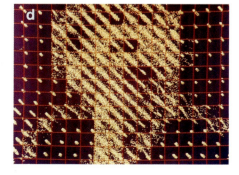

Fig. 21 d

diagonal (*upper/left* to *lower/right*) define neighbouring points with a similar grey level. A homogeneous grey level area produces a spot in the diagonal of the matrix. By comparing the co-occurrence matrices of different rectangles, regions with similar texture can be identified within the entire image compressed in x-axis; the rectangles correspond to areas of 32×32 pixels. Figure 21d shows the resulting co-occurrence matrices within these pixel area patches visualised by white dots. Note the regions with spotted, elipsoid and diffuse point clouds. Point clouds along the diagonal represent uniform grey level regions.

Figure 22d exhibits the co-occurrence matrix of the ultrasound image of an malignant melanoma (Fig. 22a). Note that that co-occurrence matrices are very sensitive to grey-level boundaries. In Fig. 22e the number of points within every matrix element was used to modulate the brightness of the clouds. This modulation makes peaks more prominent.

1.1.3. Spectrum Analysis

Due to the stratified nature of the skin and the significant signal attenuation in different skin layers, spectrum analytical methods are presently of minor use in B-scan ultrasound images. Nevertheless, frequency analytical methods have found wide application fields in duplex sonography to analyse blood flow velocities [31].

To put it into short terms, a signal (e.g. image row or line) can be described as the superimposition of a set of different sine waves with different amplitudes. An exact definition of this algorithm – the so-called Fourier transform – is beyond the scope of this text (refer to [4, 8, 35]).

1.2. Image Transformation

1.2.1. Normalization

Example: Figure 22 shows an ultrasound picture of a melanoma and its occurrence distribution graph of grey levels (histogram). We want to use this histogram for image enhancement or encoding (Fig. 22 b+c). For this, we have to see if H(L) is zero for different grey-level values "L", which means that the available levels of quantization are not used efficiently. It would then be desirable to reassign the grey-level classes in such a way that the dynamic range of the image increases. However, the full range of grey levels from 0 to 249 is already used (Fig. 22c). But many grey levels at the "light" end of the range are only used for a few points, whereas in the peak (at the "dark" end) of the histogram one grey level strongly dominates. A better way of using the available display range is to reassign values so that the resulting histogram is as flat as possible.

This procedure is called *histogram equalization*. In ultrasound images, this method improves the qualitative visual impression of the image by increasing the texture contrast nonlinearly; it has to be warned, however, that this method is unsuited for quantitative image processing. In colour flow mapping, where only a few colour levels are normally available (i.e. 16–32 levels) this method improves the contrast, making an optimal qualitative

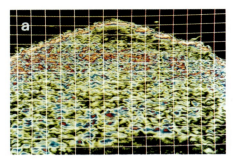

Fig. 22a–e. Statistical image analytical methods. **a** False colour-coded ultrasound image of a malignant melanoma. Small grey-level differences become apparent. **b** Occurrence distribution graph of the grey levels (histogram) of *a*. Note the logarithmic grey-level distribution. **c** This distribution becomes even more evident when the histogram is focused on the grey levels 50–250. **d** and **e** Co-occurrence matrices of the small rectangles in *a*. A 32×32 element matrix was used to represent the 32 grey-level classes.

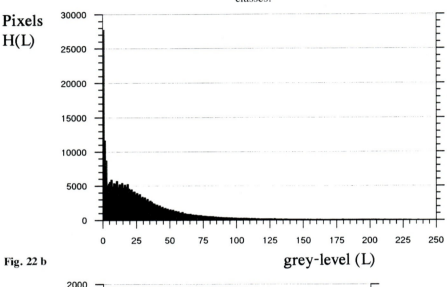

Fig. 22 b

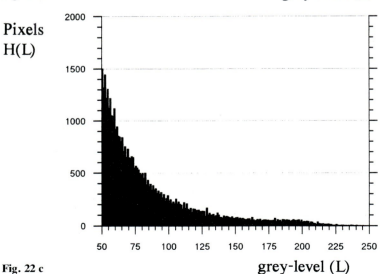

Fig. 22 c

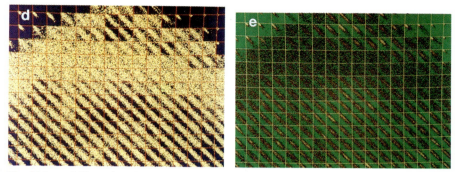

Fig. 22d, e. d Note that the echo signal attenuation at greater depth modifies the image much stronger than the changing texture in different layers of the skin. **e** Here the brightness level was modulated by the value of in the corresponding element of the matrix

sensitivity for slow and fast flow available. Such a method takes advantage of the strong contrast sensitivity of the human visual system.

Algorithm: If the image has a total of P pixels and N is the number of available brightness levels, a perfectly flat histogram must have P/N pixels at each level. If the number of picture points of some level "L" is x times that average, then that level must be mapped into x different levels ranging from Z_1 to Z_x. Thus we must introduce a rule for doing this mapping of one grey level in the old picture onto several grey levels in the new picture. There is no algorithm that works well in all applications.

Two possibilities shall be discussed here:

- *Algorithm 1:* Always map L onto the midlevel $(Z_1+Z_x)/2$. This does not result in a flat histogram, but one where brightness levels are spaced apart.
  This rule is purely heuristic (common sense). It fully uses the dynamic range, but does not produce a truly equalized histogram.

  Example. Figure 23 shows an ultrasound image of a malignant melanoma processed by midlevel histogram equalization (Fig. 23c). The corial echo reflexes have become more apparent. The false colour mapping of the image demonstrates that the skin entry echo, however, has become unsharp (Fig. 23b). Although the overall contrast of the image has increased, peak contrast (e.g. skin entry echo) has been averaged away.

- *Algorithm 2:* Assign at random one of the levels in the interval $[Z_1,Z_x]$. This can result in loss of contrast if the original histogram had two distinct peaks that were far apart.
  The motivation for choosing the latter algorithm is the wish to avoid a systematic error: when an arbitrary choice must be made, it shall be done in a random fashion.

  Example. Figure 24 shows the same ultrasound image processed by random histogram equalization (Fig. 24c). In this example, there is really no difference between Figs. 23a and 24a. Note that the false colour mapping

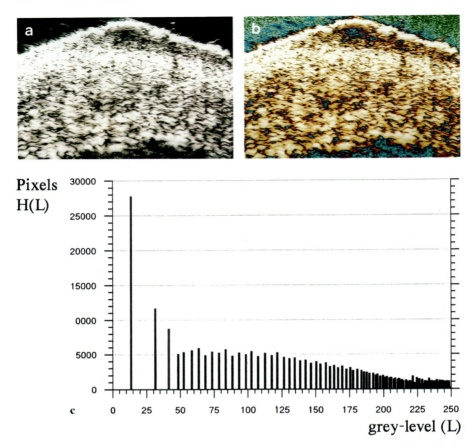

Fig. 23a–c. Histogram equalization by midlevel mapping. **a** Equalized image of Fig. 19b. **b** False colour-encoded image. **c** Grey-level distribution histogram. This algorithm does not produce a truely equalized histogram, but fully uses the dynamic grey-level range of the image

reveals the higher noise level of Fig. 24b in comparison Fig. 23b, especially in the border regions.

As has been warned earlier, this kind of processing cannot be applied to images indiscriminately, because equalization often causes a deteriorated appearance. This is especially true, when the grey-level histogram shows several peaks far apart because the peaks then disappear.

In some applications the detection of important information requires the discrimination between grey levels that are near each other. Here, the histogram equalization can expand the range of grey level contrast used in the region of interest. Alternatively, not a grey scale but a false colour table is used (see Figs. 20a, b).

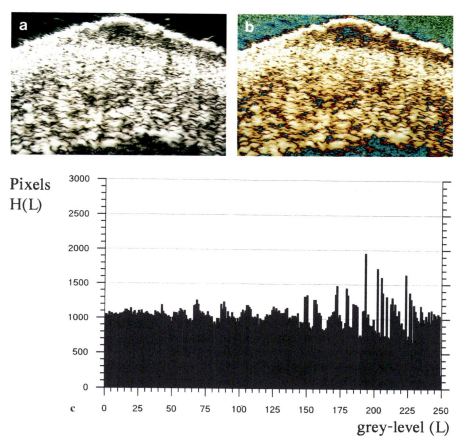

Fig. 24a–c. Histogram equalization by random mapping. **a** Equalized image of Fig. 19b. **b** False colour-coded image. Note that this image is noisier than Fig. 23b. **c** Grey-level distribution histogram. The image has a total of 512×512 points (= 262144 points/image). Since 250 grey levels are available, about 1000 points are found within the picture for every grey level after random histogram equalization

1.2.2. Filtering

Quite a lot of image processing can be performed without repeating the statistical analysis mentioned. Only some limited a priori knowledge is needed. Suppose the shape of the co-occurrence matrix of an ideal image is known and its noisy copy is to be improved. If the largest matrix elements lie along or near the main diagonal, then most pixels should have the colour of their neighbours (c.f. 1.1.2). If we wanted to eliminate noise, then each pixel of the noisy image should be replaced by a weighted sum of its neighbours to reduce the variability among adjacent pixels. We would then obtain a picture that is closer to the original.

Algorithm. The equation in Fig. 25-I describes the relation between the original image f(x,y) a weighing matrix h (x,y,i,j) and the new, filtered image g(x,y).

This algorithm is said to be a *linear filter.* This filter may change according to the localisation in the image.

Algorithm. If the weighing function h remains the same throughout the picture and is independent from the image position (x,y), then h (x,y,i,j) can be replaced by h (i,j).

These algorithms are called *space invariant filters* (Fig. 25-II). We should now study the mask H, which is defined as $H_{ij} = h(i,j)$.

When the elements of this mask have positive values (e.g. Fig. 25-IIa), we speak of a moving average filter. Such filters are extensively and successfully used to process time signals, but their significance in image processing is doubtful. When this equation is rewritten in terms of Fourier transforms (i.e. frequency spectrum analysis), it can be shown that moving average filters

I. $$g(x,y) = \sum_{i=-m}^{i=+m} \sum_{j=-m}^{j=+m} h(x,y,i,j)\, f(x+i,y+j)$$

II. $$g(x,y) = \sum_{i=-m}^{i=+m} \sum_{j=-m}^{j=+m} h(i,j)\, f(x+i,y+j)$$

IIa $$H_{average} = \begin{matrix} 1 & 1 & 1 \\ 1 & 1 & 1 \\ 1 & 1 & 1 \end{matrix}$$

IIb $$H_{Laplace} = \begin{matrix} 0 & 1 & 0 \\ 1 & -4 & 1 \\ 0 & 1 & 0 \end{matrix} \qquad H_{diag.\ Laplace} = \begin{matrix} 1 & 1 & 1 \\ 1 & -8 & 1 \\ 1 & 1 & 1 \end{matrix}$$

IIc $$H_{horiz.\ Sobel} = \begin{matrix} -1 & -c & -1 \\ 0 & 0 & 0 \\ 1 & c & 1 \end{matrix} \qquad H_{vert.\ Sobel} = \begin{matrix} 1 & 0 & -1 \\ c & 0 & -c \\ 1 & 0 & -1 \end{matrix}$$

IIc* $$P_{greylevel} = \sqrt{H_{horiz.\ Sobel}^2 + H_{vert.\ Sobel}^2}$$

Fig. 25. Image filtering methods using (**I**) linear filters, (**II**) space invariant filters. The new image g(x,y) is calculated from the old image f(x,y) using the weighing function h(i,j). In our case, the mask H has been defined as $H_{ij} = h(i,j)$. The different 3×3 matrices (masks) describe an averaging filter (**IIa**), point symmetrical edge detectors with/without diagnals (**IIb**; Laplace operator), a horizontal and vertical axis symmetrical edge detector (**IIc**; Sobel operator) and the formula which integrates both Sobel operators (**IIc***). Figs. 26 and 27 demonstrate the effect of these filters on images

attenuate certain frequencies and amplify others. During noise removal these filters smear simultaneously grey-level slopes and edges in the picture. The opposite problem exists for high-pass filters. They produce images with sharper edges, but also amplify high frequency noise.

Example. Figure 26a shows an ultrasound image processed by the moving-average filter in Fig. 25-IIa. Compared with the original picture (Fig. 19b), the edges have been smeared and the image contrast has been reduced.

When negative values are used for the elements of the mask H, gradient operators become available (see "Edge Detection").

We shall discuss here only some of the simplest edge (gradient) detectors. A common technique is to take the difference between two groups of pixels in the manner of a high-pass linear filter. To seize all conceivable orientations of the edge, several such filters are needed.

Algorithms. If we consider the mask H, then a simple point symmetrical filter is given by the Laplace operator (Fig. 25-IIb) and two simple axial filters are given by the Sobel operator (Fig. 25-IIc). Many publications have used these filters using values of 1 or 2 for "c" [1, 35].

Because these high-pass filters tend to enhance noise, this technique is of limited value for noisy images. In most cases it is preferable to use a linear filter which is symmetrical to an axis (Fig. 25-IIc) rather than a point (Fig. 25-IIb), since edge detection is superior (compare Figs. 27b, e). The latter filters are also called *directional filters*.

Examples. Figure 27c shows the result of combining the horizontal Sobel operator (Fig. 26a) with the vertical Sobel operator (Fig. 26b) using the equation in Fig. 25-IIc*.

Nonlinear image filters do not smear edges, but only remove the noise from the interior of regions. They are far more complex since the edges must be detected before applying a smoothing function. Edge detection is particularly difficult on a noisy image.

Most of these algorithms are two-part[6] filters, where for every pixel the direction of an grey-level slope or edge is estimated (part 1) thereby avoiding averaging across the edge. If no edge was detected, averaging is done (part 2; Fig. 25-IIa).

Alternatively a gradient is calculated first, giving some idea about the location of the edges. Then the original image is processed again using a linear, space-variant filter (Fig. 25-I) whose coefficients depend on the location in the gradient image, so that edges will not be smeared.

---

6 It is better to speak of "two part" than of "two pass" image processing because two different algorithms (e. g. filtering, thresholding) are used in sequence

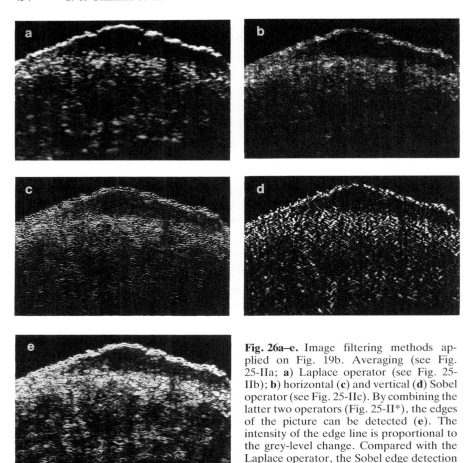

Fig. 26a–e. Image filtering methods applied on Fig. 19b. Averaging (see Fig. 25-IIa; **a**) Laplace operator (see Fig. 25-IIb); **b**) horizontal (**c**) and vertical (**d**) Sobel operator (see Fig. 25-IIc). By combining the latter two operators (Fig. 25-II*), the edges of the picture can be detected (**e**). The intensity of the edge line is proportional to the grey-level change. Compared with the Laplace operator, the Sobel edge detection is superior

1.2.3. Geometrical Modifications

Sometimes algorithms are needed to modify an image in space preparing the images for further processing. These include image mirroring techniques along the centre point or an axis (x-axis, y-axis, diagonal) and image rotation. Sometimes image compression or decompression techniques are also necessary to correct different scaling in x- and y-axis.

1.3. Segmentation

Image segmentation involves identifying areas of an image that appear uniform. The image is then subdivided into regions of uniform appearance

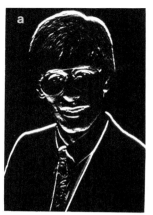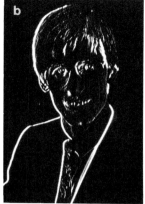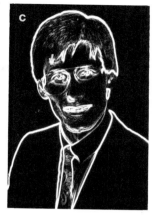

Fig. 27a–c. Image filtering methods applied on Fig. 19a. The horizontal Sobel operator detects edges in horizontal direction (**a**), the vertical Sobel Operator in vertical direction (**b**); for the algorithms see Fig. 25-IIc. By combining both (Fig. 25-IIc*), the edges of the picture can be detected (**c**). The intensity of the edge line is proportional to the grey-level gradient. In those regions where this gradient is not steep enough, contour tracing is ill-defined (*arrow*)

thereby transforming a class 1 image into a class 2 picture. Boundaries are defined as regions exhibiting greater grey-level changes than the expected image noise. The idea behind this restriction is that human visual system is highly sensitive to brightness level changes and less to absolute levels [30]. Although it is easy to define "uniformity" in terms of a grey level or a colour, it is far more difficult to specify what we mean, when we speak of a "uniform texture". When little is known about the regions we are looking for, the segmentation characteristics have to be found during processing. In this case either the statistics of the image has to be analysed (c.f. 1.1.) or groups of pixels have to be studied to check out whether they belong to a uniform region. Because the topic of segmentation is very complex we shall limit the discussion to three simple algorithms: *thresholding, edge detection and region growing*.

1.3.1. Thresholding

Algorithm. By comparing a value for each pixel with a threshold value "T", every pixel can be assigned to one of two categories, depending on whether the threshold is exceeded or not.

In the simplest case the pixel brightness level is used. The appropriate threshold value could, for example, be selected from the grey-level histogram of the picture. In fact, if an image really consists of two regions, one predominantly light and the other dark, its histogram should have two peaks (c.f. 1.1.1). Using a fixed threshold value is the simplest technique for segmentation.

Example. In Fig. 21b a threshold value "T" could be chosen between the two peaks so that the "background" region (yellow-brown region) can be defined as the set of all pixels whose value is below "T". However, the "face" and "shirt" in Fig. 21a have also been classified as background. This example illustrates that although the histogram exhibits two peaks far apart, thresholding misses the regions of interest when their brightness level lies close together. If in the photo the "face" and "shirt" had been less illuminated, simple thresholding could have separated foreground and background structures. Fig. 22b shows, that constant thresholding becomes impossiblewhen the illumination brightness varies within the image.

Automatic evaluation of a well suited threshold value can be difficult, because the presence of distinct peaks in the histogram is not common. In those cases the grey-level histogram should be evaluated only over those image regions where boundaries are assumed.

1.3.2. Edge Detection

Algorithm. These methods search for edges between regions using a gradient operator, and apply a threshold operation on the gradient to decide whether an edge or boundary has been found. Contrary to simple thresholding, a certain part of the neighbouring region around the point is taken into account. Finally, those pixels which have been identified as edges are linked to form closed curves surrounding the region of interest.

There are more elaborate edge detection schemes that overcome some of the disadvantages of the simple procedure described here at great computational cost.

Examples: Directional filters (see "Filtering") seem to be quite useful for edge detection. By combining the horizontal and vertical Sobel operator (Fig. 25-IIc*), edges in images with high contrast are easily detected (Figs. 26c, 27e). To a certain extent these edge detectors do a contour tracing, as long as the grey-level gradient is steep enough. The arrow in Fig. 27c points to a region with a poor grey level gradient.

It can be concluded that simple edge detectors are appropriate for high contrast images with little high-frequency noise. Such images cannot be segmented properly by simple grey-level thresholding.

1.3.3. Segmentation by Texture (Region Growing)

A different definition of uniformity can be set up by comparing the statistics over a region R with the statistics evaluated in parts of it. If they are comparable, then the region may be called uniform. This approach can be used to segment a region by *texture*. Co-occurrence matrices can be used to compare different regions. Alternatively, they can be described in their frequency spectrum.

Algorithm. At first the image is partitioned into a set of small regions. A uniformity test is then applied to each region, and if the test fails the region is subdivided into smaller areas. This process is repeated until all area patches are uniform. Finally the area patches are reassembled to uniform smaller regions.

Although this method seems to be elegant, this procedure leads to very small area patches in high-resolution ultrasound, so that statistical methods may fail when subdivision is done indiscriminately.

Many investigators have used statistical methods or frequency spectrum analysis for tissue characterization in ultrasound. Spectral analysis is however strongly influenced by signal distortion. In most commercial instruments, the waveform of the received echo signal has been distorted by a number of nonlinear electronic processes (amplification, demodulation and filtering). In real-time scanners, the original high-frequency information is often completely lost due to analog demodulation.

2. Oligo- and Bi-level (Class 2) Pictures

We shall deal here with images, where for every pixel only two states (point set/point not set) are available (Fig. 18). All points which are either set or not set form a separate bit map. Complex grey-level image segmentation (c.f. 1.3) may result in several bit maps, i.e. one for every region/texture type. We shall reserve the term "contour" for the discrete plane, while the term "boundary" should be used only when referring to structures in the continuous plane. Class 2 images are often related to the concept of shape, a term that is difficult to define quantitatively.

Problems are encountered when transforming a uniform region into a set of curves. Boundaries of an area in the continuous plane are easy to define. They comprise the set of all points, which have neighbourhood points both within and outside the set, no matter how small a neighbourhood of them is considered to be. The corresponding concept in the discrete plane remains paradox.

Let us focus on raster graphics, where every pixel is represented by a small square or rectangular cell. We can then introduce the following definition:

Definition: Two pixels are said to be direct neighbours (abbreviated d-neighbours) if their cells share a side, and indirect neighbours (abbreviated i-neighbours) if they touch only at a corner. The term "neighbour" denotes either type. Connectivity can then be defined as the pixel path of, for example, a contour.

The connectivity problem has produced some irritation in the literature because focusing on either "i"- or "d"-connectivity results in the logical contradiction illustrated in Fig. 28:

We are looking for the set of display cells connected. If we assume i-connectivity, then the path from A to A' is intersected by the path B to B', even though both of them lie entirely in

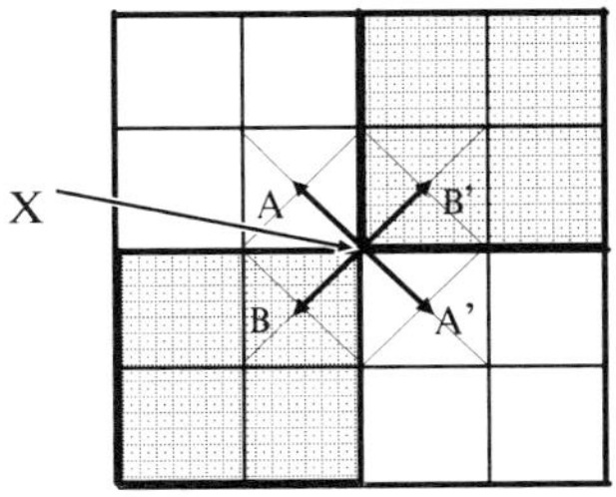

Fig. 28. The logical "contradiction" of connectivity in bi-level images is a consequence of a careless synonymous use of "pixel sets" and "raster image cell sets". However, cells may or may not include (parts of) their boundaries

disjunct sets. Thus the crossing point X must belong to both the white and the black set. If we assume d-connectivity, then neither the set of black pixels nor the set of white pixels is connected. This means that a path from A to A' (or B to B') never lies entirely within one set. Since the line segments AA' and BB' cross at the point X, this point belongs to neither set. However, we had defined that the black and white cells must completely cover the plane region. This apparent logical contradiction is a consequence of a careless synonymous use of "pixel sets" and "cell sets".

In the continuous plane, surface areas may or may not include their boundaries, and in the present example, the boundary definition is the key to connectivity. Different possibilities can be chosen: We may assume that all black cells contain their boundaries, while the white cells do not. Then the set of black cells is connected and the set of white cells is not. On raster images, we would also obtain consistent definitions if we use d-connectivity for white pixels and i-connectivity for black pixels. This choice has been popular in the literature but fails when we deal with pictures containing regions of more than two "colours" (oligo-level pictures). In those cases it makes sense to assume that wether a set of cells contains certain points of its contour is not defined by the boundary color, but by the boundary orientation.

Binary morphology and shape analysis in the discrete Class 2 picture shall now be discussed (Fig. 18).

2.1. Binary Morphology

2.1.1. Erosion and Dilatation

The erode algorithm removes a pixel from the entire perimeter of an area. It smoothes edges and removes high-frequency noise from the image. It may also separate objects when they are joined by a thin line of points. In special cases this algorithm is used several times in the picture.

The dilatate algorithm adds a pixel all around the perimeter of an area in the binary image. This algorithm is used to fill small holes or missing pixels in a region.

2.1.2. Opening (Ouverture) and Closing (Fermeture)

Both algorithms combine "erosion" and "dilatation" sequentially. It is important to notice that using the erosion algorithm and its inverse does not reproduce the original image, since isolated image points have vanished during erosion and will not reappear in the following dilatation (ouverture).

2.1.3. Thinning Algorithms

Thinning algorithms have been studied widely in picture processing and pattern recognition because they offer a way of analysis and simplyfing the shape of an uniform region.

Algorithm: All skeletal points are the centres of circles contained entirely within the uniform region R which have the property that there is not other circle with the same centre and a greater radius. The union of all skeletal points is called the *skeleton* of the region R.

Skeletons are very sensitive to noise, since a small disturbance of the boundary not only causes a disturbance in one branch but also creates new branches. Thinning algorithms are presently of little interest in high-resolution ultrasound. For a thorough discussion of these algorithms please refer to Pawlidis [35].

2.2. Shape Analysis

All pixels forming the contour of a uniform region can be connected by line segments which are part of a closed polygon. To render structure contours comparable we will assume that an observer walks clockwise along pixels belonging to a set of cells and selecting the leftmost pixel available. The initial pixel of the polygon area can be found in a number of ways, including a top-to-bottom, left-to-right scan of the image. Contour tracing terminates when the current pixel is identical with the initial pixel.

Using this algorithm, sets of points and connectivity lists can be extracted from the class 2 picture (Fig. 18). A class 3 picture is now available.

3. Class 3 Pictures and Classification

These images deal with sets of points and a connectivity list. To simplify pattern description, a whole set of different statistical structure parameters has been proposed over the last years quantifying different aspects of the overall shape of a structure. For example, different shape descriptor parameters (e.g. surface area, contour length, maximum/minimum diameter, centre of gravity, circularity) are in use. Other parameters describe the interrelation between different structure regions (e.g. number and length of touching sides).

Finally, pattern description should lead to pattern recognition. This involves making a decision on the basis of the shape of different objects. The precise psychophysiological definition of what is shape is difficult. For example, terms such as "curved" or "sharp edge" refer to shape. But how sharp must an edge be to be understood as such?

Two different approaches of shape recognition can be distinguished: in the first type the total object is classified on the basis of the overall structure. This strategy analyses the interrelation between different structure elements. Handprinted letters are a good example especially in Chinese, where strokes or other basic building elements are identified. The other approach studies the contour of the silhouette, looking for corners, protusions, intrusions and other prominent points of the contour in the class 3 picture. This strategy is suitable to classify silhouettes of different animals. In many situations both approaches must be combined.

Classification. Algorithms and data structures for numerical classification and cluster analysis is beyond the scope of this introduction to image-analytical methods. The reader is therefore referred to the standard textbooks mentioned (e.g. [19]).

References

1. Abdou IE, Pratt WK (1979) Quantitative design and evaluation of enhancement/-thresholding edge detectors. IEEE Proceedings 67: 753–763
2. Akesson A, Forsberg L, Hederström E, Wollheim E (1986) Ultrasound examination of skin thickness in patients with progressive systemic sclerosis (scleroderma). Acta Radiol Diagn 27: 91–94
3. Auer T (1991) Sonographische Phänomene der 50 MHz Sonographie an der gesunden und entzündlichen Haut. Dissertation, Ruhr-University, Bochum, FRG
4. Beth T (1984) Verfahren der schnellen Fourier-Transformation. Treubner, Stuttgart, pp 1–316
5. Breitbart EW, Rehpennig W (1983) Möglichkeiten und Grenzen der Ultraschalldiagnostik zur in vivo Bestimmung der Invasionstiefe des malignen Melanoms. Z Hautkr 58: 975–987
6. Breitbart EW, Hicks R, Rehpennig W (1986) Möglichkeiten der Ultraschalldiagnostik in der Dermatologie. Z Hautkr 61: 522–526
7. Breslow A (1975) Tumor thickness, level of invasion and node dissection in stage cutaneous melanoma. Ann Surg 182: 572–575
8. Brigham EO (1974) The fast Fourier transform. Prentice Hall, Englewood Cliffs, pp 1–251
9. Brown IA (1973) A scanning electron microscopic study of the effects of uniaxial tension on human skin. Br J Dermatol 89: 383–393
10. Buhles N, Altmeyer P (1988) Ultraschallmikroskopie an Hautschnitten. Z Hautkr 9: 926–934
11. Caletti G, Bolondi L, Labo G (1984) Ultrasonic endoscopy – the gastrointestinal wall. Scand J Gastroenterol 19 Suppl 102: 5
12. Chivers RC (1977) The scattering of ultrasound in human tissues: some theoretical models. Ultrasound Med Biol 3: 1–13
13. Chivers RC (1981) Tissue characterization. Ultrasound Med Biol 7: 1–20
14. Cole CW, Handler SJ, Burnett K (1981) The ultrasonic evaluation of skin thickness in scleredema. J Clin Ultrasound 9: 501–503
15. DiMagno EP, Buxton JL, Regan PT, Hattery RR, Wilson DA, Suarez JR, Green PS (1980) Ultrasonic endoscope. Lancet 629–631
16. el-Gammal S (1990) Experimental approaches and new developments in high frequency ultrasound in dermatology. Zentralbl Haut Geschlechtskr 157: 327
17. Greenleaf JF, Ylitalo J (1986) Doppler tomography. IEEE Ultrasonics Symposium Proceedings, pp 837–841
18. Fields S, Dunn F (1973) Correlation of echographic visualizability of tissue with biological composition and physiological state. J Acoust Soc Am 54: 809–812 L

19. Haberäcker P (1989) Digitale Bildverarbeitung. 3 rd edn, Carl Hauser, Munich pp 1–403
20. Hammentgen R (1991) Transösophageale Echokardiographie: monoplan-biplan, Atlas und Lehrbuch. Springer, Berlin, Heidelberg New York
21. Hisanaga K, Hisanaga A, Nagata K, Ichie Y (1980) High speed rotating scanner for transgastric sonography. Am J Roentgenol 135: 627–629
22. Hoffmann K, el-Gammal S, Altmeyer P (1990) B-scan Sonographie in der Dermatologie. Hautarzt 41: W7–W16
23. Hoffmann K, Stücker M, el-Gammal S, Altmeyer P (1990) 20 MHz B-scan des Basalioms. Hautarzt 41: 333–339
24. Kolosov OV, Levin VM, Mayev RG, Senjushkina TA (1987) The use of acoustic microscopy for biological tissue characterization. Ultrasound Med Biol 13: 477–483
25. Kraus W, Nake-Elias A, Schramm P (1985) Diagnostische Fortschritte bei malignen Melanomen durch hochauflösende Real-Time-Sonographie. Hautarzt 36: 386–392
26. Kraus W, Nake-Elias A, Schramm P (1986) Hochauflösende real-time-Sonographie in der Beurteilung regionaler lymphogener Metastasen vom malignen Melanomen. Z Hautkr 61:9–14
27. Kusay BS, Schwartz SL, Pandian NG, Aronovitz M, Kaplan E, Konstam MA, Connolly R, Diehl J (1989) Realtime in vivo intracardiac two-dimensional echocardiography and color flow imaging: approaches, imaging planes and echo anatomy (Abstract 2307) Circulation 80 [Suppl II]: 581
28. Lang M (1990) Untersuchungen zur Klassifikation diffuser Lebererkrankungen mit Ultraschall-Echosignalen. Dissertation, Ruhr-University, Bochum, FRG
29. Leopold GR, Woo VL, Scheible W, Nachtsheim D, Gosnik R (1979) High-resolution ultrasonography of scrotal pathology. Radiology 131: 719–722
30. Lullies, H, Trincker D (1977) Taschenbuch der Physiologie, vol III/2. Georg Fischer, Stuttgart, p 730
31. McIlroy MB, Targett RC, Roussin A, Seitz WS (1985) Doppler ultrasonic investigation of Raynaud's phenomenon: effect of temperature on blood velocity. Ultrasound Med Biol 11: 719–725
32. Müller MJ, Lorenz D, Zuna I, Lorenz WJ, van Kaide G (1989) Die Wertigkeit der computergestützten sonographischen Gewebscharakterisierung bei fokalen Läsionen der Schilddrüse. Radiologe 29: 132–136
33. Myers SL, Cohen JS, Sheets PW, Bies JR (1986) B-mode ultrasound evaluation of skin thickness in progressive systemic sclerosis. J Rheumatol. 13: 577–580
34. Newman WF, Sproull RF (1979) Principles of interactive computer graphics. 2nd ed. McGraw-Hill, Auckland
35. Pawlidis T (1987) Algorithms for graphis and image processing. Springer, Berlin Heidelberg New York
36. Pratt WK (1978) Digital image processing. Wiley, New York
37. Prince RR, Jones TB, Goddard J, Hames AE (1980) Basic concepts of ultrasonic tissue characterization. Radiol Clin North Am 48: 21–31
38. Reichert SLA, Visser CA, Koolen JJ, Chapman JV, Angelsen BAJ, Meyne NG, Dunning AJ (1990) Transesophageal examination of the left coronary artery with a 7.5 MHz annular array two-dimensional color flow doppler transducer. J Am Soc Echo 3: 118–124
39. Schmolke JK (1989) Realisierung eines Konzepts zur computertomographischen Abbildung von Bewegtzielen mittels Ultraschall-Puls-Doppler-Technik. Dissertation, University of Erlangen-Nürnberg, FRG
40. Schmolke JK, Ermert H (1988) Ultrasound pulse doppler tomography. In: McAvoy BR (ed) IEEE 1988 Ultrasonics symposium, Proceedings, Vol 2, pp 785–788
41. Schwenk WB, Schwenk WN (1989) Sonographie des Skrotalinhaltes. In: Braun B, Günther R, Schwenk B (eds) Ultraschalldiagnostik. Lehrbuch und Atlas. Ecomed, Landsberg

42. Serup J (1984) Decreased skin thickness of pigmented spots appearing in localized scleroderma (morphoea) – measurement of skin thickness by 15 MHz pulsed ultrasound. Arch Dermatol Res 276: 135–136
43. Shafir R, Itzchak Y, Heyman Z, Azizi E, Tsur H, Hiss J (1984) Preoperative ultrasonic measurements of cutaneous malignant melanoma. J Ultrasound Med 3: 203–204
44. Srivastava A, Hughes LE, Woodcock JP, Shedden EJ (1986) The significance of blood flow in cutaneous malignant melanoma demonstrated by Doppler flowmetry. Eur J Surg Oncol 12: 13–18
45. Strohm WD, Phillip J, Hagenmüller F, Classen M (1980) Ultrasonic tomography by means of an ultrasonic fibreendoscope. Endoscopy 12: 241–244
46. Walach E, Liu CN, Waag RC, Parker KJ (1986) Quantitative tissue characterization based on pulsed echo ultrasound scans. IEEE Trans Biomed Eng BME-33 7: 637–643
47. Zielke, Nauth P, Stein N, von Seelen W, Lock EW, Gaca A, Pfannenstiel P (1985) Quantitative Verfahren in der Ultraschalldiagnostik. Radiologe 25: 468–473

Subject Index

abdomen 238, 389ff
absorption 5ff, 9, 62ff
acanthosis 51, 68ff, 195, 247ff, 311
acoustic microscopy
 (→ microscopy, acoustic)
actinic elastosis (→ elastosis, actinic)
AIDS (aquired immune deficiency syndrome) 87, 100ff, 103, 190ff
– lymph nodes 100ff
aliasing
– general principle 357
– Doppler effect 147
aging, skin (→ skin aging)
analysis
– image (→ image ...)
– shape (image processing method) 439ff
– spectrum
– –, method 427
– – Doppler 141ff, 148, 292
– texture 417–419
aneurysm 164
angiography 152ff, 284
angioma 60, 173, 175, 176, 390ff
angiokeratoma 175
angiosonography 147ff, 156ff, 161ff, 404ff
– vs angiography 152ff, 284
– vs phlebography 154, 156ff
– intravascular ultrasound (IVUS) 289ff, 406ff
– intravascular flow measurement 289ff
– transesophageal echocardiography (TEE) 161ff
antigen, recall antigen test 77, 282ff
aorta 164, 165, 167
appendages, skin (→ skin appendages)
applicator 24ff, 299, 356ff, 386
– transducer (→ transducer)
– assembly (→ scanning techniques)
– holder 386
– and skin pressure 270

– coupling medium (→ coupling medium)
aquired immune deficiency syndrome (AIDS) 87, 100ff, 103, 190ff
artery 49, 114, 334
– carotid 148ff
– aorta 164, 165, 167
atopic dermatitis 48, 77, 87, 246
attenuation 7, 15ff, 27, 77ff, 407ff
– curve 408
arm
– forearm 48, 197, 252, 256ff, 284
– upper arm 188, 191, 222
arteriosclerosis 148, 152ff, 164, 167
axilla 102, 114, 127

band, echo-lucent (ELB) 50, 246, 275ff, 311ff
bandwidth (→ frequency, bandwidth)
basal cell carcinoma 72, 73, 202ff, 207ff, 314ff
– acoustic microscopy 337ff, 346, 411
– cryosurgery 277ff
– densitometry 216, 218
– inflammatory infiltrate 204ff, 210ff, 310ff
binary morphology (image processing method) 438ff
biopsy technique, skin 299–302
blood
– vessel(s) (→ artery; → vein)
– flow (→ flow, blood flow)
body regions, major
– abdomen 238, 389ff
– arm (→ arm)
– axilla 102, 114, 127
– back 192, 195, 222
– face (→ head)
– foot, sole 69, 333
– gluteal region 414
– groin 102, 234
– hand (→ hand)
– larynx (→ head)

Subject Index

- leg (→ leg; → foot; → vein)
- mediastinum 165
- neck (→ head, → carotid artery)
- shoulder 211ff
- shoulder 113
bypass, angiosonography 405

calcification 74, 198
carcinoma
- basal cell carcinoma
  (→ basal cell carcinoma)
- squamous cell carcinoma
  (→ squamous cell carcinoma)
- malignant melanoma (→ malignant melanoma)
carotid artery 148ff
cartilage 75ff
center frequency (→ frequency, center)
classes, image 421
comparative techniques 44ff
- *vs* CT (computed tomography) 111, 297, 370
- *vs* MRI (magnetic resonance imaging) 111, 297, 370
- *vs* microscopy (→ microscopy …)
contact dermatitis 58
co-occurence matrix (image processing method) 425ff
corium 42ff, 69ff, 186ff, 212, 318, 368–373
- C-scan 372
- inflammatory diseases
  (→ inflammatory diseases …)
- texture 368–373
- thickness 237
correlation (→ microscopy …)
corticosteroids 250ff, 276ff
- skin entry echo 277
- skin thickness 253ff, 277
coupling medium 24, 26, 56
- water 45, 119, 300, 410ff
- – temperature 410ff
- foil 231
- gel 231
- silicon bloc 101, 119
- and skin texture 410ff, 417
cryosurgery 278ff
- basal cell carcinoma 278
- bulla 279ff
- infiltrate, inflammatory 279
- oedema 279
cyst 178, 199

densitometry 56, 257, 414, 422ff
dermatitis
- atopic 48, 77, 87, 246
- contact 48
- stasis 50
dermatofibroma 261
diagnosis
- actinic elastosis (→ elastosis, actinic)
- aquired immune deficiency syndrome (AIDS) 87, 100ff, 103, 190ff
- basal cell carcinoma
  (→ basal cell carcinoma)
- capillary angioma 60
- carcinoma (→ tumours …)
- eczema craquelé 252
- elastosis (→ elastosis …)
- Kaposi's sarcoma, endemic 90
- Kaposi's sarcoma, epidemic 103, 190ff
- epidermolysis bullosa hereditaria 309
- dermatitis (→ dermatitis …)
- dermatofibroma 261
- granuloma, pyogenic 176
- haemangioma 173ff, 390ff
- histiocytoma 174, 196ff
- inflammatory diseases (→ inflammatory diseases …)
- lichen planus (→ lichen planus)
- lipoma 199
- leukemia, chronic lymphoblastic 89
- lymphoma (→ lymphoma …)
- malignant melanoma (→ melanoma, malignant …)
- morphea 58, 60, 231ff, 399
- mycosis fungoides 86, 311ff
- neurofibroma 73
- naevus/nevus (→ nevus …)
- osteoporosis 259ff
- psoriasis (→ psoriasis vulgaris)
- pyogenic granuloma 176
- ulcer 50
- rosacea 73, 215
- sarcoma (→ sarcoma …)
- skleroderma (→ skleroderma …)
- seborrhoic keratosis 173, 174, 194ff, 312ff, 335
- seroma 95
- skin tumours (→ tumours …)
- squamous cell carcinoma 202ff
- trichoepithelioma 52
- tumours, soft tissue 111ff
- tumours, skin (→ tumours …)
- vascular diseases
  (→ vascular system …)
- verruca seborrhoica 173, 174, 194ff, 312ff, 335
Doppler effect
- and scanning methods 404ff
- and vascular diseases
  (→ vascular system …)

- blood flow (→ flow, blood flow)
- – colour coded (→ Duplex colour flow)
- – zero crossing method   289ff
- – spectrum analysis   141ff, 148, 292
- – examination   147ff, 156ff
- – – arteries   152, 153, 404
- – – veins   154
- – general uses   3, 12, 41
  (→ angiosonography)
- – instrumentation   141ff
- – microcirculation   142ff
- – physics   139ff
- – – aliasing   147
Duplex   141, 147ff
- and vascular diseases
  (→ vascular system ...)
- grey-scale image
  (→ scanning modes, B-scan)
- colour flow image   141, 147ff, 161ff, 404ff

eccrine gland   303
echocardiography   161ff
- transesophageal (TEE)   161ff
- transthoracal (TTE)   14, 161ff, 404–5
echo-lucent band (ELB)   50, 246, 275ff, 311ff
echo phenomena   62ff
- shadow   7, 50, 66ff
- –, lateral   67ff
- shape   63ff
- boundary phenomena   64ff
- texture   65, 416ff
ecto- vs endo-sonography   402ff
eczema craquelé   252
edema   279, 283
ELB (→ echo-lucent band)
entry echo, skin (→ epidermis...)
epidermolysis bullosa hereditaria   309ff
elastosis
- actinic   72, 204, 215, 260ff, 273ff
- senile   259, 273ff
endo- vs ecto-sonography   402ff
epidermis   299ff, 317ff,
- acanthosis (→ acanthosis)
- hyperkeratosis (→ hyperkeratosis)
- parakeratosis (→ parakeratosis)
- skin entry echo   50, 68ff, 303ff, 306–7, 369–372
- stratum corneum   48, 247, 307ff
- stratum granulosum   332
- stratum Malpighii   318, 321
- stratum spinosum   318, 412
experimental approaches   267ff, 273ff, 305ff

- coupling medium
  (→ coupling medium ...)
- skin humidity   411ff
- wound (→ wound ...)
- collagen implant   262
- skin tension   57, 71ff, 185ff
- recall antigen test   77, 282ff
- corticosteroids (→ corticosteroids ...)
expert system   419

fascia, muscle   44, 58, 75ff
flow, blood flow   139ff, 141ff, 147ff, 156ff
field
- near   25ff
- far   25ff
- depth   15ff
- focal zone   16, 24ff
filtering (image processing method)   431ff
follicle, hair (→ hair ...)
foot, sole   69, 333
foramen, ovale   163ff
frequency
- bandwidth   22, 28ff, 45
- center   22, 45
- spectrum
- – vs signal penetration
  (→ penetration ...)
- – vs application fields   399ff, 401

gland
- eccrine   303
- sebaceous   43, 334, 318, 334, 378ff
gluteal region   414
granuloma, pyogenicum   176
groin   102, 234

haemangioma   173ff, 390ff
- reconstruction, three-dimensional   390ff
hair   389
- follicle   43, 50, 213, 246, 304, 333ff, 375ff
- – anagen   380ff
- – telogen   381
hand
- palm   71, 305–308
- back   309
head
- neck   121ff
- face   71, 210, 275, 278
- ear   75, 210
- larynx   114
- lip   71
histiocytoma   174, 196ff

histogram (image processing method) 422ff
histology (→ microscopy, light)
histometry (→ microscopy, light; → morphometry)
history of ultrasound   41ff, 55ff
horny material   74, 194, 213,
hyperkeratosis   195, 204, 218, 309ff

image
– analysis   34ff, 415ff
– classes   421
– class 1 (grey-scale) pictures   422ff
– class 2 (bi-/oligo-level) pictures   437ff
– class 3 pictures   439ff
– binary morphology (class 2)   438ff
– co-occurence matrix (class 1)   425ff
– densitometry (class 1)   414
– – basal cell carcinoma, statistics   216
– – malignant melanoma   428ff
– edge detection (class 1)   436
– filtering (class 1)   431ff
– geometrical transformation   434
– histogram (class 1)   422ff
– morphometry (→ morphometry)
– normalization (class 1)   417, 427ff
– processing   420ff
– segmentation (class 1)   434ff
– shape analysis (class 2)   439ff
– spectrum analysis (class 1)   427
– thresholding (class 1)   435
impedance   4ff, 45, 81, 299
implant, collagen   262
infiltrate, inflammatory   76, 248, 284, 338
inflammatory diseases   51, 88ff, 307ff, 318ff
– dermatitis (→ dermatitis ...)
– lichen planus   246, 310ff
– morphea   58, 60, 231ff, 399
– mycosis fungoides   87, 311ff
– psoriasis (→ psoriasis vulgaris)
– scleroderma (→ scleroderma ...)
intravascular ultrasound (IVUS)   289ff, 406ff, (→ angiosonography)

Kaposi's sarcoma   51, 90, 103, 190ff,
– epidemic   103, 190ff
– endemic   90
keratoma, angiokeratoma   175
keratin
– hair (→ hair)
– nail (→ nail plate)
keratosis
– hyperkeratosis (→ hyperkeratosis)

– seborrheic/seborrhoeic   173–4, 194ff, 312ff, 335

leg   50, 113, 156ff, 378ff
leukemia, chronic lymphoblastic   89
lichen planus   246, 310ff
lipoma   199
lymph node   87ff, 93ff, 100ff, 122ff, 401
– normal   87ff
– metastasis   87, 89ff, 93ff, 114ff, 133ff
– AIDS   100ff
lymphoma   89, 106, 311ff
– Hodgkin's   106
– non-Hodgkin's   106
– mycosis fungoides   87, 311ff

matrix, co-occurence (image processing method)   425ff
medium, coupling (→ coupling medium)
melanoma, malignant   89ff, 113, 119ff, 130ff, 172, 187ff, 221ff, 314ff, (→ acoustic microscopy), 350, 391ff
– and image analysis   423ff
– and texture analysis   418ff
– invasive tumour mass   76, 190, 395
– metastasis
– – skin   60, 131ff, 181ff
– – – in-transit   113
– – lymph node   87, 89ff, 93ff, 114ff, 133ff
– reconstruction, three-dimensional   392ff
– vs histology   223ff, 311
microscopy
– acoustic   325ff, 328ff
– – DM-scan   329
– – basal cell carcinoma   337, 346
– – malignant melanoma   337, 346
– – naevus, naevocellular   336
– – sapphire lens   331
– – verruca seborrhoica   335
– electron   44, 341ff
– light   44, 184ff, 223ff, 299ff, 330ff
– – skin biopsy technique   299–302
– other methods
  (→ comparative techniques ...)
morphea   58, 60, 231ff, 399
– corium   237
– subcutis   233ff
– – trabeculae   231
morphometry   135ff, 171, 184ff, 223ff, 237ff, 257ff, 345
– tumour volume and surface area   393
– tumour thickness   221
muscle fascia   58, 44, 75ff

Subject Index

musculus arrector pili   381
mycosis fungoides   87, 311ff

naevus/nevus   313ff
– blue   174, 177
– naevocellular   30, 192ff, 313ff, 336
– – echo texture   192ff, 313ff
– – skin entry echo   313ff
nail plate   42ff, 49
neck   121ff
neurofibroma   73
Nyquist criterion/sampling rate   23, 357

oedema   279, 283
orthokeratosis (→ epidermis ...)
osteoporosis   259ff
– *vs* skin thickness   259

parakeratosis   68ff, 247ff, 309ff
pattern recognition   416, 439
penetration   5ff, 62, 408
– depth   58–9, 408
phlebography   154, 156ff
phlebologic diseases   154, 156ff
– valvular insufficiency   156
– varicosis   156, 159
– vein (→ vein ...)
physics, ultrasound   3ff, 45ff
– absorption   5ff, 9, 62ff
– attenuation (→ attenuation)
– cavitation   9ff
– damping (→ attenuation)
– impedance   4ff, 81
– penetration (→ penetration ...)
– reflection   3ff, 59
– refraction   3ff, 61ff
– resolution (→ resolution)
– scattering   5, 7ff, 32ff, 62ff
– speckle   8
– tissue inhomogenity   7ff
– velocity   5, 45, 56
picture
– analysis (→ image ...)
– bi-level (Class 2)   437ff
– contour (Class 3)   439ff
– grey-level (Class 1)   422ff
– oligo-level (Class 2)   437ff
plaque, arteriosclerotic/atherosclerotic   148, 152ff, 164, 167
psoriasis vulgaris   244ff, 309ff
– acanthosis   244, 247, 309ff
– echo shadow   244, 309
– hyperkeratosis   247, 309
– infiltrate, inflammatory   248, 319
– skin entry echo   244, 309, 317ff

recall antigen test   77, 282ff
reconstruction, three-dimensional   76, 166ff, 355ff, 385ff
– algorithm   367
– – hidden line   374
– – hidden surface   381
– invasive tumour mass   76, 190, 395
– structure boundary method   365, 373ff, 375, 385ff
– volume/surface area calculations   359ff, 393
– Voxel method   365ff
reflection   3ff, 59
refraction   3ff, 61ff
resolution   8, 15ff, 32ff, 45ff, 58, 359ff
rosacea   73, 215

sarcoma
– fusocellular   113
– Kaposi's (→ Kaposi's sarcoma)
scanning techniques   12ff, 41, 46ff, 361ff
– A-scan   12, 17ff, 356
– B-scan   12, 18ff, 356, 371
– C-scan   30, 356, 372
– DM-scan   329, (→ acoustic microscopy)
– M-scan   41
– Voxel-scan   369
– linear/sector scan   13, 162, 404–6
– single transducer   13
– transducer arrays   13
scattering   5, 7ff, 32ff, 62ff
scleroderma
– circumscript (→ morphea ...)
– classification   233
– corium   234ff, 261, 318
– fascia, muscle   242
– progressive systemic   261
– skin entry echo   232ff
– skin tension   232
– skin thickness   232ff, 237, 261
– subcutis   233ff
– – trabeculae   231
sebaceous gland (→ gland, sebaceous)
segmentation (image processing method)   434ff
senile
– elastosis (→ elastosis, senile)
– skin (→ skin aging ...)
seroma   95
shadow, acoustic (→ echo phenomena, shadow)
shape
– beam profile   24ff
– three-dimensional (→ reconstruction)
shunt   164, (→ vascular system pathology)

skin
- aging   256, 271, 273ff
- - juvenile skin   42ff
- - adult skin   42
- - senile skin   44, 51, 71, 271ff
- and body regions (→ body regions)
- appendages
- - nail plate   42ff, 49
- - hair (→ hair ...)
- - gland(s) (→ gland ...)
- - M. arrector pili   381
- - vessels, blood (→ vessels, blood)
- biopsy technique   299–302
- densitometry   414
- - basal cell carcinoma   216ff
- elasticity   355, 409
- entry echo (→ epidermis ...)
- humidity   411ff
- layers   30, 42ff
- - A-scan profile   42, 80ff
- - epidermis   42ff, (→ epidermis)
- - corium (→ corium)
- - subcutis (→ subcutis)
- - muscle fascia (→ muscle fascia)
- - bone   44, 275
- - cartilage   75ff
- pathology
- - bulla   274, 309
- - calcification   74, 198
- - horny material   74, 194, 213
- - inflammatory infiltrate
  (→ infiltrate)
- - oedema   48, 248, 284
- thickness   48, 81ff, 171, 237ff, 256ff
- tumours (→ tumours)
signal, ultrasound
- post-amplification, digital   30, (→
  image, normalization)
- pre-amplification   316
  (→ time-gain control)
- transformation, analog-to-digital   357,
  412ff
- - Nyquist sampling rate   23, 357
- - quantisation   357, 412
- - sampling   357, 412
- - aliasing   357ff
- demodulation   413ff
- - filtering   413
- - -, effect of   414
sound... (→ ultrasound ...)
squamous cell carcinoma   202ff
- vs basal cell carcinoma   204
subcutis   42ff, 74ff, 82, 186ff, 212, 318,
  389ff
subepidermal band (→ echo-lucent band)
system, expert   419

test, recall antigen   77, 282ff
TEE (→ echocardiography)
three-dimensional reconstruction
  (→ reconstruction)
thresholding (image processing method)
  435
thrombus, atrial   164
time-gain control   15ff, 299
- principles   15, 408ff
- curves   16
- using 50 MHz   23
tissue
- damage   9ff
- - by heat   9
- - by cavitation   9
- ultrasound phenomena   3ff
  (→ physics, ultrasound)
tomography, computed (CT)
  (→ comparative techniques ...)
transducer
- technology   26ff, 298ff, 316ff
- sapphire lens (→ microscopy, acoustic)
- beam profile   24ff
- bandwidth   22, 28ff, 45
- center frequency   22, 45
- tissue penetration (→ penetration)
- Nyquist Criterion   23, 357
- ultrasound field (→ field ...)
- coupling medium
  (→ coupling medium ...)
trichoepithelioma   52
TTE (→ echocardiography)
tumours
- benign   171ff, 192ff
- invasive tumour mass   76, 190, 395
- volume (→ reconstruction...)
- malign   187ff, 315, 392ff
- skin   171ff, 181ff, 202ff, 207ff, 312ff,
  336ff
- soft tissue   111ff

ulcer, leg   50
ultrasound
- vs other techniques (→ comparative
  techniques ...)
- frequency spectra   401
- history of   41ff, 55ff
- new concepts   399ff
- phenomena (→ echo phenomena)
- speed (→ velocity, ultrasound)

Valsalva maneuver   154
valvular insufficiency   156ff
varicosis   156, 159
vascular system   147ff, 156ff, 161ff, 289ff

– function
– – flow measurement   289ff
– – shunt   164
– – turbulence   148
– – Valsalva maneuver   154
– – valvular insufficiency   156ff
– anatomy
– vessel wall   293, 334, 406
– vessels (→ artery ...; → vein ...)
– pathology   147, 156, 161
– – aneurysm   164
– – atherosclerotic plaque   148, 152ff, 164, 167
– – stenosis   150
– – thrombus   154, 164
– – varicosis   156, 159
– sonography (→ angiosonography)
vein
– femoral   154, 158
– iliac   154
– saphenous   157ff
velocity of ultrasound   5, 45, 56
– in skin   48
verruca seborrhoica   173, 174, 194ff, 312ff, 335
vessel, blood
– high-resolution B-scan   70
– artery (→ artery ...)
– vein (→ vein ...)
voxel reconstruction   365ff

wound
– healing   260, 267ff, 277ff
– – after punch biopsy   267ff
– – after cryosurgery   277ff
– volume   267ff, 281ff
– – *vs* time   269ff